BSAVA
SMALL ANIMAL FORMULARY
5th Edition

Editor-in-Chief:
Bryn Tennant BVSc PhD CertVR MRCVS
Capital Diagnostics, SAC Veterinary Services,
Bush Estate, Penicuik, Midlothian EH26 0QE

Published by:
British Small Animal Veterinary Association
Woodrow House, 1 Telford Way
Waterwells Business Park, Quedgeley
Gloucester GL2 2AB

A Company Limited by Guarantee in England.
Registered Company No. 2837793.
Registered as a Charity.

Copyright © 2005 BSAVA

First edition 1994
Second edition 1997
Third edition 1999
Reprinted with corrections 2000
Fourth edition 2002
Reprinted with corrections 2003
Fifth edition 2005

A catalogue record for this book is available from the British Library

ISBN 0 905214 88 9

The publishers and contributors cannot take responsibility for information
provided on dosages and methods of application of drugs mentioned in this
publication. Details of this kind must be verified by individual users from the
appropriate literature.

Typeset and printed by Fusion Design, Wareham, Dorset, UK

ii

Other titles from BSAVA:

Manual of Advanced Veterinary Nursing
Manual of Canine & Feline Behavioural Medicine
Manual of Canine & Feline Clinical Pathology
Manual of Canine & Feline Dentistry
Manual of Canine & Feline Emergency and Critical Care
Manual of Canine & Feline Endocrinology
Manual of Canine & Feline Gastroenterology
Manual of Canine & Feline Haematology and Transfusion Medicine
Manual of Canine & Feline Infectious Diseases
Manual of Canine & Feline Nephrology and Urology
Manual of Canine & Feline Neurology
Manual of Canine & Feline Wound Management and Reconstruction
Manual of Canine & Feline Oncology
Manual of Companion Animal Nutrition and Feeding
Manual of Exotic Pets
Manual of Ornamental Fish
Manual of Psittacine Birds
Manual of Rabbit Medicine and Surgery
Manual of Raptors, Pigeons and Waterfowl
Manual of Reptiles
Manual of Small Animal Anaesthesia and Analgesia
Manual of Small Animal Cardiorespiratory Medicine and Surgery
Manual of Small Animal Dermatology
Manual of Small Animal Diagnostic Imaging
Manual of Small Animal Fracture Repair and Management
Manual of Small Animal Ophthalmology
Manual of Small Animal Reproduction and Neonatology
Manual of Veterinary Care
Manual of Veterinary Nursing
Manual of Wildlife Casualties

Forthcoming titles:

Manual of Canine & Feline Abdominal Surgery
Manual of Canine & Feline Articular Surgery
Manual of Canine & Feline Head, Neck and Thoracic Surgery
Manual of Canine & Feline Lameness Diagnosis

For information on these and all BSAVA publications
please visit our website: www.bsava.com

Contents

Editorial Panel

Preface to the fifth edition

The *BSAVA Small Animal Formulary* is now in its fifth edition. The continued publication of this book by BSAVA is a testament to the value placed on it by the members of BSAVA and the continued positive feedback received over the past few years. I am grateful for all the comments that have been made and any comments on this new edition are welcome, particularly information on rarely used drugs. Please post or e-mail comments to me at Bryn.Tennant@sac.co.uk.

The three years since the last edition have seen changes in prescribing practices, the arguments on which have long been played out. However, the use of 'off-label' drugs continues to draw comments. Many of the drugs listed in the formulary are unlicensed for the species we treat. If they are to be used ahead of a licensed product there must be a clear and definable clinical advantage to their use. Some comments on prescribing off-label drugs have been added to the section on prescribing and I urge you to read them, though an in-depth discussion on when to use 'off-label' drugs is beyond the scope of this book. I have also added a brief section outlining some health and safety considerations relating to medicines being potential carcinogens and teratogens. Again, I suggest you read this section.

We have added some new monographs, and as usual some drugs have come off the market and are no longer available. See the Appendix for lists of new and deleted drugs. I have also trimmed down the number of trade names listed for human products. Where a non-proprietary (generic) unlicensed product is available, I have generally only listed that and deleted other trade names. For the licensed products all trade names have been retained and the omission of any specific product is purely accidental. All monographs were updated in the period July–December 2004.

In the fourth edition we adopted the rINN system of naming drugs. This system has now been adopted by most publishers in the human and veterinary fields. We have continued to indicate the original British Approved Names in the monographs.

Each monograph has again been read by a member of the Editorial Panel (listed on page ii). Their names will be familiar to many of you, as most are involved in referral practice. The collective knowledge of the panel gained from their extensive clinical experience ensures that the information provided is as accurate as possible. I am very grateful to all the panel members for providing their contributions in a timely and efficient manner. They are all very busy and for them to give up their time to this project, for the benefit of BSAVA members, is very much appreciated by myself and I am sure by those who use this book every day. I must also thank the publishing team at BSAVA for their editorial and administrative assistance.

Bryn Tennant
November 2004

Foreword

The *BSAVA Small Animal Formulary* is sent free of charge to all BSAVA members as each new edition is published. This is the fifth edition of the Formulary and once again it has been revised to ensure, as far as is reasonably possible, that the information herein is up to date, useful and easy to extract.

The last edition was published three years ago and the new one will enable practitioners to replace their cherished, care-worn and well-thumbed fourth editions with the new updated version.

The prescription and dispensing of veterinary medicines are issues that will profoundly affect the profession as major changes to this important aspect of clinical work are expected in the next few years. We must continue to demonstrate a commitment to the careful and responsible use of medicines to indicate to the Regulatory Authorities that we uphold the highest standards of pharmacy practice. For this reason, in addition to the drug monographs, ancillary information on these issues has been included.

Once again, grateful thanks are due from the Association to the Editor-in-chief, Bryn Tennant, and his editorial team, for their continued diligent and patient involvement in this important publication.

Ian Mason BVetMed PhD CertSAD DipECVD MRCVS
BSAVA President 2004–5

INTRODUCTION

How to use the Formulary

The Formulary has three sections. This Introduction covers the use of the Formulary and includes information on prescribing, health and safety considerations, storage and dispensing of products (drugs). The second section contains the drug monographs. The Appendices provide useful information, including antibiotic selection, dosing animals with renal or hepatic disease, lymphoma protocols and common sedative combinations. There are two indices. The first lists products according to their therapeutic use, whilst the main index lists all the products and their trade names alphabetically. Trade names are printed in italics.

The information given for each product is provided for guidance only.

Veterinary surgeons using this publication are warned that many of the drugs and doses listed are not currently authorized by the Veterinary Medicines Directorate (VMD) or the European Agency for the Evaluation of Medicinal Products (EMEA) (either at all or for a particular species), or manufacturers' recommendations may be limited to particular indications.

For information on a drug, look up the generic name in the A–Z section, where you will find listed:

* Generic name, and in brackets other names, the trade name(s), common name and/or synonym. The list of trade names is not necessarily comprehensive, and the mention or exclusion of any particular commercial product is not a recommendation or otherwise as to its value. **The trade names of products authorized for use in one or more of the species indicated in the monograph are shown in bold type. Non-authorized products are in plain type and are asterisked**. Note that an indication that a product is authorized does not necessarily mean that it is authorized for all species listed in the monograph; check individual data sheets. Veterinary medicinal products must be administered in accordance with the prescribing cascade, as set out in the Medicines (Restrictions on the Administration of Veterinary Medicinal Products) Regulations 1994 as amended (see below). The pharmaceutical categorization of each drug is indicated in italics.
* Indications: detailing the drug class and/or main indications for its use
* Forms: listing forms available
* Dose: indicating recommended doses. The dosages are those recommended by the manufacturers in their data sheets and package inserts, **or** are based on those given in published articles or textbooks, **or** are based on clinical experience. These recommendations should be used only as guidelines and should not be considered appropriate for every case. Clinical judgement

must take precedence. 'Birds' includes psittacines and raptors. 'Reptiles' includes chelonians, lizards and snakes. 'Small mammals' includes rodents, lagomorphs and small carnivores.

- Adverse effects and contraindications: indicating the more important adverse effects and contraindications to the use of a product. This information draws attention to those effects that may be of clinical significance and is not intended to be a comprehensive list of all adverse effects. The information is taken from published veterinary and human references and not just from product literature.
- Drug interactions: listing those interactions which may be of clinical significance. The information is taken from human and veterinary literature.

For further information on veterinary licensed products see *Compendium of Data Sheets for Veterinary Products* published by NOAH. For details on human licensed products see the *British National Formulary*, available online at www.BNF.org.

Any suspected adverse reactions should be reported both to the company holding the marketing authorization for the product concerned and to the Veterinary Medicines Directorate at Woodham Lane, New Haw, Addlestone, Surrey Freepost KT 4503.

Guidance on prescribing

The prescribing cascade
The prescribing 'cascade' contained in the Medicines (Restrictions on the Administration of Veterinary Medicinal Products) Regulations 1994 sets out the conditions that must be met. These Regulations provide that when no authorized veterinary medicinal product exists for a condition in a particular species, and in order to avoid unacceptable suffering, veterinary surgeons exercising their clinical judgement may prescribe for one or a small number of animals under their care in accordance with the following sequence:

1. A veterinary medicine authorized for use in another species, or for a different use in the same species ('off-label' use).
2. A medicine authorized in the UK for human use.
3. A medicine to be made up at the time on a one-off basis by a veterinary surgeon or a properly authorized person.

'Off-label' use of medicines
'Off-label' use is the use of medicines outside the terms of their marketing authorization (MA). It may include medicines authorized outside the UK that are used in accordance with an import certificate issued by the VMD. A veterinary surgeon with detailed knowledge of the medical history and clinical status of a patient, may reasonably prescribe a medicine 'off-label' in accordance with the prescribing cascade. Authorized medicines have been scientifically assessed

against statutory criteria of safety, quality and efficacy when used in accordance with the authorized recommendations on the product literature. Use of an unauthorized medicine provides none of these safeguards and may, therefore, pose potential risks that the authorization process seeks to minimize.

Medicines may be used 'off-label' for a variety of reasons including:

- No authorized product available for the condition or specific subpopulation being treated
- Need to alter the duration of therapy, dosage, route of administration etc., to treat the specific condition presented
- An authorized product has proved ineffective in the circumstances of a particular case (all cases of suspected lack of efficacy of authorized veterinary medicines should be reported to the VMD).

Responsibility for the use of a medicine 'off-label' lies solely with the prescribing veterinary surgeon. He or she should inform the owner of the reason why a medicine is to be used 'off-label' and record this reason in the patient's clinical notes. When electing to use a medicine 'off-label' always:

- Discuss all therapeutic options with the owner
- Use the cascade to determine your choice of medicine
- Obtain signed informed consent if an unauthorized produce is to be used, ensuring that all potential problems are explained to the clients
- Administer unauthorized medicines against a patient-specific prescription. Do not administer to a group of animals if at all possible.

An 'off-label' medicine must show a comparative clinical advantage to the authorized product in the specific circumstances presented (where applicable). Medicines may be used 'off-label' in the following ways (this is not an exhaustive list):

- Authorized product at an unauthorized dose
- Authorized product for an unauthorized indication
- Authorized product used outwith the authorized age range
- Authorized product administered by an unauthorized route
- Authorized product used to treat an animal in an unauthorized physiological state, e.g. pregnancy (i.e. an unauthorized indication)
- Product authorized for use in humans or a different animal species to that being treated.

Adverse effects may or may not be specific for a species, and idiosyncratic reactions are always a possibility. If no adverse effects are listed, consider data from different species. When using novel or unfamiliar drugs, consider pharmaceutical and pharmacological interactions. In some species, and with some diseases, the ability to metabolize/excrete a drug may be impaired/enhanced. Use the lowest dose that might be effective and the safest route of administration. Ensure that you are aware of the clinical signs that may suggest toxicity.

Information on 'off-label' use may be available from:

- The manufacturer of the medicine
- Formularies and textbooks
- Clinical papers in refereed journals
- Online sources: e.g. http://www.bnf.org.uk
  http://www.ingenta.com
  http://www.ncbi.nlm.nih.gov/entrez/query.fcgi/
  http://www.fda.gov/cder

Drug storage and dispensing

A code of practice on the storage and dispensing of medicines is available (Code of practice. Sale or supply of animal medicines by veterinary surgeons. *The Veterinary Record* 1990 **127**, 236–240). Loose tablets or capsules that are re-packaged from bulk containers should be dispensed in child-resistant containers and supplied with a package insert (if one exists). Preparations for external application should be dispensed in coloured fluted bottles. Oral liquids should be dispensed in plain glass bottles with child-resistant closures.

The label should include:

- The owner's name and address
- Date
- Product name (and strength)
- Total quantity of the product supplied in the container
- Instructions for dosage
- Practice name and address
- The wording 'Keep out of reach of children' and 'For animal treatment only'.

The words 'For external use only' should be included on labels for products for topical use. All labels should be typed.

Drug categorization for prescription purposes

Distribution categories

Retail supply of veterinary medicinal products is restricted according to which of four distribution categories they are legally classified under:

- Prescription Only Medicines (*POM*) may be supplied only by veterinary surgeons for animals under their care or by registered pharmacists in accordance with a veterinary prescription
- Pharmacy (*P*) products may be supplied only by veterinary surgeons for animals under their care or by registered pharmacists, without requiring a veterinary prescription

- Pharmacy and Merchants List (*PML*) products may be supplied by veterinary surgeons for animals under their care, by registered pharmacists or by registered agricultural merchants
- General Sales List (*GSL*) products may be supplied by any retail outlet, including supermarkets and pet shops.

Controlled Drugs

Controlled Drugs are regulated by the Misuse of Drugs Act 1971 and the Misuse of Drugs Regulations 1985. These regulations classify such drugs into 5 schedules, numbered in decreasing order of severity of control.

Schedule 1: Includes LSD, cannabis, lysergide and other drugs that are not used medicinally. Possession and supply are prohibited except in accordance with Home Office Authority.

Schedule 2: Includes etorphine, morphine, papaveretum, pethidine, diamorphine (heroin), cocaine and amphetamine. Record all purchases and each individual supply (within 24 hours). Registers must be kept for 2 calendar years after the last entry. Drugs must be kept under safe custody (locked secure cabinet), except secobarbital. Drugs may not be destroyed except in the presence of a person authorized by the Secretary of State. You could be prosecuted for failure to comply with this act.

Schedule 3: Includes buprenorphine, pentazocine, the barbiturates (e.g. pentobarbital and phenobarbital but not secobarbital – now Schedule 2) and others. Buprenorphine, diethylpropion and temazepam must be kept under safe custody (locked secure cabinet); it is advisable that all Schedule 3 drugs are locked away. Retention of invoices for 2 years is necessary.

Schedule 4: Includes butorphanol, most of the benzodiazepines (temazepam is now in Schedule 3), and androgenic and anabolic steroids (e.g. clenbuterol). Exempted from control when used in normal veterinary practice.

Schedule 5: Includes preparations (such as several codeine products) which, because of their strength, are exempt from virtually all Controlled Drug requirements other than the retention of invoices for 2 years.

Note: Prescriptions for Schedule 2 and 3 Controlled Drugs (with the exception of phenobarbital and temazepam) must be written in longhand by the prescribing veterinary surgeon and meet the prescription requirements of the Misuse of Drugs Regulations 1985. It is not acceptable to use typewriting nor the handwriting of any other person.

Writing a prescription

Good prescription principles include the following. Only 1, 8, 10 and 12 are legal requirements, the remainder are good practice:

1. Print or write legibly in ink or otherwise so as to be indelible. Sign in ink with your normal signature. Include the date on which the prescription was signed.
2. Use product or approved generic name for drugs **in capital letters – do not abbreviate.** Ensure the full name is stated, to include the pharmaceutical form and strength.
3. State duration of treatment where known and the total quantity to be supplied.
4. Write out microgram/nanogram – **do not abbreviate**.
5. Always put a 0 before an initial decimal point (e.g. 0.5 mg), but avoid the unnecessary use of a decimal point (e.g. 3 mg not 3.0 mg).
6. Give precise instructions concerning route/dose/formulation. Directions should preferably be in English without abbreviation. It is recognized that some Latin abbreviations are used; for details see page 9.
7. Any alterations invalidate the prescription – rewrite.
8. Prescriptions for Schedule 2 and most Schedule 3 Controlled Drugs **must** be entirely handwritten and include the total quantity in both words and figures, the form and strength of the drug.
9. The prescription should not be repeated more than three times without re-checking the patient.
10. Both the prescriber's and the client's names and addresses.
11. The directions that the prescriber wishes to appear on the labelled product. It is good practice to include the words 'For animal treatment only'.
12. A declaration that 'This prescription is for an animal under my care' or words to that effect.

The following is a standard form of prescription used:

From: *Address of practice*	*Telephone No.*
	Date
Animal's name	*Owner's name*
	Owner's address
Rx *Print name, strength and formulation of drug*	
Total quantity to be supplied	
Amount to be administered	
Frequency of administration	
Duration of treatment	
For animal treatment only	
For an animal under my care	
Non-repeat/repeat X *1, 2 or 3*	
	Name and Signature of veterinary surgeon

Health and safety in prescribing

Many medicines can be toxic to humans as well as animals. Toxicity may be mild or severe and includes carcinogenic and teratogenic effects. Warnings are given in the monographs. However, effects are not always well characterized and idiosyncratic reactions may occur. It is good practice for everyone to wear gloves and safety glasses when splitting tablets or aspirating potentially toxic liquids and to avoid inhaling powders by wearing a mask or working in a laminar-flow cabinet when handling powders, liquids or broken tablets. Avoid breaking tablets of cytotoxic drugs. The carcinogenic potential of medicines is something that many prescribers and users of drugs may not be aware of. Below are lists of medicines included in the *BSAVA Formulary* that are known or potential carcinogens. The lists are not all-inclusive: they include only those substances that have been evaluated. Most of the drugs are connected only with certain kinds of cancer. The relative carcinogenicity of the agents varies considerably and some do not cause cancer at all times or under all circumstances. Some may only be carcinogenic if a person is exposed in a certain way (for example, ingesting as opposed to touching the drug). For more detailed information, refer to the International Agency for Research on Cancer (IARC) or the National Toxicology Program (NTP) (information is available on their respective websites).

Drugs known to be human carcinogens:

Azathioprine
Busulfan
Chlorambucil
Cyclophosphamide
Ciclosporin
Oestrogens: non-steroidal and steroidal (Note: This applies to the group of compounds as a whole and not necessarily to all individual compounds within the group)
Melphalan

Drugs reasonably anticipated to be human carcinogens:

Androgenic (anabolic) steroids
Chloramphenicol
Cisplatin
Doxorubicin
Dantron
Metronidazole
Phenoxybenzamine
Phenytoin
Progesterone

Many drugs have the potential to cause injury to fetuses. Care must be taken in dosing pregnant animals. In addition, women of childbearing potential should avoid direct contact with the drugs listed below. The following list contains drugs that have been proven to be capable of acting as teratogens in animals and/or humans:

- ACE inhibitors – benazepril, enalapril, lisinopril, ramipril
- Albendazole
- Androgens
- Antibiotics – doxycycline, rifampin, streptomycin, trimethoprim
- Antifungals – ketoconazole, fluconazole, itraconazole, griseofulvin, flucytosine
- Antineoplastic drugs – busulfan, carboplatin, cisplatin, cytarabine, doxorubicin, fluorouracil, vincristine, vinblastine
- Antithyroid drugs – carbimazole/methimazole
- Desferrioxamine
- Diltiazem
- Finasteride
- Lithium
- Methotrexate
- Misoprostol
- Penicillamine
- Phenytoin
- Vitamin A
- Warfarin

In addition there are a few drugs that probably pose a risk to pregnant women and animals but have not been conclusively shown to be teratogens:

- Antibiotics – aminoglycosides, sulphonamides
- Anabolic steroids
- Antineoplastic drugs – chlorambucil, crisantaspase, cyclophosphamide, melphalan
- Beta-blockers
- NSAIDs

Abbreviations used in prescription writing

a.c.	before meals
ad. lib.	at pleasure
amp.	ampoule
b.i.d	twice a day
cap.	capsule
g	gram
h	hour
i.m.	intramuscular
i.p.	intraperitoneal
i.v.	intravenous
m^2	square metre
mg	milligram
ml	millilitre
o.m.	in the morning
o.n.	at night
p.c.	after meals
p.r.n	as required
q	every, e.g. q8h = every 8h
q.i.d./q.d.s	four times a day
q.s.	a sufficient quantity
s.c.	subcutaneous
Sig:	directions/label
stat	immediately
susp.	suspension
tab	tablet
t.i.d./t.d.s.	three times a day

Note: . Directions should preferably be in English without abbreviation. It is recognized that some Latin abbreviations are used when prescribing, but these should be limited to those listed above.

Other abbreviations used in the Formulary

ACE	angiotensin converting enzyme
ACTH	adrenocorticotrophic hormone
AV	atrioventricular
BW	body weight
CBC	complete blood count
CHF	congestive heart failure
CNS	central nervous system
COX	cyclo-oxygenase
CRF	chronic renal failure
CSF	cerebrospinal fluid
d	day
DIC	disseminated intravascular coagulation
ECG	electrocardiogram
EPI	exocrine pancreatic insufficiency
GI	gastrointestinal
h	hour
Hb	haemoglobin
i.m.	intramuscular
i.p.	intraperitoneal
i.t.	intratracheal
i.v.	intravenous
min	minute
p.o.	by mouth, orally (*per os*)
PU/PD	polyuria/polydipsia
RBC	red blood cell
SLE	systemic lupus erythematosus
STA	Special Treatment Authorization
VPC	ventricular premature contraction
WBC	white blood cell

DRUG LISTINGS AND MONOGRAPHS

The trade names of products licensed for use in dogs and/or cats are shown in bold type. Trade names of non-licensed products are in plain type and asterisked.

Acarbose (Glucobay*) *POM*

Indications: Acarbose inhibits alpha-glucosidases in the brush border of the small intestine, delaying post-prandial glucose peak by delaying carbohydrate digestion. It has a small but significant effect, reducing blood glucose. It improves control of glycaemia in diabetic animals responding poorly to insulin and dietary management.

Forms: *Oral:* 50 mg, 100 mg tablets.

Dose:
Cats: 12.5–25 mg/cat p.o. q12h.
Dogs: 12.5–25 mg/dog p.o. q12h (increase to 50 mg/dog q12h if no effect after 2 weeks and can titrate dose to 100 mg/dog although side effects will occur).

Adverse effects and contraindications: Diarrhoea is common (particularly at high doses), weight loss may occur and abnormal liver function tests, hepatitis and jaundice have been reported in man. Contraindicated in man during pregnancy or with concurrent inflammatory bowel disease.

Drug interactions: It has a synergistic effect with **sulphonylureas**.

Acepromazine maleate (ACP) *POM*

Indications: Acepromazine is a phenothiazine used alone or with opioid drugs for sedation or pre-anaesthetic medication in dogs, cats and rabbits. ACP is used in the management of aortic thromboembolism in cats. In small mammals it is used alone to provide sedation or as a pre-anaesthetic medication, or in combination with ketamine to provide anaesthesia. The duration of its sedative effect is dose-dependent; normal doses last from 1 to 4 hours. It is a suitable sedative for use in animals undergoing GI contrast studies as it has minimal effect on transit time.

Forms:
Injectable: 2 mg/ml solution.
Oral: 10 mg, 25 mg tablets.

Dose:
Cats: 0.05–0.2 mg/kg i.v., i.m., s.c. or 1–3 mg/kg p.o. Unreliable sedation when used alone. Co-administration of opioids and/or alpha$_2$ agonists lowers dose requirements. Up to 0.4 mg/kg in the management of thromboembolism.
Dogs: 0.01–0.1 mg/kg i.v., i.m., s.c. or 1–3 mg/kg p.o. Use lower doses i.v. Higher doses do not always increase sedation, but do increase adverse effects. Co-administration of opioids and/or alpha$_2$ agonists lowers dose requirements.
Small mammals: Ferrets: 0.2 mg/kg i.m., s.c., p.o.; Guinea pigs: 2.5–5 mg/kg i.m., s.c., p.o.; Rats: 2.5 mg/kg i.m., s.c., p.o.; Gerbils: 3 mg/kg i.m., s.c., p.o.; Hamsters: 5 mg/kg i.m., s.c., p.o.; Mice: 1–5 mg/kg i.m., s.c., p.o.
Reptiles: 0.1–0.5 mg/kg i.m.

See Sedation protocols, pages 297–301.

Adverse effects and contraindications: Cats, animals with liver dysfunction and giant breeds of dog should receive doses at the lower end of the dosage range; even low doses have been associated with prolonged effects of the drug. Rarely, an animal may develop profound hypotension following administration of phenothiazines. In these cases treatment with fluids (Hartmann's or colloid) and either phenylephrine or noradrenaline is indicated if hypotension is life-threatening. Doses above 0.01 mg/kg may precipitate hypotension in hypovolaemic animals. Some Boxers may collapse temporarily when normal doses are given by i.v. injection. Aggressive behaviour has been reported (very rarely) with the use of ACP. Do not leave dogs receiving ACP for the first time alone with other animals or children. The use of ACP in the management of sound phobias in dogs, such as firework or thunder phobia, is discouraged by behaviourists.

Drug interactions: Other CNS depressant agents (barbiturates, narcotics, anaesthetics) may cause additive CNS depression if used with acepromazine. **Quinidine** given with phenothiazines may cause additional cardiac depression. **Anti-diarrhoeal mixtures** (e.g. **kaolin/ pectin**, **bismuth salicylate**) and **antacids** may cause reduced GI absorption of oral phenothiazines. Increased blood levels of both drugs may result if **propranolol** is administered with phenothiazines. As phenothiazines block alpha-adrenergic receptors, concomitant use with **adrenaline** may lead to unopposed beta activity, thereby causing vasodilation and tachycardia.

Acetazolamide (Diamox*) *POM*

Indications: Acetazolamide is a carbonic anhydrase inhibitor which is primarily used for the treatment of acute glaucoma. It reduces the production of bicarbonate in aqueous humour and the water secreted with it, thus lowering intraocular pressure.

Forms:
Injectable: 500 mg solution.
Oral: 250 mg, 500 mg tablets.

Dose: *Dogs:* 5–10 mg/kg i.v. single dose or 2–10 mg/kg p.o.
q8–12h.

Adverse effects and contraindications: These appear to be dose-related and include weakness, vomiting, diarrhoea, panting, metabolic acidosis, diuresis, anorexia and potassium depletion. Topical carbonic anhydrase inhibitors are preferred in dogs and cats. Cats are particularly susceptible to the adverse effects of systemic carbonic anhydrase inhibitors. Avoid in this species.

Drug interactions: Primidone absorption may be inhibited by oral acetazolamide. Acetazolamide alkalinizes urine, thus the excretion rate of weak bases may be decreased, but weak acids increased. Concomitant use of **corticosteroids** may exacerbate potassium depletion causing hypokalaemia.

Acetylcysteine (Ilube*: Parvolex*) *POM*

Indications: Acetylcysteine is a mucolytic that decreases the viscosity of bronchial secretions. It also reduces the extent of liver injury following paracetamol overdose by maintaining glutathione levels in the liver. It may be useful in the treatment of keratoconjunctivitis sicca (KCS) (dry eye), or in melting corneal ulcers where the drug has an anticollagenase action. In the eye it may be used in conjunction with hypromellose.

Forms:
Injectable: 200 mg/ml solution.
Topical: 5% ophthalmic solution.

Dose:
Cats, Dogs:
- Mucolytic: Either nebulize 50 mg as a 2% (dilute with saline) solution over 30–60 minutes or instil directly into the trachea 1–2 ml of a 20% solution.
- Paracetamol poisoning: After inducing emesis, use immediately if ingestion occurred within 24 hours. Either give 150 mg/kg by i.v. infusion in 200 ml 5% glucose over 15 minutes, followed by 50 mg/kg i.v. infusion in 500 ml over 4 hours, then 100 mg/kg i.v. infusion in 1000 ml over 16 hours or give 140 mg/kg loading dose p.o., then 70 mg/kg p.o. q4h for 17 doses unless initial serum paracetamol levels indicate a non-toxic level. Oral solution should be diluted to a 5% solution and given via a stomach tube as it tastes unpleasant.
- KCS: 1 drop of the ophthalmic solution topically to the eye q6–8h.

- Melting corneal ulcers: 1 drop of the ophthalmic solution q1–4h in the affected eye for 24–48h. Topical autologous serum is more effective for the treatment of a melting corneal ulcer and is preferred to acetylcysteine.

Rabbits, Birds: Mucolytic: Either nebulize 50 mg as a 2% (dilute with saline) solution over 30–60 minutes or instil directly into the trachea 1–2 ml of a 20% solution.

Adverse effects and contraindications: Acetylcysteine has caused hypersensitivity and bronchospasm when used in the pulmonary tree. When given orally for paracetamol poisoning it may cause GI effects (nausea, vomiting) and rarely urticaria. Foul taste makes oral dosing difficult, therefore, administration via nasogastric tube is best.

Drug interactions: Use of **activated charcoal** for paracetamol poisoning is controversial as it may also absorb acetycysteine.

Aciclovir (Zovirax*) POM

Indications: Aciclovir is a pyrimidine analogue that inhibits thymidine incorporation into viral DNA. In man it is used in the management of ocular herpesvirus infections (herpes simplex virus 1). Aciclovir has very low effectiveness against feline herpesvirus 1 (FHV-1) *in vitro*, and its clinical use is questionable. *In vitro* studies show the combination of aciclovir and recombinant human interferon (IFN)-α to be effective against FHV-1; *in vivo* efficacy is not known.

Forms: *Topical:* 3% ointment.

Dose: *Cats:* Apply a small amount q4–6h for a maximum of 3 weeks.

Adverse effects and contraindications: It may have an initial stinging effect; reduce frequency application if necessary.

ACTH – see Tetracosactide

Adrenaline (Epinephrine*) POM

Indications: Adrenaline is an endogenous catecholamine that exerts alpha- and beta-adrenergic activity. It increases heart rate and the strength of myocardial contraction, increasing cardiac output. It has a variable effect on peripheral vascular smooth muscle; renal blood flow may increase or decrease depending on other factors. Bronchial smooth muscle relaxes and so airway resistance in status asthmaticus is reduced. Its widespread metabolic effects, e.g. glycogenolysis, lipolysis, gluconeogenesis, increase plasma glucose. Exogenous adrenaline is used for resuscitation in cardiac arrest, status asthmaticus and to offset the effects of histamine released in severe anaphylactoid reactions.

Forms:
Injectable (Adrenaline)*:* 1:1000 (1 mg/ml).
Ophthalmic (Eppy)*:* 1% eye drop.

Dose:
Cats: 20 µg/kg of a **1:10,000** solution (100 µg/ml) i.v., i.m.
Dogs: 20 µg/kg of a **1:1000** solution (1000 µg/ml) diluted to 5–10 ml in normal saline given by the i.v., intratracheal, intraosseous or intracardiac routes. **For dogs <10 kg use a 1:10,000 solution.**
Use lower doses for treating bronchoconstriction. The i.v. route is preferred if hypotension accompanies an anaphylactic reaction. Repeat doses may be required at 2–5 minute intervals.

When preparing injection, **do not confuse 1:1000 with 1:10,000 concentrations**. Do not use if it is pink, brown or contains precipitate. Adrenaline is sensitive to light and air, and is unstable in 5% dextrose.

Adverse effects and contraindications: By increasing myocardial work, adrenaline threatens myocardial oxygen balance and produces arrhythmias. Although useful in asystole it can cause ventricular fibrillation. These may be ameliorated by administering oxygen, and slowing the heart with beta$_1$ antagonists. The duration of action of adrenaline is normally short (2–5 minutes). Adverse effects include tachycardia, arrhythmias, dry mouth and cold extremities. Beware of using adrenaline in patients with diabetes mellitus, hypertension or hyperthyroidism. Repeated injections can cause necrosis at the injection site. Use with caution in hypovolaemic animals. It is not a substitute for fluid replacement therapy.

Drug interactions: Toxicity may occur if used with other **sympatho-mimetic amines** because of additive effects. The effects of adrenaline may be potentiated by **antihistamines** and **thyroxine**. **Propranolol** may block the beta effects of adrenaline, thus facilitating an increase in blood pressure. **Alpha blocking agents** or **diuretics** may negate or diminish the pressor effects of adrenaline. When adrenaline is used with drugs that sensitize the myocardium (e.g. **halothane**, **high doses of digoxin**) monitor for signs of arrhythmias. Try to avoid the use of adrenaline in halothane-anaesthetized animals. Hypertension may result if adrenaline is used with **oxytocic agents.**

Albendazole (Albex*) *PML*

Indications: Albendazole is a benzimidazole anthelmintic used to treat *Toxacara cati, Trichuris vulpis, Uncinaria stenocephala, Ancylostoma caninum, Taenia pisiformis, Taenia hydatigena, Echinococcus granulosus, Taeniaformis hydatigena, Aelurostrongylus abstrusus, Angiostrongylus vasorum, Capillaria* spp., *Paragonimus kellicoti* and *Oslerus osleri* infections. Albendazole is also effective in

Giardia infections and may be useful in the management of
Encephalitozoon cuniculi infection.

Forms: *Oral:* 25 mg/ml, 100 mg/ml suspensions.

Dose:
Cats, Dogs: 25 mg/kg p.o. q12h for 5–10 days.
Small mammals: Rabbits: *Encephalitozoon cuniculi* 15 mg/kg p.o.
q24h; 30 mg/kg p.o. for ocular encephalitozoonosis. Its use for
E. cuniculi is anecdotal and extrapolated from man. Drug of choice is
fenbendazole.
Reptiles: 50–75 mg/kg p.o. q24h for 1–5 days.

Adverse effects and contraindications: Albendazole has been
reported to cause bone marrow toxicosis (pancytopenia) in a cat and
dog; use with caution in these species. Some benzimidazoles including
albendazole have been shown to be teratogenic. Do not use at mating or
during early pregnancy.

Alfaxalone/Alfadolone (Alphaxolone/Alphadolone)
(**Saffan**) *POM*

Indications: Alfaxalone and alfadolone are steroid-based intravenous
anaesthetics licensed for use in cats and monkeys. They may be used
(unlicensed) in various small animals. Low doses given i.m. produce
sedation, not anaesthesia.

Forms: *Injectable:* 9 mg alfaxalone/ml plus 3 mg alfadolone/ml
solution in polyethoxylated castor oil (Cremaphor EL).

Dose:
Cats: 9 mg (0.75 ml)/kg i.v. or 12–18 mg (1–1.5 ml)/kg i.m. Drug
effects are least erratic when the quadriceps muscle group is used.
Small mammals: Ferrets: 9–12 mg (0.5–0.75 ml)/kg i.v., i.m.; Rabbits:
6–9 mg/kg i.v. or 9 mg/kg i.m.; Rodents: 20 mg/kg i.m. or 120 mg/kg i.p
except Guinea Pigs: 40 mg/kg i.m. or i.p.
Birds: 5–10 mg/kg i.v., i.m., s.c.
Reptiles: 6–9 mg/kg i.v. or 15 mg/kg i.m.

Adverse effects and contraindications: Saffan causes fatal
anaphylactic reactions in dogs (due to histamine release) caused by
the cremaphor vehicle; **do not use in dogs**. Cats may exhibit oedema
and flushing of the paws and ears although such reactions usually
subside within a few hours. Rarely, laryngeal, pulmonary or cerebral
oedema may occur. Prompt therapy with antihistamines,
corticosteroids or diuretics may alleviate associated clinical signs. If
given i.v. to birds, transient apnoea may be seen. In small mammals
analgesia is insufficient for major surgery. Respiratory arrest may
occur with higher dose rate.

Drug interactions: Barbiturates must not be used in animals sedated with alfaxalone/alfadolone.

Alfentanil (Rapifen*) *POM* Scheduled 2 Controlled Drug

Indications: Alfentanil is a pure mu (OP3) agonist of the phenyl-piperidine series. Its high lipid solubility confers a rapid onset (15–30 seconds) and a short duration of action (3–7 minutes). It shows slight cumulative properties only after repeated injections or prolonged infusions. As an analgesic drug it is 10–20 times more potent than morphine in man and is given by repeated doses or infusion to dogs to provide profound intra-operative analgesia. The dose of propofol required for induction of anaesthesia is reduced considerably if alfentanil is given immediately before or with the anaesthetic. It is a potent respiratory depressant.

Forms: *Injectable:* 0.5 mg/ml, 5.0 mg/ml solution.

Dose: *Dogs:* 0.001–0.005 mg/kg i.v. may be used to provide intra-operative analgesia. A solution made from 10 ml of 0.5 mg/ml alfentanil in 490 ml Hartmann's solution, infused at 1 ml/10 kg/min, is equivalent to 0.001 mg/kg/min. Infusion rates of 0.001–0.0025 mg/kg/min are required for profound analgesia. Adding 50 mg ketamine (0.5 ml) to the solution and infusing at the same rate increases the anaesthetic-sparing effect and improves the quality of post-operative analgesia.

Adverse effects and contraindications: Rapid injection can cause severe bradycardia, even asystole. This may be prevented by slow injection or the prior or co-injection of atropine (0.04 mg/kg). Alfentanil is a potent respiratory depressant; IPPV must be imposed whenever alfentanil is used.

Drug interactions: The dose requirement for alfentanil is reduced by drugs with CNS depressant effects. Alfentanil reduces the dose requirements of concurrently administered **anaesthetics**, including inhaled anaesthetics, by at least 50%.

Alimemazine (Trimeprazine) (Vallergan*) *POM*

Indications: Alimemazine is a phenothiazine antihistamine. It has antihistamine, antimuscarinic and anti-emetic effects and is indicated for the management of pruritus and allergies. It has been advocated for the short-term management of mild sound phobias in dogs and for control of mild anxiety conditions in dogs including anxiety related to car travel.

Forms: *Oral:* 10 mg tablets; 1.5 mg/ml, 6 mg/ml syrups.

Dose: *Cats, Dogs:* 0.5–2 mg/kg p.o. q12h.

Adverse effects and contraindications: Alimemazine causes sedation which may be excessive in cats (beware its use in this species). It may also cause depression, hypotension and extrapyramidal reactions (rigidity, tremor, weakness, restlessness).

Drug interactions: Quinidine when given with phenothiazines may cause additive cardiac depression. **Propranolol** may cause increased blood levels of phenothiazines. Phenothiazines block alpha-adrenergic receptors, therefore, concurrent **adrenaline** administration leads to unopposed beta activity, which can result in vasodilation and increased heart rate.

Allopurinol (Allopurinol*) *POM*

Indications: Allopurinol is a xanthine oxidase inhibitor that decreases formation of uric acid by blocking the conversion of hypoxanthine to xanthine, and of xanthine to uric acid. It is used prophylactically in dogs in the treatment of recurrent uric acid uroliths and hyperuricosuric calcium oxalate urolithiasis and, in combination with meglumine antimonate, to treat leishmaniasis. Published data suggests long-term treatment with allopurinol is an effective way of maintaining clinical remission in dogs with leishmaniasis but does not eliminate the organism from the bone marrow. In birds and reptiles it is used in the treatment of hyperuricaemia and gout, and the management of renal disease.

Forms: *Oral:* 100 mg, 300 mg tablet.

Dose:
Dogs:
- Uric acid urolithiasis: 10 mg/kg p.o. q8h for 1 month, then 10 mg/kg p.o. q24h.
- Leishmaniasis: 30 mg/kg p.o. q24h with meglumine antimonate for up to 3 months, then 20 mg/kg p.o. q24h for one week each month.

Birds: 10 mg/kg p.o. q12h, 10 mg tablet/30 ml drinking water.
Reptiles: 10–20 mg/kg p.o. q24h.

Adverse effects and contraindications: Use with caution in patients with impaired renal function.

Drug interactions: In man allopurinol may enhance the effects of **azathioprine** and **theophylline**.

Alphaxolone/Alphadolone – see Alfaxolone/Alfadolone

Alprazolam (Xanax*) *POM*

Indications: Alprazolam, a benzodiazepine, is used in the treatment of anxiety-related disorders in dogs and cats, e.g. short-term management of fears and phobias including fear related to car travel. Primarily used in treatment of feline cases but it can be useful as a short-term drug for the management of canine noise phobia during exposure to the fear-inducing stimulus. In addition, it can be used during a long-term behavioural therapy programme for canine sound phobias in order to avoid relapses due to exposure to an intensely fear-inducing stimulus during treatment. Alprazolam may be given with sertraline or selegeline in these circumstances.

Forms: *Oral:* 0.25 mg, 0.5 mg tablets.

Dose:
Cats: 0.125–0.25 mg/kg as required up to twice a day.
Dogs: 0.01–0.1 mg/kg as required up to twice a day.

Adverse effects and contraindications: Drowsiness and mild transient incoordination may develop. Human patients report dizziness. In cats there have been reports of increased friendliness. Alprazolam is contraindicated in the long-term treatment of canine and feline behavioural disorders due to risks of disinhibition and interference with memory and learning. A paradoxical increase in activity is possible following oral administration. Alprazolam appears to be less hepatotoxic than diazepam, possibly because it is not metabolized into nordiazepam or any other active metabolite, as is the case with diazepam and clorazepate.

Drug interactions: These are as for diazepam.

Aluminium antacids (Aluminium Hydroxide*; Asilone*; Gastrocote*; Maalox*; Mucogel*; Topal*) *GSL*

Indications: Aluminium antacids lower serum phosphate levels in cats and dogs with hyperphosphataemia by binding phosphate (PO_4^{3-}) in the GI tract, making it unavailable for absorption. They neutralize gastric acid and are used in the management of gastritis. Frequent administration is necessary to prevent rebound acid secretion.

Forms: *Oral:* Various products are available as tablets or gel. Aluminium hydroxide alone – 500 mg tablet, 4% w/w gel. Other human products are compound preparations containing a variety of other compounds including MgO, $Mg(OH)_2$, alginates and dimeticone. Aluminium hydroxide content varies.

Dose: *Cats*, *Dogs*: Initially 10–30 mg/kg p.o. q8h (tablets) or 5–10 ml p.o. q8h (gel) with or immediately after meals. Monitor serum phosphate levels at 10–14 day intervals and adjust dosage accordingly to achieve normal serum levels.

Adverse effects and contraindications: Constipation may occur. Phosphate-binding agents are usually used only if low phosphate diets are unsuccessful. Thoroughly mix the drug with food to disperse it throughout the GI tract and to increase its palatability. Long-term use (many years) of oral aluminium products in man has been associated with aluminium toxicity. This is unlikely to be a problem in veterinary medicine.

Drug interactions: Do not administer **tetracycline** products orally within 2 hours of aluminium salts.

Amantadine (Lysovir*; Symmetrel*) POM

Indications: Amantadine is a tricyclic amine that can be used as an adjunct analgesic for the treatment of chronic pain. In dogs it has been used to control neuropathic pain in cancer patients that is poorly controlled by opioids. Some dogs with osteoarthritis may benefit from its addition to the therapeutic plan. Support for the use of amantadine in this area is anecdotal.

Forms: *Oral:* 100 mg capsule, 10 mg/ml syrup.

Dose: *Dogs:* 3 mg/kg p.o. q24h. This is an empirical dose and based on very few reports.

Adverse effects and contraindications: In man minor GI and CNS effects have been reported.

Amethocaine – see Tetracaine

Amikacin (Amikin*) POM

Indications: Amikacin is an aminoglycoside antibiotic active against many Gram-negative bacteria including some that may be resistant to gentamicin. Aminoglycosides require an oxygen-rich environment to be effective, thus they are ineffective in low-oxygen sites (abscesses, exudates), making all obligate anaerobic bacteria resistant. They are bactericidal and their mechanism of killing is concentration-dependent, leading to a marked post-antibiotic effect, allowing pulse-dosing regimens to limit toxicity.

Forms: *Injectable:* 50 mg/ml, 250 mg/ml solutions.

Dose:
Cats, Dogs: 5–10 mg/kg i.v., i.m., s.c. q8h or 10–15 mg/kg i.v., i.m., s.c. q24h (possibly less nephrotoxic). Doses up to 30 mg/kg i.v., i.m., s.c. q24h have been recommended by some authors for managing septic shock, although there is an increased risk of adverse effects with such high doses. Intravenous doses should be given slowly, generally over 30–60 minutes.
Birds: 10–20 mg/kg i.m., s.c. q8–12h.
Reptiles: 2.5–5 mg/kg i.m. q72h @ 25°C.

Adverse effects and contraindications: In common with other aminoglycosides, amikacin is nephrotoxic and ototoxic, and can potentiate neuromuscular blockade. Monitoring serum amikacin levels should be considered to ensure therapeutic levels and minimize toxicity, particularly in neonates, geriatric patients and those with reduced renal function. Amikacin should be reserved for use in gentamicin-resistant infections or where gentamicin resistance is a high probability. Use with caution in birds as it is toxic.

Drug interactions: Avoid the concurrent use of other nephrotoxic, ototoxic or neurotoxic agents (e.g. **amphotericin B**, **cisplatin**, **furosemide**). Increase monitoring and adjust dosages when these drugs must be used with amikacin. Aminoglycosides may be inactivated by **beta-lactam antibiotics** (e.g. **penicillins**, **cephalosporins**) or **heparin**; do not give these drugs in the same syringe. The effect of non-depolarizing muscle relaxants (e.g. **atracurium**, **pancuronium**, **tubocurarine**, **vecuronium**) may be enhanced by aminoglycosides. Synergism may occur when aminoglycosides are used with **penicillins** or **cephalosporins** (*Streptococcus faecalis*) or with **ticarcillin** (*Pseudomonas aeruginosa*).

Amiloride (Amiloride*) *POM*

Indications: Amiloride is a potassium-sparing weak diuretic used in the management of oedema. It causes retention of potassium and is a more effective alternative to giving potassium supplementation with thiazide or loop diuretics.

Forms: *Oral:* 5 mg tablets; 1 mg/ml solution.
Also present in compound preparations with hydrochlorothiazide and furosemide.

Dose: ***Cats, Dogs:*** Doses in companion animals have not been widely reported. 0.1 mg/kg p.o. q12h is used in man.

Adverse effects and contraindications: Avoid its use if renal insufficiency, diabetes mellitus or hyperkalaemia present. Hypotension, hyperkalaemia and hyponatraemia may develop with its use.

Drug interactions: Avoid the concomitant administration of **potassium**.

Amino acid solutions (Aminoplasmal*; **Duphalyte;**
Freamine*; HeplexAmine*; Nephramine*; Synthamin*; Viamin*) *POM*

Indications: Amino acid solutions supply essential amino acids for protein production. They are used parenterally in patients requiring nutritional support.

Forms: *Injectable:* Crystalline amino acid solutions with added electrolytes for i.v. use only. There are many products available that contain various concentrations of amino acids (6.4–24.9%) and electrolytes.
Aminoplasmal: 8.03%, 16.06% amino acids + K^+, Mg^{2+}, Na^+, Cl^-, HCO_3^-
Freamine: 9.73%, 13.0%, 15.3% amino acids + Na^+, Cl^-, HCO_3^-
HeplexAmine: 8% + Na^+, Cl^-, HCO_3^-
Nephramine: 6.4% essential amino acids only + Na^+, Cl^-, HCO_3^-
Synthamin: 9.1%, 14% amino acid + K^+, Mg^{2+}, Na^+, Cl^-, HCO_3^-
Viamin: 9.4%, 13.5% amino acids + K^+, Mg^{2+}, Na^+, Cl^-, HCO_3^-

Duphalyte contains small quantities of many amino acids and some electrolytes. Its main use is in the prevention and treatment of dehydration and electrolyte imbalances. It is not suitable as a sole source of amino acids in animals requiring nutritional support.

Dose:
Cats: 5–8 g protein/100 kcal (418 kJ) illness energy requirements.
Duphalyte: 10 ml/kg by slow i.v. infusion or s.c.
Dogs: 3–6 g protein/100 kcal (418 kJ) illness energy requirements.
Duphalyte: 10 ml/kg by slow i.v. infusion or s.c.

Illness energy requirement = (70 x body weight$^{0.75}$) x illness factor. The illness factor ranges 1.3–2 in dogs and 1.4–1.5 in cats.

Adverse effects and contraindications: If amino acid solutions that do not contain electrolytes are used, an electrolyte mixture should be added to the parenteral fluid mixture. Amino acid solutions are hypertonic and should not be administered undiluted into a peripheral vein; dilute with fat if given through a peripheral vein to provide partial parenteral nutrition. If mixed with glucose as part of a total parenteral nutrition package, administer through a central vein into the cranial vena cava.

Aminophylline (Aminophylline*) *POM*

Indications: Aminophylline is a stable mixture of theophylline and ethylenediamine. The latter increases the water solubility of theophylline. Aminophylline is a spasmolytic agent and has a mild diuretic action. It is used to dilate bronchi and in the management of pulmonary oedema.

Forms:
Injectable: 25 mg/ml solution.
Oral: 100 mg tablet.
For modified-release preparations see Theophylline.
100 mg of aminophylline is equivalent to 79 mg of theophylline.

Dose:
Cats: 6.6 mg/kg p.o. q12h or 2–5 mg/kg slowly i.v. (diluted) for emergency bronchodilation.
Dogs: 9–11 mg/kg slowly i.v. (diluted) for emergency bronchodilation, i.m., p.o. q6–8h.
Aminophylline causes intense local pain when given i.m. and is very rarely used or recommended via this route.

Adverse effects and contraindications: These include nausea, vomiting, increased gastric acid secretion, diarrhoea, polyphagia, PU/PD and cardiac arrhythmias. Hyperaesthesia may be seen in cats. Administer with caution in patients with severe cardiac disease, gastric ulcers, hyperthyroidism, renal or hepatic disease, severe hypoxia or severe hypertension. Theophylline has a low therapeutic index and should be dosed on a lean body weight basis. Most adverse effects are related to the serum level and may be symptomatic of toxic levels.

Drug interactions: Do not mix aminophylline in a syringe with other drugs. Agents that may increase the serum levels of theophylline include **cimetidine, erythromycin** and **allopurinol. Phenobarbital** may decrease the serum concentration of theophylline. Theophylline may decrease the effects of **phenytoin** and **pancuronium**. Theophylline and **beta-adrenergic blockers** (e.g. **propranolol**) may antagonize each other's effects. Theophylline with **halothane** may cause an increased incidence of cardiac dysrhythmias and with **ketamine** an increased incidence of seizures.

Amiodarone (Cordarone X*) *POM*

Indications: Amiodarone is a class 3 anti-dysrhythmic drug, used in veterinary medicine for treatment of refractory tachydysrhythmias. It prolongs the duration of the action potential in the atria and ventricles, inhibits sympathetic nervous system action, slows the sinus rate, prolongs sinus node recovery time, and prolongs the absolute and relative refractory periods in the AV node and His–Purkinje system. It may be useful in ventricular pre-excitation syndromes because it can prolong AV nodal and anomalous pathway absolute refractory periods. It has slow GI absorption, a slow onset of action and a long elimination half-life.

Forms: *Oral:* 100 mg, 200 mg tablets.

Dose: *Dogs:* 10–15 mg/kg q12h p.o. for 7 days, then 5–7.5 mg/kg q12h for 14 days; thereafter 7.5 mg/kg q24h.

Adverse effects and contraindications: Amiodarone causes bradycardia, AV block and prolongation of the QT interval. It is a negative inotrope and can cause hypotension. GI (vomiting) and systemic side-effects (hypothyroidism, pulmonary fibrosis and corneal deposits) have been reported in man. Anorexia, hepatotoxicity and positive Coombs' test results have been reported in dogs. T4 level decreases with amiodarone administration, but clinically apparent hypothyroidism is rare.

Drug interactions: Amiodarone may significantly increase serum levels and/or pharmacological effects of **anti-coagulants**, **beta-blockers**, **calcium-channel blockers**, **ciclosporin**, **digoxin**, **lidocaine**, **methotrexate**, **procainamide**, **quinidine** and **theophylline**. **Cimetidine** may increase serum levels of **amiodarone**.

Amitraz (Aludex) *POM*

Indications: Amitraz is used to treat generalized mite infestations including demodicosis, sarcoptic mange and cheyletiellosis (unlicensed use). It increases neuronal activity through its action on octopamine receptor sites in mites.

Forms: Topical: 5% w/v concentrated liquid

Dose: *Dogs, Ferrets:* Demodicosis: Use a 0.05% solution – 1 ml Aludex in 100 ml water. Other mites, including *Sarcoptes*: Use a 0.025% solution – 1 ml Aludex in 200 ml water.

Make up sufficient to allow complete immersion of paws and total wetting of the coat. Pour over affected parts, working into skin with sponge or soft brush. Do not rinse off. Treat q5–7d until neither live mites nor viable eggs are present in three consecutive scrapes at weekly intervals or for 3 weeks after resolution of signs.

Small mammals: Rodents: 0.007% solution–1.4 ml Aludex in 1000 ml water. Apply with a cotton bud q14d for 3–6 treatments.

Caution: Wear waterproof gloves and apron to protect exposed skin when mixing solution and when treating. Avoid handling the animal immediately after treatment. The concentrate is flammable until diluted with water. Do not store diluted product.

Adverse effects and contraindications: A small number of dogs may develop transient lethargy and depression following treatment, which is exacerbated by chilling. These signs can be alleviated by washing in soapy water and administering an alpha$_2$ antagonist, e.g. atipamezole. Contraindicated in pregnant or lactating animals, in chihuahuas and in dogs suffering from heat stress. Amitraz is not licensed for use in the cat or small mammals. Amitraz is harmful to fish.

Amitriptyline (Amitriptyline*) *POM*

Indications: Amitriptyline is a tricyclic antidepressant that blocks noradrenaline and serotonin re-uptake in the brain, thereby increasing the effects of these neurotransmitters. It has been used in the management of pruritus and psychogenic disorders where there is a component of anxiety, including canine acral lick dermatitis, urine marking in cats, feline lower urinary tract disorders and feline hyperaesthesia.

Forms: *Oral:* 10 mg, 25 mg, 50 mg tablets; 5 mg/ml, 10 mg/ml solution.

Dose:
Cats: 0.25–1 mg/kg p.o. q24h.
Dogs: 1–2 mg/kg p.o. q12–24h.

Adverse effects and contraindications: A variety of adverse effects have been reported in man, including sedation, dry mouth, diarrhoea, vomiting, excitability, arrhythmias, hypotension, syncope, increased appetite, weight gain and, less commonly, seizures and bone marrow disorders.

Drug interactions: There is an increased risk of arrhythmias if amitriptyline is administered concurrently with **anaesthetics** and **anti-arrhythmics**. Tricyclics antagonize the effects of **anti-epileptics**. There is enhancement of sedative effects if used with other sedative drugs. Do not use in combination with monoamine oxidase inhibitors.

Amlodipine (Istin*) *POM*

Indications: Amlodipine is a 2nd generation dihydropyridine calcium-channel blocker, with predominant effects in the peripheral vasculature. It is a mild negative cardiac inotrope and chronotrope. It is used to treat systemic hypertension in cats and appears to be safe even when there is concurrent renal failure. Amlodipine has been used in dogs with systemic hypertension and in normotensive dogs with refractory cardiac failure, to reduce cardiac afterload.

Forms: *Oral:* 5 mg, 10 mg tablets.

Dose:
Cats: 0.625–1.25 mg/cat p.o. q24h.
Dogs: 0.05–0.1 mg/kg p.o. q12–24h.

Adverse effects and contraindications: To date no adverse effects have been reported at the recommended doses. Amlodipine is metabolized in the liver and dosage should be reduced when there is hepatic dysfunction. Amlodipine should be avoided in cardiogenic shock and pregnancy.

Drug interactions: Little is known regarding drug interactions and its pharmacokinetics in animals. Hepatic metabolism may be impaired by drugs such as **cimetidine**. Hypotension is a risk if combined with other anti-hypertensives, e.g. **ACE inhibitors**, **diuretics** and **beta-blockers**.

Amoxicillin (Amoxycillin) (Amoxinsol; Amoxycare; Amoxypen; Betamox; Bimoxyl; Clamoxyl; Duphamox; Vetremox; Vetrimoxin) POM

Indications: Amoxicillin is an acid-stable, beta-lactamase-susceptible aminopenicillin. It binds to penicillin-binding proteins involved in cell wall synthesis, thereby decreasing bacterial cell wall strength and rigidity, and affecting cell division, growth and septum formation. As animal cells lack a cell wall, the beta-lactam antibiotics are extremely safe. Beta-lactam antibiotics are active against certain Gram-positive and Gram-negative aerobic organisms and many obligate anaerobic organisms but not against those that produce penicillinases, e.g. *Escherichia coli*, *Staphylococcus aureus*. The more difficult Gram-negative organisms (*Pseudomonas* spp. and *Klebsiella* spp.) are usually resistant. Amoxicillin is excreted well in bile and urine.

Forms:
Injectable: 50 mg/ml suspension; 250 mg, 500 mg powder for reconstitution (Amoxil).
Oral: 40 mg, 100 mg, 150 mg, 200 mg tablets; 750 mg powder which when reconstituted provides 50 mg/ml; 25 g, 75 g of 100% amoxicillin powder for incorporation into drinking water; 20 mg/ml paste.
Refrigerate oral suspension after reconstitution – discard if solution becomes dark or after 7 days.

Dose:
Cats, Dogs: 7 mg/kg i.m. q12h or 11–22 mg/kg p.o. q8–12h. (Doses of 16–33 mg/kg i.v. q8h are used in man to treat serious infections.)
Small mammals: Ferrets: 100–150 mg/kg i.m., s.c. q12h; Rats, Mice: 100–150 mg/kg i.m., s.c. q12h.
Birds: 150 mg/kg i.m., s.c. q8–12h (q24h for long-acting preparations); Pigeons: 200 mg/l drinking water (Vetremox pigeon) q24h for 3–5d; Waterfowl: 1 g/l drinking water (amoxinsol soluble powder) alternate days for 3–5d, 300–500 mg/kg soft food for 3–5d.
Reptiles: (most species): 5–10 mg/kg i.m., p.o. q12–24h; chelonians: 5–50 mg/kg i.m., p.o. q12h.

Dose and dosing interval are determined by infection site, formulation used (long-acting depot *versus* rapidly acting soluble), severity of disease and organism. Amoxicillin can be given with food without substantial effects on its bioavailability. Amoxicillin is a bactericidal drug with time-dependent mode of killing. This means it is important to maintain tissue concentrations above MIC throughout the interdosing interval.

Adverse effects and contraindications: Avoid the use of oral antibiotic agents in critically ill patients as absorption from the GI tract may be unreliable. Nausea, diarrhoea and skin rashes are the commonest adverse effects. **Do not administer penicillins to hamsters, guinea pigs, gerbils, chinchillas or rabbits.**

Drug interactions: Avoid the concurrent use of amoxicillin with bacteriostatic antibiotics (e.g. **tetracycline**, **erythromycin**, **chloramphenicol**). Do not mix in the same syringe as **aminoglycosides**.

Amoxicillin/Clavulanate (Augmentin*; Nisamox; Synulox) POM

Indications: Amoxicillin is combined with a beta-lactamase inhibitor (clavulanate). This combination is active against Gram-positive and Gram-negative aerobic organisms and many obligate anaerobic organisms. Penicillinase-producing *E. coli* and *Staphylococcus* spp. are susceptible but difficult Gram-negative organisms such as *Pseudomonas aeruginosa* and *Klebsiella* spp. are often resistant.

Forms:
Injectable: 175 mg/ml suspension (140 mg amoxicillin, 35 mg clavulanate); 600 mg powder (500 mg amoxicillin, 100 mg clavulanate), 1.2 g powder (1 g amoxicillin, 200 mg clavulanate) for reconstitution (Augmentin).
Oral: 50 mg palatable tablet (40 mg amoxicillin, 10 mg clavulanate); 250 mg palatable tablet (200 mg amoxicillin, 50 mg clavulanate); 500 mg palatable tablets (400 mg amoxicillin, 100 mg clavulanate); powder which when reconstituted contains 50 mg/ml (amoxicillin 40 mg, clavulanate 10 mg) in a palatable solution.
Tablets are wrapped in foil, moisture-resistant packaging; do not remove until to be administered. Refrigerate oral suspension after reconstitution – discard if solution becomes dark or after 10 days.

Dose:
Cats, Dogs: 8.75 mg/kg (combined) i.v. q8h, i.m., s.c. q24h or 12.5–25 mg/kg (combined) p.o. q8–12h. Doses up to 25 mg/kg i.v. q8h are used to treat serious infections in man.
Small mammals: Ferrets: 12.5–20 mg/kg i.m., s.c. q12h.
Birds: 35 mg/kg i.v. q8–12h, i.m., s.c. q24h, 125 mg/kg p.o. q8h or 500 mg/l drinking water (poultry).
Dose and dosing interval determined by infection site, severity and organism.

Adverse effects and contraindications: Avoid oral antibiotic agents in critically ill patients as absorption from the GI tract may be unreliable. Such patients may require i.v. formulation. Nausea, diarrhoea and skin rashes are the commonest adverse effects. **Do not administer to hamsters, guinea pigs, gerbils, chinchillas and rabbits.**

Drug interactions: Avoid the concurrent use of amoxicillin with bacteriostatic antibiotics (e.g. **tetracycline**, **erythromycin**). Do not mix in the same syringe as **aminoglycosides**. Do not use with **allopurinol** in birds.

Amphotericin B (Abelcet*; AmBisome*; Amphocil*; Fungilin*; Fungizone*) POM

Indications: Amphotericin B is a polyene fungicidal antibiotic used to treat serious systemic mycoses, fungal septicaemia or fungal urinary tract infections. *Candida* is particularly susceptible to this agent. The drug is not absorbed following oral administration and is used by this route in man to treat intestinal candidiasis. Amphotericin has also been used to treat leishmaniasis. Various reports suggest elimination of this parasite from the bone marrow from some but not all affected dogs can be achieved with this treatment. Amphotericin is highly plasma protein-bound and penetrates into body fluids and tissues relatively poorly.

Forms:
Injectable: 50 mg/vial powder for reconstitution.
Oral: 100 mg tablets (Fungilin).
Loss of drug activity is negligible for at least 8 hours in room light. After reconstitution the preparation is stable for 1 week if refrigerated and stored in the dark. Do not dilute in saline.
Abelcet, AmBisome, Amphocil are lipid formulations that are less toxic.

Dose:
Cats, Dogs:
- Systemic use: 0.25–1 mg/kg i.v. q24–48h. Administer slowly over 4–6 hours. Dilute the initial solution in 50 ml of 5% dextrose to give a final concentration of 0.1 mg/ml. Alternatively, 0.25–1 mg/kg may be dissolved in 5–20 ml of 5% dextrose and given rapidly i.v. 3 times/week. Start at the lower end of the dose range and increase gradually as the patient tolerates therapy. Several months of therapy are often necessary. A total cumulative dose of 4–8 mg/kg is recommended by some authors. Lipid formulations are far less toxic than conventional formulations for i.v. use because the drug is targeted to macrophages, but these preparations are much more expensive.
- Leishmaniasis: Use lipid-formulated products. 1–2.5 mg/kg twice weekly for 8 injections. Increase dose rate gradually – total dose >10 mg/kg.
- Irrigation of bladder: 200 mg amphotericin/litre of sterile water infused at a rate of 5–10 ml/kg into the bladder lumen daily for 5–15 days.

Small mammals: Ferrets: 0.4–0.8 mg/kg i.v. q7d for treatment of blastomycosis; Rabbits: 1 mg/kg i.v. q24h.
Birds: 1–1.5 mg/kg q8h i.v. for 7 days, or 1–1.5 mg/kg in 2 ml sterile water q24h intratracheally for 12 days then every other day for 5 weeks. For oral fungal disease apply q8h topically in mouth.
Reptiles: Nebulization of 5 mg in 150 ml saline for 1h q12h for 7 days.

Adverse effects and contraindications: These include hypo-kalaemia, leading to cardiac arrhythmias, phlebitis, hepatic failure, renal failure, vomiting, diarrhoea, pyrexia, muscle and joint pain, anorexia and anaphylactoid reactions. Nephrotoxicity is a major concern; do not use other nephrotoxic drugs concurrently. Risk of nephrotoxicity may be reduced if a fluid high in sodium is administered at the same time as the drug treatment is given. Adverse effects of fever, vomiting, etc. may be decreased by pre-treating with aspirin, diphenhydramine or an anti-emetic. Amphotericin B is very toxic to birds when administered systemically; avoid i.v. use if at all possible.

Drug interactions: Physically incompatible with **electrolyte solutions**. Amphotericin may increase the toxic effects of **cisplatin, fluorouracil, doxorubicin** and **methotrexate**. **Flucytosine** is synergistic with amphotericin B *in vitro* against *Candida, Cryptococcus* and *Aspergillus*.

Ampicillin (**Amfipen**; **Ampicaps**; **Ampicare**; **Ampitab**; Penbritin*)
POM

Indications: Ampicillin is an acid-stable, beta-lactamase-susceptible aminopenicillin. It binds to penicillin-binding proteins involved in cell wall synthesis, thereby decreasing bacterial cell wall strength and rigidity, and affecting cell division, growth and septum formation. As animal cells lack a cell wall the beta-lactam antibiotics are extremely safe. They are active against many Gram-positive and Gram-negative aerobic organisms and obligate anaerobes, but not against those that produce penicillinases, e.g. *Escherichia coli* and *Staphylococcus aureus*. The difficult Gram-negative organisms such as *Pseudomonas aeruginosa* and *Klebsiella* spp. are usually resistant. Ampicillin is excreted well in bile and urine.

Forms:
Injectable: Ampicillin sodium 250 mg, 500 mg powders for reconstitution (human licensed product only); 150 mg/ml suspension.
Oral: Ampicillin 50 mg, 125 mg tablets; 250 mg, 500 mg capsules.

Dose:
Cats, Dogs:
Routine infections: 10–40 mg/kg i.v., i.m., s.c., p.o. q6–8h.
CNS or serious bacterial infections: 40 mg/kg i.v. q6h is recommended
Small mammals: Ferrets: 25 mg/kg i.m., s.c. q12h; Rats, Mice: 25 mg/kg i.m., s.c. q12h, 50–200 mg/kg p.o. q12h.
Birds: 50–100 mg/kg i.v., i.m. q8–12h or 1–2 g/litre drinking water, 2–3 g/kg soft feed.
Reptiles: 20 mg/kg s.c., i.m. q24h @ 26°C.

Dose and dosing interval determined by infection site, severity and organism. Ampicillin is a bactericidal drug with time-dependent mode of killing. This means it is important to maintain tissue concentrations above MIC throughout the interdosing interval.

Adverse effects and contraindications: Avoid the use of oral antibiotic agents in critically ill patients as absorption from the GI tract may be unreliable. Nausea, diarrhoea and skin rashes are the commonest adverse effects. After reconstitution the sodium salt will retain adequate potency for up to 8 hours if refrigerated, but use within 2 hours if kept at room temperature. **Do not administer penicillins to hamsters, guinea pigs, gerbils, chinchillas or rabbits.**

Drug interactions: The absorption of ampicillin is reduced in the presence of **food**. Avoid the concurrent use of ampicillin with bacterio-static antibiotics (e.g. **tetracycline**, **erythromycin**, **chloramphenicol**). Do not mix in the same syringe as **aminoglycosides**.

Amprolium (Coxoid) GSL

Indications: Amprolium is a coccidiostat used in the treatment of coccidiosis in homing/racing pigeons.

Forms: *Oral:* 3.84% solution for dilution in water.

Dose: *Pigeons:* 28 ml of the concentrate in 4.5 litres of drinking water for 7 days. In severe outbreaks continue with half strength solution for a further 7 days. Medicated water should be discarded after 24 hours.

Drug interactions: Do not use with or mix with any other medicinal product or substance having a similar effect.

Antibacterial immunoglobulin (Stegantox) POM

Indications: Stegantox is a polyclonal purified endotoxin-specific IgG prepared from horses immunized with extracts of several *Salmonella* species, *Escherichia coli* (several serotypes), *Klebsiella pneumoniae*, *Pseudomonas aeruginosa*, *Serratia marcescens* and *Shigella flexneri*. Stegantox neutralizes and opsonizes bacterial endotoxins, is bactericidal in the presence of complement and enhances phagocytosis of Gram-negative bacteria. It is indicated in the management of endotoxaemia, which may occur in severe septic conditions. It is likely to be most effective early in the disease prior to damage to organs by endotoxins. It will not reverse toxic effects present prior to treatment. It must be used in conjunction with appropriate therapy for the specific condition.

Forms: *Injectable:* 10 mg vial.

Dose: *Cats, Dogs:* 10 mg/20 kg slow i.v. repeated once only with at least 24 hours between doses.

Adverse effects and contraindications: All antisera have the potential to produce anaphylactoid reactions, particularly if the patient has previously received products containing horse protein. Repeated doses may lead to hypersensitivity reactions. Adrenaline or antihistamines may be used to manage these adverse effects.

Anti-diarrhoeal mixtures (BCK; Forgastrin) *GSL*

Indications: Adsorbents form a protective coating on the GI wall and adsorb toxins. Bismuth may be active against gastric spiral bacteria (e.g. *Helicobacter* spp.), and may have an anti-secretory activity in the small intestine. *See also Kaolin, Bismuth, Sterculia, Charcoal.*

Forms: *Oral:* BCK: Oral granules containing 40 mg/g bismuth, 50 mg/g calcium phosphate, 400 mg/g charcoal, 430 mg/g kaolin.
Forgastrin: Oral powder containing 25 mg/g bismuth, 270 mg/g charcoal.

Dose: *Cats, Dogs:* 5–15 ml p.o. q8–12h.

Adverse effects and contraindications: Beware long-term use of bismuth compounds (unless chelates) as absorbed bismuth can be neurotoxic.

Drug interactions: Anti-diarrhoeal adsorbents may decrease the absorption of **lincomycin** and **clindamycin**.

Antivenom (Farillon*) *POM*

Indications: European viper venom antitoxin is used in the management of snake bites by the European Viper.

Forms: *Injectable:* available from Farillon Ltd, 01708 379000.

Dose: *Cats, Dogs:* 10 ml concentrated antivenom per animal, diluted in 5 ml of 0.9% NaCl/kg body weight. Administer by i.v. infusion over 30 minutes or i.v. injection over 10–15 minutes. Repeat after 1–2 hours if signs persist.

Adverse effects and contraindications: Anaphylactic reactions may develop.

Apomorphine (APO-go*) *POM*

Indications: Apomorphine is a dopaminergic drug used to induce self-limiting emesis within a few minutes of administration in dogs.

Forms: Injectable: 10 mg/ml solution

Dose: *Dogs:* 40–100 µg/kg s.c., i.m. (s.c. route is more effective).

Adverse effects and contraindications: Induction of vomiting is contraindicated if the dog is unconscious, fitting, or has a reduced cough reflex, or if the poison has been ingested for more than 2 hours, or if the ingesta contains paraffin, petroleum products or other oily or volatile organic products, due to the risk of inhalation. Induction of emesis is contraindicated if strong acid or alkali has been ingested, due to the risk of further damage to the oesophagus. Apomorphine may induce excessive vomiting, respiratory depression and sedation.

Apraclonidine (Iopidine*) *POM*

Indications: Apraclonidine is a topical selective alpha$_2$ adrenoceptor agonist used to reduce intraocular pressure in cases of glaucoma in man. However, its effect in dogs is inconsistent and it is unlikely to be effective as the sole agent in most forms of canine glaucoma. It may be most useful in alleviating pressure rises after intraocular surgery.

Forms: *Topical:* 0.5% solution, preservative-free 1% solution (single-dose vials).

Dose: *Dogs:* 1 drop q8h for short-term use only.

Adverse effects and contraindications: Causes mydriasis, blanching of conjunctival vessels and bradycardia in dogs. In man dry mouth and ocular irritation are reported. Commercial preparations are considered too toxic for use in cats. Do not use in dogs with uncontrolled cardiac disease.

Artificial tears – see Hypromellose

Ascorbic acid – see Vitamin C

Aspirin (Acetyl salicylic acid) (Aspirin*) *P*

Indications: Aspirin is an NSAID that inhibits COX-1 enzyme, thereby limiting prostaglandin production. NSAIDs have antipyretic, analgesic, anti-inflammatory and anti-platelet effects. Aspirin is used to control mild to moderate pain and to prevent arterial thromboembolization.

Forms: *Oral:* 300 mg tablet.

Dose:
Cats: 10–25 mg/kg p.o. q48h; a suggested dosing schedule for chronic therapy (anti-inflammatory or anti-platelet) in an average sized cat is $^1/_4$ of a 300 mg tablet p.o. on Monday, Wednesday and Friday.
Dogs:
- Antipyretic/analgesic: 10 mg/kg p.o. q12h.
- Anti-inflammatory: 10–25 mg/kg p.o. q8–12h.
- Rheumatoid arthritis: 42 mg/kg p.o. q3d.

Note: Some texts recommend a very low dose of 0.5 mg/kg p.o. q24h to inhibit platelet cyclooxygenase (and therefore platelet function) without preventing the beneficial effects of prostacyclin production.

Adverse effects and contraindications: Adverse effects are dose-related and reflect the pathophysiological changes expected with reduced prostaglandin synthesis. The commonest adverse effect is GI irritation and ulceration. Cytoprotection from gastric ulceration is provided by misoprostol. Renal papillary necrosis (renal failure) is the second most common adverse effect, particularly if hypotension, dehydration or other nephrotoxic drugs are present. Blood dyscrasias and hepatotoxicity may be seen rarely. Do not use if gastric or duodenal ulceration is suspected, in haemorrhagic syndromes, or in cases of renal failure. Severe toxicity (usually with an acute overdose) may present with vomiting, pyrexia, metabolic acidosis, depression, coma, seizures and GI bleeding. Treatment of acute toxic ingestion includes emptying the gut, treating the acidosis, alkalinizing urine with sodium bicarbonate, and supportive therapy.

Drug interactions: Do not use with **corticosteroids**, or with other **NSAIDs**. In man there is an increased risk of convulsions if NSAIDs are administered with **fluoroquinolones**. NSAIDs may antagonize the hypotensive effects of **anti-hypertensives** (e.g. **beta-blockers**). The concomitant use of **diuretics** may increase the risk of nephrotoxicity.

Atenolol (Atenolol*; Tenormin*) *POM*

Indications: Atenolol is a cardioselective beta adrenoceptor antagonist (beta-blocker) that is relatively specific for beta$_1$ adrenoceptors; at high doses it inhibits beta$_2$ adrenoceptors. It blocks the chronotropic and inotropic effects of beta-adrenergic stimulation, thereby slowing the heart. Its bronchoconstrictor, vasodilatory and hypoglycaemic effects are less marked. At levels in excess of therapeutic doses atenolol has a quinidine-like stabilizing effect on the heart. Indications include cardiac arrhythmias (atrial fibrillation, supraventricular tachycardia), hyperthyroidism, hypertrophic cardiomyopathy, aortic stenosis and systemic hypertension.

Forms: *Oral:* 25 mg, 50 mg, 100 mg tablets.

Dose:
Cats: 6.25–12.5 mg/cat p.o. q24h.
Dogs: 0.5–2 mg/kg p.o. q12h.

Adverse effects and contraindications: Adverse effects are most frequently seen in geriatric patients with chronic heart disease or in patients with rapidly decompensating cardiac failure. They include bradycardia, impaired AV conduction, myocardial depression, heart failure, syncope, glucose intolerance, bronchospasm, diarrhoea and peripheral vasoconstriction. The use of atenolol is contraindicated in patients with supraventricular bradycardia and AV block and relatively contraindicated in animals with congestive heart failure. Although the use of atenolol is not contraindicated in patients with diabetes mellitus, insulin requirements should be monitored as atenolol may enhance the hypoglycaemic effect of **insulin**. Depression and lethargy are occasionally seen and are a result of atenolol's high lipid solubility and its penetration into the CNS. It is recommended to withdraw therapy gradually in patients who have been receiving the drug chronically.

Drug interactions: As the beta effects of **sympathomimetics** (e.g. **adrenaline**, **phenylpropanolamine**, **terbutaline**) may be blocked by atenolol, the unopposed alpha effects may result in severe hypertension and a decreased heart rate. The hypotensive effect of atenolol is enhanced by **anaesthetic agents** that depress myocardial activity, **phenothiazines**, **anti-hypertensive** drugs (e.g. **hydralazine**, **prazosin**), **diazepam**, **diuretics** and other **anti-arrhythmics**. There is an increased risk of severe hypotension, heart failure and AV block if atenolol is used with **calcium-channel blockers** (e.g. **diltiazem**, **verapamil**). Concurrent **digoxin** administration potentiates bradycardia. The metabolism of atenolol is accelerated by **thyroid hormones**, thus the dose of atenolol may need to be decreased when initiating **carbimazole** therapy. Atenolol enhances the effects of **muscle relaxants** (e.g. **suxamethonium**, **tubocurarine**). Hepatic enzyme induction by **phenobarbital** may increase the rate of metabolism of atenolol. The bronchodilatory effects of **theophylline** may be blocked by atenolol.

Atipamezole (Antisedan) *POM*

Indications: Atipamezole is a selective alpha$_2$ adrenoceptor antagonist, capable of inhibiting and abolishing the sedative and analgesic effects of medetomidine and other alpha$_2$ agonists. There is incomplete reversal of adverse cardiovascular and respiratory effects.

Forms: *Injectable:* 5 mg/ml solution.

Dose:
Cats: 0.5 mg/cat i.m. Usually 2.5 times the preceding dose of medetomidine or half the volume of medetomidine given.
Dogs: 0.05–0.2 mg/kg i.m. Usually 5 times the preceding dose of medetomidine given or the same volume of medetomidine given.
Small mammals: 1 mg/kg i.m., i.p., s.c.
Birds: 0.25 mg/kg i.m.

Note: When alpha$_2$-mediated cardiovascular collapse is imminent, atipamezole may be given i.v.
See Sedation protocols, pages 297–301.

Adverse effects and contraindications: Atipamezole, like other alpha$_2$ antagonists, will antagonize alpha$_2$-mediated analgesia. It should only be used in cases where post-operative pain will not be present, or in animals that have received another class of analgesic, e.g. NSAIDs, local anaesthetics or opioid agonists. The use of atipamezole is not recommended during pregnancy. In dogs a transient hypotensive effect has been observed during the first 10 minutes post-injection. Occasionally vomiting and panting are seen post-injection. Wear gloves when administering atipamezole.

Atracurium (Tracrium*) POM

Indications: Atracurium is a non-depolarizing muscle relaxant with an intermediate duration of action (15–35 minutes). It is popular because its non-enzymatic elimination makes its action independent of renal and/or hepatic function.

Forms: *Injectable:* 10 mg/ml solution.

Dose: *Cats, Dogs:* 0.5 mg/kg i.v. initially, then increments of 0.2 mg/kg i.v.

Adverse effects and contraindications: Neuromuscular blocking agents **must not be used** if the provision of adequate anaesthesia and analgesia cannot be guaranteed and the means for adequate lung ventilation are unavailable. Atracurium has minimal autonomic nervous effects and is relatively safe to administer to animals with hepatic or renal failure. Although it is non-cumulative after repeated doses, antagonism of neuromuscular block is recommended.

Drug interactions: Aminoglycosides, **clindamycin** and **lincomycin** may potentiate the effect of atracurium. Duration of action is longer when **isoflurane** (rather than halothane) is used to maintain anaesthesia.

Atropine (**Atrocare**; Atropine*) POM

Indications: Atropine is a short-acting antimuscarinic (parasympatholytic) drug producing mydriasis and cycloplegia, tachycardia, bronchodilation and general inhibition of GI function. It is used to prevent or correct bradycardia and bradyarrhythmias, to dilate pupils, in the management of organophosphate and carbamate toxicities, and in conjunction with anticholinesterase drugs during antagonism of neuromuscular block.

Forms:
Ophthalmic: 0.5%, 1% solution in single use vials, 5 ml bottle; 1% ointment.
Injectable: 0.6 mg/ml.

Dose:
Cats, Dogs:
• Ophthalmic: 1 drop, or a small amount of ointment in affected eye q8–12h to cause mydriasis, then once q24–72h to maintain mydriasis.
• To treat bradyarrhythmias: 0.02–0.04 mg/kg i.v. Low doses may produce paradoxical heart rate slowing before the desired response supervenes.
• Pre-anaesthetic use: 0.04 mg/kg i.m., s.c.; 0.02 mg/kg i.v.
• Organophosphate poisoning: Dose to effect 0.2–0.5 mg/kg ($^1/_4$ i.v., $^3/_4$ i.m., s.c.), repeat prn; or 0.1–0.2 mg/kg ($^1/_2$ i.v., $^1/_2$ i.m.) then i.m. q6h.
• Neuromuscular blockade antagonism: Atropine 0.04 mg/kg with edrophonium (0.5–1.0 mg/kg).
Small mammals: 0.04 mg/kg i.m., s.c. In rabbits endogenous atropinase levels may make repeated injections q10–15min necessary.
Birds:
• Pre-anaesthetic: 0.04 mg/kg i.m., s.c.
• Organophosphate poisoning: 0.2–0.5 mg/kg i.v., i.m. q4h.
Reptiles: 0.01–0.04 mg/kg i.m., i.p.

Adverse effects and contraindications: Routine use of atropine for pre-anaesthetic medication is no longer popular as atropine can promote ventricular arrhythmias that are more malignant than those it is held to prevent. If in doubt, monitor the heart rate and ECG and treat bradyarrythmias only if they arise. Adverse effects of atropine and its derivatives include sinus tachycardia, ventricular arrhythmias, blurred vision, mydriasis, photophobia, cycloplegia, increased intraocular pressure, vomiting, abdominal distension, ileus, urinary retention and the drying of bronchial secretions. Bradyarrhythmias may develop at low doses or transiently after initial administration (especially if given i.v.). Bitter taste after topical application of a solution in cats, and some dogs, can result in hypersalivation. The topical ophthalmic ointment formulation is therefore preferred in cats. Its use is contraindicated in glaucoma and lens luxation. Atropine reduces tear production and should be avoided in KCS. Atropine should only be used for therapeutic purposes, and not as a diagnostic aid in ocular conditions.

Drug interactions: Atropine is compatible (for at least 15 minutes) when mixed with various medications. Atropine is not compatible with bromides, iodides, sodium bicarbonate, other alkalis or noradrenaline. The following may enhance the activity of atropine: **antihistamines**, **procainamide**, **quinidine**, **pethidine**, **benzodiazepines** and **phenothiazines**. The adverse effects of atropine may be potentiated by **primidone**, **disopyramide** and prolonged **corticosteroid** use (may increase intraocular pressure). Atropine may enhance the actions of **thiazide diuretics** and **sympathomimetics** and antagonize the actions of **metoclopramide**. Atropine may aggravate some signs seen with amitraz toxicity, leading to hypertension and gut stasis.

Auranofin (Ridaura*) *POM*

Indications: Auranofin is an oral gold salt used in the management of active progressive autoimmune diseases (e.g. pemphigus complex, immune-based arthritides). It may suppress the disease process and may require up to 4 months to show a full response.

Forms: *Oral:* 3 mg tablet.

Dose: *Dogs:* 0.05–0.2 mg/kg p.o. q12h. Maximum daily dose 9 mg/day. Seek specialist advice before use.

Adverse effects and contraindications: The use of auranofin is contraindicated in patients with diabetes mellitus, SLE, haematological, hepatic, renal or cardiac disorders. Toxic effects include diarrhoea (commonest), mucous membrane haemorrhage or ulceration, renal proximal tubule damage, blood dyscrasia, encephalitis, neuritis and hepatitis. Monitor haematology q14d initially then q28–56d.

Aurothiomalate (Myocrisin*) *POM*

Indications: Aurothiomalate is a gold salt used for the treatment of autoimmune diseases (e.g. pemphigus complex, immune-based arthritides) but not SLE. It may suppress the disease process and it may require up to 2 months for a full response to be seen.

Forms: *Injectable:* 20 mg/ml, 40 mg/ml, 100 mg/ml suspensions/solutions.

Dose:
Cats: 1 mg/cat i.m. on day 1; 2 mg/cat i.m. on day 7; then 1 mg/kg i.m. q7–28d.
Dogs: 5 mg/dog i.m. on day 1; 10 mg/dog i.m. on day 7 (max. 1 mg/kg), then 1 mg/kg i.m. q7–28d.
Administer by deep i.m. injection. Seek specialist advice before use.

Adverse effects and contraindications: Contraindications to its use include diabetes mellitus, SLE, haematological, hepatic, renal or cardiac disorders. Toxic effects include mucous membrane ulceration or haemorrhage, blood dyscrasias, renal proximal tubule damage, encephalitis, neuritis and hepatitis. Monitor haematology q14d initially then q28–56d.

Azathioprine (Azathioprine*; Imuran*) *POM*

Indications: Azathioprine is an immunosuppressive agent with similar actions to those of mercaptopurine. It is metabolized to 6-mercaptopurine *in vivo*. Azathioprine suppresses cell-mediated immunity, alters antibody production and inhibits cell growth. It is used in the management of immune-mediated diseases.

Forms: *Oral:* 25 mg, 50 mg tablets.

Dose: *Dogs:* 2 mg/kg p.o. q24h until remission achieved then
0.5–2 mg/kg p.o. q48h.
Often used in conjunction with corticosteroid therapy.

Adverse effects and contraindications: Bone marrow suppression
is the most serious adverse effect. This may be influenced by the
activity of thiopurine acetyltransferase, which is involved in the
metabolism of the drug and which can vary between individuals due
to genetic polymorphism. Cats in particular often exhibit a reaction
that results in a severe, non-responsive fatal leucopenia and
thrombocytopenia. Its use in cats cannot be recommended. In
animals with renal impairment, the dosing interval should be
extended.

Drug interactions: Enhanced effects and increased azathioprine
toxicity when used with allopurinol.

Azidothymidine – see Zidovudine

Azithromycin (Zithromax*) *POM*

Indications: Azithromycin is an azalide derived from the macrolide
erythromycin. It has a slightly greater activity than the parent
compound and, in man, has a longer tissue half-life than erythromycin,
shows better oral absorption and is better tolerated. It has bactericidal
or bacteriostatic properties, dependent upon the drug concentration
and the organism's susceptibility. It binds to the 50S ribosome,
inhibiting peptide bond formation. Azithromycin is indicated as an
alternative to penicillin in allergic individuals, as it has a similar,
although not identical, antibacterial spectrum. It is active against
Gram-positive cocci (some *Staphylococcus* spp. are resistant),
Gram-positive bacilli, some Gram-negative bacilli (*Haemophilus* and
Pasteurella spp.), mycobacteria, obligate anaerobes, *Chlamydophila*
spp., *Mycoplasma* spp. and *Toxoplasma*. Some strains of
Actinomyces, *Nocardia* and *Rickettsia* are also inhibited. Most strains
of the Enterobacteriaceae (*Pseudomonas* spp., *E. coli*, *Klebsiella* spp.)
are resistant. It is particularly useful in the management of respiratory
tract infections, mild to moderate skin and soft tissue infections, and
non-tubercular mycobacterial infections. It has not proved possible to
eliminate *Chlamydophila felis* from chronically infected cats using
azithromycin even with once daily administration.

Forms: *Oral:* 250 mg capsule; 200 mg/ml suspension (reconstitute
with water).

Dose:
Cats: 5 mg/kg p.o. q48h.
Dogs: 5–10 mg/kg p.o. q12–24h.
Doses are empirical and subject to change as experience with the drug is gained. More work is needed to optimize the clinically effective dose rate.

Adverse effects and contraindications: There is little information on the use of this drug in animals and its pharmacokinetics have not been studied closely in the dog and cat. However, in man similar adverse effects to those of erythromycin are seen, i.e. vomiting, cholestatic hepatitis, stomatitis and glossitis, but the effects are generally less marked than with erythromycin. Use with great care in animals with hepatic dysfunction. Reduce its dose in animals with renal impairment. Azithromycin activity is enhanced in an alkaline pH; administer on an empty stomach.

Drug interactions: Azithromycin may increase the serum levels of **methylprednisolone, theophylline** and **terfenadine**. The absorption of **digoxin** may be enhanced.

AZT – see Zidovudine

Barium sulphate contrast media (Baritop[1]*; BIPS[2]*; E-Z[3]*; HD[5]*; Micropaque[4]*) *POM*

Indications: Barium sulphate is a positive contrast agent, appearing radiopaque on a radiograph. Its use is restricted to examination of the GI tract, as it is neither absorbed by the intestine nor acted on by alimentary secretions. It is osmotically inactive and so does not draw fluid into the intestinal lumen. The particles of barium sulphate in colloidal suspension provide excellent mucosal detail. Barium paste is of particular use in evaluation of the oesophagus, as it adheres to the mucosa. Liquid barium may be used for any region of the GI tract. It may be mixed with food to delineate dilations or strictures of the oesophagus but is usually used alone when investigating the stomach, or small or large intestine. BIPS (barium-impregnated polyethylene spheres) are designed to detect GI obstructions, and to give an estimate of gastric emptying time and intestinal transit time.

Forms: Ready prepared colloidal suspension; powder for reconstitution with water to form a paste or liquid suspension, or mixed with food;

ready prepared paste; BIPS: 4 small or 1 large capsule containing 10 large (5 mm diameter) and 30 small (1.5 mm diameter) spheres. Manufacturers: [1] Sanochemia UK; [2] Medical I.D. Systems; [3] E-Z-EM; [4] Guerbet Laboratories; [5] Mallinkrodt Medical.

Dose: Depends on the contrast examination being performed. Readers are referred to standard radiography texts for details of procedures.

Adverse effects and contraindications: Barium is non-absorbable and may lead to granulomatous reactions or adhesions if leakage occurs into the thoracic or abdominal cavities through a perforation. Iodine-containing contrast media may be preferable if oesophageal or GI perforation is suspected. Aspiration of barium during administration or as a consequence of regurgitation or vomiting can lead to aspiration pneumonia.

Benazepril (Fortekor) POM

Indications: Benazepril is an ACE inhibitor that inhibits conversion of angiotensin I to angiotensin II. It is indicated to reduce afterload on the heart when there is cardiac insufficiency and in cases of hypertension, and may be of benefit in certain cases of renal disease, particularly protein-losing glomerulopathies. Benazepril is rapidly converted by the liver to the active drug benazeprilat. Unlike enalapril, benazepril has significant hepatic metabolism and may not need dose adjustment in renal failure. *See Enalapril for further comments.* Benazepril is licensed for use in dogs, and is licensed for the management of cats with chronic renal insufficiency.

Forms: *Oral:* 5 mg, 20 mg tablets.

Dose:
Cats (chronic renal insufficiency): 0.5–1 mg/kg p.o. q24h.
Dogs (heart failure): 0.25–0.5 mg/kg p.o. q24h.

Adverse effects and contraindications: Potential adverse effects include hypotension, hyperkalaemia and renal impairment. Dosage should be reduced if there are signs of hypotension (weakness, disorientation). Although no teratogenic effects have been reported, it is not recommended for breeding dogs, or pregnant or lactating bitches as it apparently crosses the placenta and enters milk.

Drug interactions: Concomitant usage with potassium-sparing diuretics, e.g. **spironolactone,** or **potassium** supplements could result in hyperkalaemia. There may be an increased risk of nephrotoxicity when used with **NSAIDs**. Concomitant administration of other anti-hypertensives could cause hypotension.

Benzoyl peroxide (Paxcutol) POM

Indications: Benzoyl peroxide is a topical keratolytic and antimicrobial agent used to treat pyodermas and seborrhoeic dermatitis. In the treatment of folliculitis it has a useful follicle-flushing effect.

Forms: *Topical:* 2.5% shampoo.

Dose: *Dogs:* To be used as a shampoo q24h to q30d.

Adverse effects and contraindications: Irritant to eyes and mucous membranes. May be irritant to skin. Reduction in contact time may reduce irritancy.

Betamethasone (Betnesol*; **Betsolan**; **Fuciderm**; Maxidex*; **Norbet**; **Oterna**; **Vetsovate**) *POM*

Indications: Betamethasone is a glucocorticoid anti-inflammatory drug. It has an anti-inflammatory potency 8.75 times greater than prednisolone. On a dose basis, 0.12 mg betamethasone is equivalent to 1 mg prednisolone. Betamethasone has a long duration of activity and therefore is not suitable for long-term daily or alternate-day use.

Forms:
Injectable: 2 mg/ml suspension for i.m. use; 2 mg/ml solution for i.v. use.
Oral: 0.25 mg tablet.
Eye and ear drops: 0.1% betamethasone solution.
Topical: Betamethasone is present in varying concentrations in several topical preparations with or without antibacterials.

Dose:
Cats:
- Ocular: 1 drop of ophthalmic solution to affected eye q6–8h.
- Skin: Apply cream to affected area q8–12h.
- Anti-inflammatory: 0.04 mg/kg i.v. q3w prn for up to 4 injections.
- Shock: up to 0.08 mg/kg i.v.
Dogs:
- Ocular: 1 drop of ophthalmic solution to affected eye q6–8h.
- Skin: Apply cream to affected area q8–12h.
- Anti-inflammatory: 0.04 mg/kg i.v., i.m. q3w prn for up to 4 injections, 0.025 mg/kg p.o. q24h.
- Shock: 0.08 mg/kg i.v.
Small mammals: 0.1 mg/kg s.c. q24h.

Caution: Wear gloves when applying cream.

Adverse effects and contraindications: Prolonged use of glucocorticoids suppresses the hypothalamic–pituitary axis resulting in adrenal atrophy. Animals on chronic corticosteroid therapy should be given tapered decreasing doses when discontinuing the drug. Catabolic effects of glucocorticoids lead to weight loss and cutaneous atrophy. Iatrogenic hyperadrenocorticism may develop. Vomiting, diarrhoea and GI ulceration may develop. Glucocorticoids may increase glucose levels and decrease serum T3 and T4 values. Do not use in pregnant animals. Systemic corticosteroids are generally contraindicated in patients with renal disease and diabetes mellitus. Impaired wound healing and delayed recovery from infections may be seen. Topical corticosteroids are contraindicated in ulcerative keratitis.

Drug interactions: There is an increased risk of GI ulceration if used concurrently with **NSAIDs**. Glucocorticoids antagonize the effect of **insulin**. **Phenobarbital** and **primidone** may accelerate the metabolism of corticosteroids. There is an increased risk of hypokalaemia when used concurrently with **acetazolamide, amphotericin** and **potassium-depleting diuretics (furosemide, thiazides)**.

Betaxolol (Betoptic*) POM

Indications: Betaxolol is a beta$_1$-selective beta-blocker used to reduce raised intraocular pressure in glaucoma.

Forms: Topical: 0.25%, 0.5% solution; 0.25% suspension.

Dose: Dogs: 1 drop/eye q8–12h used alone or adjunctively with, for example, a topical carbonic anhydrase inhibitor.

Adverse effects and contraindications: The use of betaxolol in man is precluded in patients with cardiac failure or heart block. It is known to cause bradycardia in dogs.

Bethanechol chloride (Myotonine*) POM

Indications: Bethanechol is a muscarinic agonist (cholinergic or parasympathomimetic) that increases urinary bladder detrusor muscle tone and contraction. It may be of value in the management of urinary retention.

Forms: Oral: 10 mg, 25 mg tablets.

Dose:
Cats: 1.25–5 mg/cat or 0.1–0.2 mg/kg p.o. q8h.
Dogs: 5–25 mg/dog p.o. q8h.

Adverse effects and contraindications: Adverse effects include vomiting, diarrhoea, GI cramping, anorexia, salivation and bradycardia (with overdosage). Treat overdoses with atropine. Best given on an empty stomach to avoid GI distress. Bethanechol does not initiate a detrusor reflex and is ineffective if the bladder is areflexic. As it may increase urethral resistance, do not use when urethral resistance is increased unless in combination with agents that reduce urethral outflow pressure (e.g. phenoxybenzamine).

Bisacodyl (Dulcolax*) *GSL*

Indications: Bisacodyl is a mild stimulant laxative that increases intestinal motility.

Forms: *Oral:* 5 mg tablet.

Dose:
Cats: 2–5 mg/cat prn.
Dogs: 5–20 mg/dog prn.

Bismuth (BCK; De-Noltab*; **Genetrix diarrhoea tablets**; Pepto-Bismol*) *P/GSL*

Indications: Bismuth is a gastric cytoprotectant with activity against spiral bacteria. Tripotassium dicitratobismuthate (bismuth chelate) is effective in healing gastric and duodenal ulcers in man, due to its direct toxic effects on gastric *Helicobacter pylori* and by stimulating mucosal prostaglandin and bicarbonate secretion. It is often used in conjunction with an H_2 receptor antagonist and appropriate antibacterial therapy.

Forms: *Oral:*
BCK, granules containing 39.2 mg/g bismuth subnitrate, 49 mg/g calcium phosphate, 400 mg/g charcoal, 422 mg/g kaolin.
Pepto-Bismol, bismuth subsalicylate suspension.
De-Noltab 120 mg bismuth chelate tablet.
Genetrix 32.5 mg bismuth carbonate, 65 mg catechu, 210 mg chalk, 16.5 mg rhubarb powder.

Dose: *Cats, Dogs:* BCK: 5–15 ml p.o. q8–12h; Pepto-Bismol: 1 ml/kg p.o. q4–6h; De-Nol/De-Noltab: <30 kg BW 2.5 ml or $1/_2$ tab p.o. q6h, >30 kg BW 5 ml or 1 tab p.o. q6h.
Dogs: Genitrix: 1–3 tablets/dog q4h.

Adverse effects and contraindications: Avoid long-term use (except chelates) as absorbed bismuth is neurotoxic. Bismuth chelate is contraindicated in renal impairment. Nausea and vomiting reported in man.

Drug interactions: Absorption of **tetracyclines** is reduced by bismuth.

Bowel cleansing solutions (Klean-Prep*; Movicol*) *POM*

Indications: Bowel cleansing solutions contain polyethylene glycol, as an osmotic laxative, and balanced electrolytes to maintain isotonicity and prevent net fluid loss or gain. When administered orally they rapidly induce diarrhoea, emptying the bowel prior to endoscopic examination.

Forms: Solutions or powder to be mixed with water.

Dose: *Dogs:* Prior to lower GI examination: 22–33 ml/kg p.o. by stomach tube twice or three times, at least 4 hours apart.

Adverse effects and contraindications: Occasional vomiting is seen, especially if the maximum volume is administered. Inhalation can cause severe, and even fatal, aspiration pneumonia. Do not administer to heavily sedated patients or animals with a reduced gag reflex.

Brinzolamide (Azopt*) *POM*

Indications: Brinzolamide is a topical carbonic anhydrase inhibitor used in the control of glaucoma. It can be used alone or in combination with other topical glaucoma drugs. It may be better tolerated than dorzolamide.

Forms: *Topical drops:* 10 mg/ml.

Dose:
Cats: 1 drop/eye q12h.
Dogs: 1 drop/eye q6–8h.

Adverse effects and contraindications: Brinzolamide may cause less ocular irritation than dorzolamide. Do not use when severe hepatic or renal disease is present.

Bromhexine (Bisolvon) *POM*

Indications: Bromhexine is a bronchial secretolytic used to aid the management of respiratory diseases.

Forms:
Injectable: 3 mg/ml solution.
Oral: 10 mg/g powder.

Dose:
Cats: 3 mg/cat i.m. q24h; 1 mg/kg p.o. q24h.
Dogs: 3–15 mg/dog i.m. q12h; 2–2.5 mg/kg p.o. q12h.
Small mammals: 0.3 mg/animal p.o. q24h.
Birds: 3–6 mg/kg i.m.

Bromide – see Potassium bromide

Bromocriptine (Bromocriptine*; Parlodel*) *POM*

Indications: Bromocriptine stimulates dopamine receptors in the CNS and inhibits release of prolactin by the pituitary. It has been used in the management of false pregnancy and pituitary-dependent hyperadrenocorticism (PDH), although for the latter its efficacy is very low and adverse effects are common.

Forms: *Oral:* 1 mg, 2.5 mg tablets; 5 mg, 10 mg capsules.

Dose: *Dogs:*
- PDH: 0.05 mg/kg p.o. q12h.
- False pregnancy: 0.01 mg/kg p.o. q12h for 10 days or 0.03 mg/kg q24h for 16 days.

Adverse effects and contraindications: Vomiting, anorexia, depression and behavioural changes may be seen.

Drug interactions: Metoclopramide may antagonize its hypoprolactinaemic effect.

Budesonide (Budenofalk*; Entocort CR*) *POM*

Indications: Budesonide is a novel steroid given orally or as an enema. It is available as an uncoated powder suitable for inhalant use in man or as enteric coated microspheres released in the intestine. It is metabolized approximately 90% on its first pass through the liver. Budesonide's potential use is in the therapy of idiopathic inflammatory bowel disease as an anti-inflammatory/immunosuppressive steroid with minimal systemic adverse effects.

Forms: 3 mg capsule (Entocort CR, Budenofalk), 0.02 mg/ml enema (Entocort).

Dose:
Cats: Not to exceed 1 mg p.o. q8h.
Dogs: Not to exceed 3 mg p.o. q8h.
Note: These dosages have been extrapolated from human medicine, and the correct dose of either form and their efficacy are unknown.

Adverse effects and contraindications: There is little information on the use of this drug in veterinary medicine. Iatrogenic hyperadrenocorticism may develop with its use. Elevation in liver enzymes, hepatomegaly, lethargy and polyuria/polydipsia have been noted. Adrenal suppression has been documented in dogs and iatrogenic hypoadrenocorticism is a potential risk if it is withdrawn rapidly following prolonged use.

Bupivacaine (Marcain*) *POM*

Indications: Bupivacaine is a long-acting amide-linked local anaesthetic (duration of activity up to 8 hours), used where a prolonged action is required, e.g. extradural analgesia, or intercostal nerve blocks following thoracic surgery. Onset of action is slower than lidocaine; there is a latent period of 20–30 minutes when used for extradural analgesia. Low concentrations, e.g. 0.25%, may produce analgesia without muscle relaxation. High concentrations, e.g. 0.75%, are likely to produce analgesia and muscle relaxation.

Forms: *Injectable:* 2.5, 5.0 and 7.5 mg/ml solutions.

Dose: *Cats, Dogs:*
Perineural: 1–2 ml of a 0.5% solution.
Extradural: 1.6 mg/kg (analgesia to level of L4), 2.3 mg/kg (analgesia to level of T11–T13).
Interpleural: 0.5–5 ml of 0.5% solution instilled by thoracostomy tube and allowed to bathe incision site provides useful analgesia after intercostal thoracotomy. Occasionally elicits signs of discomfort.

Adverse effects and contraindications: Do not use for intravenous regional anaesthesia. Inadvertent intravascular injection may precipitate severe cardiac arrythmias that are refractory to normal treatment.

Buprenorphine (**Vetergesic**) *POM* Schedule 3 Controlled Drug

Indications: Buprenorphine is a long-acting partial mu-opioid agonist/ antagonist drug used to relieve moderate pain. Its onset of action is slow (15–30 minutes), intensity and duration of effect are variable (3–8 hours in most cases). As a partial agonist it antagonizes the effects of full agonists (morphine, pethidine). May be mixed with acepromazine to produce neuroleptanalgesia for minor procedures, or pre-anaesthetic medication. *See Sedation protocols, pages 297–301.* Buprenorphine is most effective when given before noxious stimulation (pre-emptive analgesia) and in conjunction with other analgesic drugs. Its sedative and euphoric effects are less marked than those of morphine.

Forms: *Injectable:* 0.3 mg/ml solution.

Dose:
Cats, Dogs: 0.006–0.02 mg/kg i.v., i.m., s.c. q8h or prn.
Small mammals: Ferrets: 0.05 mg/kg s.c. q6–12h; Rabbits: 0.05–0.1 mg/kg i.m., s.c. q6–12h; Guinea pigs, Rats, Gerbils and Hamsters: 0.01–0.05 mg/kg i.m., s.c. q6–12h; Mice: 0.05–0.1 mg/kg i.m., s.c. q6–12h.
Birds: 0.1 mg/kg i.v., i.m.
Reptiles: 0.01 mg/kg i.m. q24–48h.
See Sedation protocols, pages 297–301.

Adverse effects and contraindications: Attempts to treat severe pain with buprenorphine may be unsuccessful. In these circumstances, increasing doses may diminish, rather than improve the quality of analgesia, and so alternative analgesics, e.g. local anaesthetics or NSAIDs, should be considered. As with other opioid drugs, buprenorphine may constrict branches of the pancreatic duct and so should not be used in cases of pancreatitis. It is metabolized in the liver; some prolongation of effect may be seen with impaired liver function. Buprenorphine crosses the placenta and may exert sedative effects in neonates born to bitches treated prior to parturition.

Drug interactions: Buprenorphine should not be given to animals which have received pure mu agonists (e.g. **morphine**, **pethidine**), unless antagonism of analgesia is desirable and/or justified. It may potentiate the sedative and ventilatory depressant effects of other **CNS depressants**. In rabbits and guinea pigs it can be used to reverse the effects of fentanyl.

Buserelin (Receptal*) *POM*

Indications: Buserelin is a synthetic releasing hormone analogue for both luteinizing and follicle stimulating hormones (LH-RH, GnRH, LH/FSH-RH). It is used to supplement LH in cases of ovulation failure or delay and to induce lactation post-partum. In males, it may stimulate the secretion of testosterone and is indicated in the management of genital hypoplasia and reduced libido. In ferrets it may be used in the management of signs of oestrus. In rabbits it is used to induce ovulation post-partum for insemination and to improve conception rates.

Forms: *Injectable:* 4 µg/ml solution.

Dose:
Cats: 2 µg/cat i.m. once.
Dogs: 4 µg/dog q24–48h i.m.
Small mammals: Ferrets: 1.5 µg/ferret i.m. q24h for 2 days; Rabbits: 0.8 µg/rabbit s.c. at time of insemination or mating.

Adverse effects and contraindications: Anaphylactic reactions may occasionally occur.

Buspirone (Buspar*) *POM*

Indications: Buspirone blocks serotonin (5-hydroxytryptamine) receptors. It is used in the management of mild to moderate anxiety-related behaviour problems, including urine spraying in cats when associated with mild anxiety.

Forms: *Oral:* 5, 10 mg tablets.

Dose:
Cats: 0.5–1.0 mg/kg p.o. q8–12h. For urine spraying: 5 mg/cat twice daily for a minimum of 2 weeks; if patient responds continue treatment for 8 weeks and then gradually withdraw. If no response, cease treatment.
Dogs: 1–2 mg/kg p.o. q8–12h.

Adverse effects and contraindications: Contraindicated in states of renal or hepatic impairment and in epileptics. Potential effects include disinhibition and increased friendliness (in cats). Caution is advised if buspirone is to be used in multi-cat households due to reports of paradoxical increases in intra-specific aggression in association with buspirone medication.

Busulfan (Busulphan) (Myleran*) *POM*

Indications: Busulfan is an antineoplastic alkylating agent used to manage chronic granulocytic leukaemia and polycythaemia vera.

Forms: *Oral:* 0.5 mg, 2 mg tablets.

Dose: *Cats, Dogs:* 2–6 mg/m^2 p.o. q24h initially until remission achieved then at a reduced dosage/frequency as required to maintain remission.
See page 293 for conversion of body weight to surface area (m^2).

Adverse effects and contraindications: Frequent haematological assessment is required as excessive myelosuppression may result in irreversible bone marrow aplasia. Hyperpigmentation of the skin, progressive pulmonary fibrosis and hepatotoxicity may occur.

Butorphanol (Torbugesic; Torbutrol) *POM*

Indications: Butorphanol is a synthetic partial opioid agonist/ antagonist with an intermediate duration of action. It is a potent antitussive and suppresses mild to moderate pain. Its sedative and euphoric effects are less marked than those of morphine. Analgesic effects are seen within 15 minutes and persist for up to 3 hours. Sedative effects may be recognized for up to 3 hours. Butorphanol may be mixed with acepromazine to produce neuroleptanalgesia for minor procedures, or pre-anaesthetic medication. Butorphanol is most effective when given before noxious stimulation and in conjunction with other non-opioid analgesics.

Forms:
Injectable: 10 mg/ml solutions.
Oral: 5 mg, 10 mg tablets.

Dose:
Cats: 0.05–0.6 mg/kg i.m., s.c. prn, otherwise q6–8h.
Dogs:
• Antitussive: 0.05–0.1 mg/kg i.m., s.c. or 0.5–1 mg/kg p.o. q6–12h.
• Analgesic: 0.05–0.6 mg/kg i.v., i.m., s.c. prn, otherwise q6–8h.
• Anti-emetic prior to chemotherapy: 0.2–0.6 mg/kg s.c.
Small mammals: Ferrets: 0.25–0.4 mg/kg s.c. q4–6h. In ferrets use with xylazine to provide sedation. Rabbits: 0.1–0.5 mg/kg s.c q4h. In rabbits can use with mecletomidine and ketamine to provide sedation and anaesthesia. Chinchilla: 0.5–2 mg/kg s.c. q4h; Guinea pigs: 1 mg/kg s.c. q4h; Rats, Gerbils, Hamsters, Mice: 1–5 mg/kg s.c. q4h.
Birds: 2–4 mg/kg i.m., i.v. q4–6h.
Reptiles: Pre-anaesthetic, analgesia: 0.4–1.5 mg/kg s.c., i.m.
See Sedation protocols, pages 297–301.

Adverse effects and contraindications: Butorphanol may cause sedation, ataxia, anorexia and rarely diarrhoea. Use with caution in patients with hypothyroidism, severe renal insufficiency, Addisons' disease and patients with increased CSF pressure. Butorphanol may constrict branches of the pancreatic duct and so should not be used in cases of pancreatitis. Prolonged activity may occur when high doses are administered to patients with either impaired hepatic or renal function. Adverse or prolonged effects may be treated with naloxone provided the antagonism of analgesia is justified.

Drug interactions: The depressant activity of butorphanol may be potentiated by **barbiturates**, **phenothiazines** and **tranquillizers**. Butorphanol may potentiate the sedative and ventilatory depressant effects of other CNS depressants. Concomitant use of butorphanol with **metoclopramide** may lead to antagonism as each drug has opposing effects on GI motility. The concurrent use of **pancuronium** may cause conjunctival changes.

Butylscopolamine (Hyoscine)/Metamizole (Dipyrone)
(Buscopan*; **Buscopan Compositum**) *POM*

Indications: Butylscopolamine is a quarternary ammonium antimuscarinic advocated as a long-acting GI antispasmodic. Metamizole is a pyrazoline drug with anti-inflammatory, analgesic and antipyretic effects.

Forms:
Injectable: Buscopan Compositum, 4 mg/ml butylscopolamine and 500 mg/ml metamizole. Buscopan 20 mgl/ml butylscopolamine only.
Oral: Buscopan 10 mg butylscopolamine only.

Dose: *Dogs:* 0.1 ml/kg i.v., i.m. (compositum) 0.5 mg/kg i.m., p.o. q12h (butylscopolamine alone).

Adverse effects and contraindications: Adverse effects of butylsco-polamine include a dry mouth, blurred vision, hesitant micturition and constipation at doses acting as gut neuromuscular relaxants. The i.m. route may cause a local reaction. Adverse effects associated with metamizole include hepatitis, nephropathy, blood dyscrasia and GI disturbances. Because of the seriousness of the adverse effects, it should be used as a second-line agent for the treatment of pyrexia and rarely as an anti-inflammatory. Its use in cats is strongly discouraged.

Drug interactions: Metamizole should not be given to dogs that have been treated with a **phenothiazine**, as hypothermia may result.

Cabergoline (Dostinex*; **Galastop**) *POM*

Indications: Cabergoline is a potent anti-prolactin drug. It is used in the management of pseudopregnancy and galactostasis in lactating bitches, and, in combination with prostaglandin $F_{2\alpha}$ analogue (e.g. dinoprost), to terminate unwanted pregnancy in the bitch. Pregnancy termination takes place by resorption of the fetuses. Cabergoline is specifically indicated for the treatment of aggression associated with pseudopregnancy in entire bitches and with elevated prolactin levels in speyed bitches.

Forms: *Oral:* 500 μg tablets; 50 μg/ml non-aqueous solution.

Dose: *Dogs:*
• Pseudopregnancy, abortion: 5 μg/kg p.o. q24h.
If used to terminate pregnancy with prostaglandin $F_{2\alpha}$ analogue, continue use until abortion is complete. Assess serum progesterone concentrations to determine if abortion is complete.
If used to manage pseudopregnancy, use for 5 days.
Use for 10–14 days to control prolactin-related aggression in bitches.
• Galactostasis: 2.5–5 μg/kg q24h for 4–6 days.

Adverse effects and contraindications: In man, reported adverse effects include nausea, vomiting, constipation, postural hypotension and, rarely, exacerbation of behavioural changes. These have yet to be reported in dogs.

Drug interactions: Metoclopramide antagonizes the hypoprolactinaemic effects.

Calcitonin (Salcatonin) (Forcaltonin*; Miacalcic*) *POM*

Indications: Synthetic or recombinant salmon calcitonin is used to lower plasma calcium concentration in patients with hypercalcaemia. The drug inhibits bone resorption and intestinal resorption of calcium and enhances calciuresis although its effects are weak and short-acting.

Forms: *Injectable:* 50 IU/ml, 100 IU/ml, 200 IU/ml solutions.

Dose:
Cats: 4 IU/kg i.m. q12h.
Dogs: 4–8 IU/kg i.m., s.c. q8–24h.

Adverse effects and contraindications: Data concerning its use in small animals are limited. In man, nausea, anorexia and vomiting are most frequently encountered. Resistance to the effects of the drug develop in a small percentage of people treated.

Calcium borogluconate (Calcibor*) *PML*

Indications: Calcium borogluconate is used to treat hypocalcaemia.

Forms: *Injectable:* 200 mg/ml solution equivalent to 15 mg/ml calcium.

Dose:
Cats, Dogs: 50–150 mg calcium borogluconate/kg = 0.5–1.5 ml/kg of a 10% solution i.v. over 20–30 minutes (equivalent to 0.225–0.675 mEq calcium/kg or 3.8–11.4 mg calcium/kg). Monitor the ECG and stop if a bradycardia develops. An additional 1–1.5 g/kg (4.5–6.75 mEq/kg) may need to be administered i.v. over the next 24 hours. 150–750 mg/kg/day (0.675–3.375 mEq/kg/day) p.o. divided q8h; adjust dose by monitoring serum calcium and phosphorus levels.
Serum calcium levels and renal function tests should be assessed.
Birds: Egg retention, hypocalcaemia: 150–200 mg/kg i.m., s.c. Use with oxytocin for egg retention.
Reptiles: Egg retention: 100 mg/kg i.m. Use with oxytocin or vasotocin. Hypocalcaemia: 100–200 mg/kg i.v., i.m., s.c. as indicated.

Adverse effects and contraindications: Do not administer perivascularly. Mild to severe tissue reactions may develop following i.m. or s.c. administration. Venous irritation and hypotension may develop after i.v. administration. Intravenous use in dehydrated reptiles and birds may precipitate gout.

Drug interactions: Do not add calcium salts to i.v. solutions containing **bicarbonate**, **carbonate**, **phosphate**, **sulphate** or **tartrate salts**. Patients on **digoxin** therapy may develop arrhythmias if receiving i.v. calcium.

Calcium chloride (Calcium chloride*) *POM*

Indications: Calcium chloride is used in the treatment of hypocalcaemia and as a positive inotrope in the management of cardiac arrest.

Forms: *Injectable:* 100 mg/ml (10%) solution; contains 1.36 mEq Ca/ml.

Dose:
Cats, Dogs:
- Hypocalcaemia: 5–10 mg/kg or 0.05–0.1 ml/kg of a 10% solution i.v. (equivalent to 0.068–0.136 mEq/kg).
- Cardiac arrest: 1–2 ml of a 10% solution i.v. to effect; monitor the ECG.
Birds: 150–200 mg/kg i.v., i.m. q8h.

Adverse effects and contraindications: Do not administer perivascularly. Mild to severe tissue reactions may develop following i.m. or s.c. administration. Venous irritation and hypotension may develop after i.v. administration.

Drug interactions: As for calcium borogluconate.

Calcium edetate – see Edetate calcium disodium

Calcium gluconate (Calcium gluconate*) *POM*

Indications: Calcium gluconate is used in the management of hypocalcaemia and hyperkalaemia. Calcium gluconate is preferred to calcium chloride in the treatment of acute hypocalcaemia.

Forms:
Injectable: 100 mg/ml solution; contains 0.45 mEq Ca/g.
Oral: 600 mg tablets.
Note: 11.2 mg calcium gluconate contains 1 mg calcium.

Dose: *Cats, Dogs:*
- Hypocalcaemia: 50–150 mg calcium gluconate/kg or 0.5–1.5 ml/kg of a 10% solution i.v. over 20–30 minutes (equivalent to 0.225–0.675 mEq Ca/kg or 4.5–14 mg Ca/kg). Monitor the ECG and stop if a bradycardia develops. An additional 1–1.5 g/kg (4.5–6.75 mEq/kg) may need to be administered i.v. over the next 24 hours.
150–750 mg/kg/day (0.675–3.375 mEq/kg/day) p.o. divided q8h; adjust dose by monitoring serum calcium and phosphorus levels. Serum calcium levels and renal function tests should be assessed.
- Hyperkalaemia: 0.5–1.5 ml of a 10% solution/kg i.v. slowly once.
Birds: Hypocalcaemia, egg retention: 50–100 mg/kg slow i.v., i.m. (diluted). Use with oxytocin for egg retention.
Reptiles: Hypocalcaemia, egg retention: 50–100 mg/kg i.m., s.c. Use with oxytocin for egg retention.

Adverse effects and contraindications: Do not administer perivascularly. Mild to severe tissue reactions may develop following i.m. or s.c. administration. Venous irritation and hypotension may develop after i.v. administration.

Drug interactions: As for calcium borogluconate.

Carbimazole (Neo-Mercazole*) *POM*

Indications: Carbimazole is a thioglyoxaline that is metabolized to the active drug methimazole. Methimazole interferes with the synthesis of thyroid hormones by inhibiting peroxidase-catalysed reactions (blocks oxidation of iodide), the iodination of tyrosyl residues in thyroglobulin, and the coupling of mono- or di-iodotyrosines to form T3 and T4. There is no effect on iodine uptake and they do not inhibit peripheral de-iodination of T4 to T3. It is used to control thyroid hormone levels in cats with hyperthyroidism, although methimazole is available as a licensed product.

Forms: *Oral:* 5 mg tablet.

Dose: *Cats:* 5 mg/cat p.o. q8h. Increase dose if no response by 3 weeks. Adjust dose on the basis of serum thyroxine levels once a euthyroid state is achieved.

Adverse effects and contraindications: Vomiting, rashes, alopecia, jaundice, anorexia, lymphopenia and leucopenia are rarely seen. Carbimazole must be discontinued for at least 2 weeks prior to ^{131}I treatment.

Carbomer 980 (Geltears*; Liposic*; Viscotears*) *P*

Indications: Carbomer 980 (polyacrylic acid) is a mucomimetic. It is used as a tear replacement and is beneficial for the management of KCS. It has longer corneal contact time than the aqueous tear substitutes.

Forms: *Topical:* 0.2% gel.

Dose: *Cats, Dogs:* 1 drop/eye(s) q4–6h.

Adverse effects and contraindications: It is tolerated well and ocular irritation is unusual.

Carboplatin (Carboplatin*; Paraplatin*) *POM*

Indications: Carboplatin is an analogue of cisplatin. Carboplatin binds to DNA to form intra- and interstrand cross links and DNA–protein cross links. It is used as a cell cycle non-specific antineoplastic agent.

It improves survival times when used as an adjunct to amputation in dogs with appendicular osteosarcoma and may have some efficacy in certain carcinomas.

Forms: *Injectable:* 10 mg/ml solution (stable at 5°C for >24h).

Dose: Seek specialist advice before use.
Cats: 200 mg/m^2 i.v. q4 weeks.
Dogs: 300 mg/m^2 i.v. q4 weeks.
The drug is highly irritant and must be administered via a preplaced intravenous catheter. It is usually injected into the side port of a freely running i.v. infusion of 0.9% NaCl over a 10–15 minute period. *See page 293 for conversion of body weight to surface area (m^2).* Do not use needles or i.v. sets containing aluminium as precipitation of the drug may occur.

Caution: Carboplatin is a potent cytotoxic drug. It should only be prepared and administered by trained personnel. Reconstitution or transfer to syringes or infusion bags should be carried out in designated areas, preferably a laminar flow cabinet. Personnel must be protected with suitable clothing, gloves, mask and eye shield. In the event of contact with skin or eyes, the affected area should be washed with copious amounts of water or normal saline. Medical advice should be sought if the eyes are affected. Pregnant women should be excluded from handling cytotoxic agents.

Adverse effects and contraindications: The adverse effects of carboplatin include myelosuppression, nephrotoxicity, nausea, vomiting, electrolyte abnormalities, ototoxicity, neurotoxicity and anaphylactic reactions. However, compared to cisplatin, carboplatin shows reduced nephrotoxicity, neurotoxicity and emetogenicity.

Drug interactions: Concomitant use of **aminoglycosides** or **other nephrotoxic agents** may increase the risk of nephrotoxicity and ototoxicity.

Carnidazole (Spartix) *GSL*

Indications: Carnidazole is active against *Trichomonas columbae*, the cause of pigeon canker. It should be used in conjunction with good loft hygiene, including disinfection of feed and water bowls.

Forms: *Oral:* 10 mg tablet.

Dose: *Pigeons:* 10 mg/adult pigeon, 5 mg/young pigeon. A single dose is usually sufficient, although treatment can be repeated 3 days later. Treat all birds in the loft simultaneously. **Not to be used in pigeons intended for human consumption.**
Other birds: 20–30 mg/kg p.o. once.

Carprofen (Rimadyl) *POM*

Indications: Carprofen is an NSAID that preferentially inhibits COX-2 enzyme thereby limiting the production of prostaglandins involved in inflammation. It is a poor inhibitor of COX-1 enzyme and as such is safer than some other NSAIDs. Carprofen has antipyretic, analgesic, anti-inflammatory and anti-platelet effects. It is used to control mild to moderate pain and inflammation associated with the musculoskeletal system. Its analgesic activity is enhanced if administered pre-emptively.

Forms:
Injectable: 50 mg/ml.
Oral: 20 mg, 50 mg tablets.

Dose:
Cats: 4 mg/kg i.v., s.c. pre-operatively. ONE single further dose of carprofen, at 2 mg/kg i.v., s.c., may be administered. The use of a 1 ml graduated syringe is recommended in order to measure the dose accurately.
Dogs: 4 mg/kg i.v., s.c. pre-operatively, reducing to 2 mg/kg p.o. q12h post-operatively for up to 7 days, then to 2 mg/kg p.o. q24h after 7 days depending upon response.
Small mammals: 4 mg/kg i.v., i.m., s.c.
Birds: 5 mg/kg i.m., s.c., p.o. q24h.
Reptiles: 1–5 mg/kg i.v., i.m., s.c. q24h.

Adverse effects and contraindications: As carprofen preferentially inhibits the COX-2 enzyme, adverse effects are less severe than with some other NSAIDs. General adverse effects associated with NSAID use include GI irritation and ulceration, renal papillary necrosis, particularly if hypotension, dehydration or other nephrotoxic drugs are present, nausea, diarrhoea and fluid retention, which may precipitate cardiac failure. Although these are less likely to develop following the use of carprofen it is prudent not to use this drug if gastric or duodenal ulceration is suspected, in haemorrhagic syndromes, in cardiac or renal failure or in dehydrated, hypovolaemic or hypotensive patients (increased risk of nephrotoxicity). There is an increased risk of toxicity in dogs under 6 weeks. **Do not give to pregnant animals.**

Drug interactions: Carprofen is highly protein-bound and may displace other protein-bound drugs, thereby increasing the risk of toxicity. Do not administer concurrently with or within 24 hours of other **NSAIDs**. Avoid the concurrent use of **NSAIDs** with other potentially nephrotoxic agents, e.g. **aminoglycosides**.

Carvedilol (Eucardic*) *POM*

Indications: Carvedilol is a 3rd generation non-selective beta-blocker/alpha$_1$-blocker with ancillary anti-oxidant effects. It therefore combines the potential benefit of a non-selective beta-blocker with the afterload reduction properties of an alpha$_1$-blocker. The anti-oxidant properties may decrease the oxidant stress associated with progressive heart failure. It is indicated as an adjunct to diuretics, ACE inhibitors and digoxin/pimobendan in the management of symptomatic chronic heart failure. There is currently limited data on the pharmacokinetics and pharmacodynamics of carvedilol in dogs.

Forms: *Oral:* 3.125 mg, 6.25 mg, 12.5 mg, 25 mg tablets.

Dose: *Dogs:* Suggested target dose of 0.4 mg/kg p.o. q24h, to avoid overzealous beta blockade in dogs with heart disease. Start at lower dose and gradually increase dose at 2-week intervals to achieve target dose, if tolerated.

Adverse effects and contraindications: There is little information on the use of this drug in dogs. The adverse effects are likely to be similar to propranolol, namely bradycardia, impaired AV conduction, myocardial depression, heart failure, syncope, bronchospasm, diarrhoea and peripheral vasoconstriction. Its use is contraindicated in patients with supraventricular bradycardia, AV block and acute or decompensated heart failure. A reduction in the glomerular filtration rate with carvedilol use may exacerbate any pre-existing renal impairment.

Drug interactions: Severe hypertension may develop when carvedilol is given with sympathomimetics (e.g. **adrenaline, noradrenaline**). Asystole, severe hypotension and heart failure develop in humans when carvedilol is given with **verapamil**. Enhanced hypotensive effects may develop when carvedilol is given with **phenothiazines, nitroprusside, calcium-channel blockers** and **alpha blockers.** Hypotensive effect of carvedilol antagonized by **NSAIDs**. Carvedilol may enhance the hypoglycaemic effect of insulin. There is the possibility of an increase in systemic vascular resistance developing when carvedilol is administered concomitantly with **dobutamine**. There is an increased risk of AV block and bradycardia when beta-blockers given with **diltiazem** or **cardiac glycosides**. Carvedilol increases plasma concentration of **ciclosporin**.

Cefalexin (Cephalexin) (Cefaseptin; Ceporex; Rilexine) POM

Indications: Cefalexin is an orally active 1st generation cephalosporin antibiotic, a member of the beta-lactam group, which is resistant to some bacterial beta-lactamases, particularly those produced by staphylococcal organisms. Cefalexin binds to proteins involved in bacterial cell wall synthesis, thereby decreasing cell wall strength and rigidity, and affecting cell division. It is active against several Gram-positive and Gram-negative organisms (e.g. *Staphylococcus* spp., *Pasteurella* spp. and *Escherichia coli*). *Pseudomonas* spp. and *Proteus* spp. are often resistant to cefalexin.

Forms:
Injectable: 180 mg/ml suspension.
Oral: 50 mg, 75 mg, 120 mg, 250 mg, 300 mg, 500 mg, 600 mg tablets; granules which, when reconstituted, provide a 100 mg/ml oral syrup.

Dose:
Cats, Dogs: 10–30 mg/kg i.m., s.c., p.o. q8–12h.
Small mammals: 15–30 mg/kg i.m. q8–12h.
Birds: 35–100 mg/kg p.o. q6–8h.
Reptiles: 40–80 mg/kg i.m. q24h @ 30°C.
In severe or acute conditions in all the above species, the dose may be doubled or given at more frequent intervals.
Dose and dosing interval are determined by infection site, severity of disease and organism. Cefalexin is a bactericidal drug with a time-dependent mode of killing. It is important to maintain tissue concentrations above the MIC throughout the inter-dosing interval.

Adverse effects and contraindications: Patients hypersensitive to penicillin agents may also be sensitive to cephalosporins (cross hypersensitivity occurs in <10% of human patients). Vomiting and diarrhoea are the commonest adverse effects; administration with food may reduce these effects. Cefalexin may cause enterotoxaemia in rodents and lagomorphs, although it is used in rabbits. It may cause pain on injection.

Drug interactions: The bactericidal activity of cephalosporins may be affected by the concomitant use of **bacteriostatic agents** (e.g. **erythromycin**, **oxytetracycline**). There may be an increased risk of nephrotoxicity if cephalosporins are used with **amphotericin** or **loop diuretics** (e.g. **furosemide**); monitor renal function. Do not mix in the same syringe as **aminoglycosides**.

Cefalonium (Cephalonium) (Cepravin) *POM*

Indications: Cefalonium is a broad spectrum antibacterial active against Gram-positive and Gram-negative bacteria. It is used to treat bacterial keratoconjunctivitis. This product is not licensed for use in the cat.

Forms: *Topical:* 8% ointment.

Dose: *Cats, Dogs:* Apply to the affected eye q12–24h until the infection has resolved.

Cefotaxime (Cefotaxime*) *POM*

Indications: Cefotaxime is a 3rd generation cephalosporin antibiotic, a member of the beta-lactam group, which is resistant to many bacterial beta-lactamases. Its mode of action is as for cefalexin. It has an increased activity against many Gram-negative organisms (not *Pseudomonas* spp.) but lesser activity against many Gram-positive organisms than 1st and 2nd generation cephalosporins. Its use is reserved for patients suffering from acute sepsis or serious infections where cultures are pending and the animal is not a good candidate for intensive aminoglycoside therapy (pre-existing renal dysfunction).

Forms: *Injectable:* 500 mg, 1 g, 2 g powder for reconstitution.

Dose:
Cats, Dogs: 30–80 mg/kg i.v., i.m. or s.c. q6h; increase dosing interval in patients with severe renal disease.
Birds: 50–100 mg/kg i.m. q6–8h.
Reptiles: 20–40 mg/kg i.m. q24h.
Cefotaxime is a time-dependent bactericidal antibiotic. It is important to maintain tissue concentrations above the MIC.

Adverse effects and contraindications: Patients hypersensitive to penicillin agents may also be sensitive to cephalosporins (cross-sensitivity occurs in <10% of human patients). The reconstituted solution is stable for 10 days when refrigerated. It may produce pain on injection.

Drug interactions: The bactericidal activity of cephalosporins may be affected by the concomitant use of **bacteriostatic agents** (e.g. **oxytetracycline**, **erythromycin**). There may be an increased risk of nephrotoxicity if cephalosporins are used with **amphotericin** or **loop diuretics** (e.g. **furosemide**); monitor renal function. Do not mix in the same syringe as **aminoglycosides**.

Cefoxitin (Mefoxin*) *POM*

Indications: Cefoxitin is a cephamycin antibiotic, a member of the beta-lactam group, but resistant to bacterial beta-lactamases. Its mode of action is as for cefalexin. It is active against Gram-negative bacteria including the gut-dwelling obligate anaerobe *Bacteroides fragilis,* which is resistant to many antibacterial drugs. It is not effective against *Pseudomonas aeruginosa.* Cefoxitin is recommended for the treatment of abdominal sepsis such as peritonitis.

Forms: *Injectable:* 1 g powder for reconstitution.

Dose: *Cats, Dogs:* 30–40 mg/kg i.v., i.m., s.c. q6–8h.
Cefoxitin is a time-dependent bactericidal antibiotic. It is important to maintain tissue concentrations above the MIC.

Adverse effects and contraindications: Patients hypersensitive to penicillin agents may also be sensitive to cefoxitin (cross hypersensitivity occurs in <10% of human patients). It may cause pain on injection. Bleeding problems have been reported in man due to drug-induced hypoprothrombinaemia.

Drug interactions: The bactericidal activity of cefoxitin may be affected by the concomitant use of **bacteriostatic agents**. There may be an increased risk of nephrotoxicity if cefoxitin is used with **amphotericin** or **loop diuretics** (e.g. **furosemide**); monitor renal function. Do not mix in the same syringe as **aminoglycosides**.

Ceftazidime (Fortum*; Kefadim*) *POM*

Indications: Ceftazidime is a 3rd generation cephalosporin antibiotic, a member of the beta-lactam group, but resistant to bacterial beta-lactamases. Its mode of action is as for cefalexin. It has an increased activity against many Gram-negative organisms but less activity against many Gram-positive organisms when compared to 1st and 2nd generation cephalosporins. Ceftazidime has very good activity against *Pseudomonas* spp. Its use is reserved for patients with acute sepsis or serious infections where cultures are pending and the animal is not a good candidate for intensive aminoglycoside therapy (pre-existing renal dysfunction).

Forms: *Injectable:* 250 mg, 500 mg, 1 g, 2 g powder for reconstitution.

Dose:
Cats, Dogs: 20–50 mg/kg i.v. q8–12h.
Birds: 75–100 mg/kg i.v., i.m. q8h.
Reptiles: 20 mg/kg i.m. q72h.
Ceftazidime is a time-dependent bactericidal antibiotic. It is important to maintain tissue concentrations above the MIC.

Adverse effects and contraindications: Patients hypersensitive to penicillin agents may also be sensitive to cephalosporins (cross-hypersensitivity occurs in <10% of human patients).

Drug interactions: The bactericidal activity of cephalosporins may be affected by the concomitant use of **bacteriostatic agents** (e.g. **oxytetracycline**, **erythromycin**). There may be an increased risk of nephrotoxicity if cephalosporins are used with **amphotericin** or **loop diuretics** (e.g. **furosemide**); monitor renal function. Do not mix in the same syringe as **aminoglycosides**.

Cefuroxime (Zinacef *; Zinnat*) *POM*

Indications: Cefuroxime is a 2nd generation cephalosporin antibiotic, a member of the beta-lactam group, but resistant to some bacterial beta-lactamases. Its mode of action is as for cefalexin. It has an increased activity against many Gram-negative organisms but less activity against many Gram-positive organisms when compared to 1st generation cephalosporins. Cefuroxime has good activity against a wider spectrum of the members of the Enterobacteriaceae but not *Pseudomonas* spp. Many obligate anaerobes are also susceptible. Because of this broad spectrum of activity, the 2nd generation cephalosporins have many uses but may be particularly indicated for surgical prophylaxis in prolonged and difficult orthopaedic procedures. The sodium salt of this drug is not stable in the GI tract and so can only be used parenterally.

Forms: *Injectable:* 250 mg, 1.5 g powder for reconstitution (sodium salt). Infusion kits are also available.

Dose:
Cats, Dogs: 20–50 mg/kg i.v., i.m. or s.c. q8–12h.
Reptiles: 100 mg/kg i.m. daily for 10 days at 30°C.
Cefuroxime is a time-dependent bactericidal antibiotic. It is important to maintain tissue concentrations above the MIC.

Adverse effects and contraindications: Patients hypersensitive to penicillin agents may also be sensitive to cephalosporins (cross-hypersensitivity occurs in <10% of human patients). Cephalosporins can be toxic to guinea pigs and hamsters and should be avoided in these species. It may cause pain on i.m. and s.c. injection.

Drug interactions: The bactericidal activity of cephalosporins may be affected by the concomitant use of **bacteriostatic agents** (e.g. **oxytetracycline**, **erythromycin**). There may be an increased risk of nephrotoxicity if cephalosporins are used with **amphotericin** or **loop diuretics** (e.g. **furosemide**); monitor renal function. Do not mix in the same syringe as **aminoglycosides**.

Cephalexin – see Cefalexin

Cephalonium – see Cefalonium

Charcoal (BCK; Carbomix*; Liqui-Char-Vet) P

Indications: Charcoal is an adsorbent used for treating intoxication with organophosphates, carbamates, chlorinated hydrocarbons, strychnine, ethylene glycol, inorganic and organic arsenical and mercurial compounds, and polycyclic organic compounds (most pesticides). It is useful in minimizing the effects of dermal toxicants that may be ingested following grooming.

Forms: *Oral:* 50g activated charcoal powder or premixed slurry (50 g/240 ml); 40% w/w granules (BCK).

Dose: *Cats, Dogs:* 0.5–4 g of activated charcoal/kg as a slurry in water by stomach tube; usually followed by a saline cathartic 20–30 minutes later. Repeat dosing prn if emesis or massive ingestion occurs. As a general rule administer at a dose of at least 10 times the volume of intoxicant ingested.

Caution: Activated charcoal powder floats, covering everything in the area; prepare very carefully as it will stain permanently.

Adverse effects and contraindications: Activated charcoal should not be used prior to the use of emetics.

Drug interactions: Activated charcoal reduces the absorption and therefore efficacy of orally administered drugs.

Chlorambucil (Leukeran*) *POM*

Indications: Chlorambucil is an antineoplastic immunosuppressive alkylating agent of the nitrogen mustard type, used to manage lymphoproliferative, myeloproliferative and immune-mediated diseases.

Forms: *Oral:* 2 mg tablet.

Dose: *Cats, Dogs:* For treatment of chronic lymphocytic leukaemia: 2–6 mg/m^2 p.o. q24h initially until remission achieved, then at reduced dosage/frequency as required to maintain remission. Often used with prednisolone 40 mg/m^2 p.o. q24h for 7d then 20 mg/m^2 q48h. *See page 293 for conversion of body weight to surface area (m^2).*

Adverse effects and contraindications: Adverse effects include anorexia, nausea, vomiting, leucopenia, thrombocytopenia and anaemia (rarely).

Drug interactions: Drugs that stimulate hepatic cytochrome P450 system increase the cytotoxic effects of chlorambucil. **Prednisolone** has a synergistic effect in the management of lymphoid neoplasia.

Chloramphenicol (Chloramphenicol*; **Chloromycetin**; Kemicetine*) *POM*

Indications: Chloramphenicol is a bacteriostatic antibiotic that acts by binding to the 50S ribosomal subunit of susceptible bacteria, preventing bacterial protein synthesis. Unlike erythromycin, lincomycin, clindamycin and tylosin, chloramphenicol also has an affinity for mitochondrial ribosomes of rapidly proliferating mammalian cells (e.g. bone marrow), which may result in bone marrow suppression. Chloramphenicol has a broad spectrum of activity against Gram-positive (including *Streptococcus* spp.and *Staphylococcus* spp.), Gram-negative (including *Brucella* spp., *Salmonella* spp. and *Haemophilus* spp.) and obligate anaerobic bacteria (including *Clostridium* spp. and *Bacteroides fragilis*). Other sensitive organisms include *Chlamydophila* spp., *Mycoplasma* spp. (it is unreliable in the treatment of ocular mycoplasmosis) and *Rickettsia* spp. Resistant organisms include *Nocardia* spp. and *Mycobacterium* spp. Acquired resistance may occur in the Enterobacteriaceae. It is a highly lipophilic and non-polar drug and so penetrates many tissues including the CNS and prostate.

Forms:
Injectable: 1 g powder for reconstitution for i.v., i.m., s.c. use.
Topical: Ophthalmic 1% ointment (with or without hydrocortisone), 0.5% solution; Otic 5% solution.
Oral: 250 mg capsules.

Dose:
Cats, Dogs:
Ophthalmic: 1 drop q4–8h.
Otic: Apply 2–12 drops to affected ear q6–12h.
Systemic: Cats 15–30 mg/kg i.v., i.m., s.c., p.o. q12h; Dogs 25–60 mg/kg i.v., i.m., s.c., p.o. q8–12h. For CNS infections 10–15 mg/kg p.o. q4–6h is recommended in some texts.
Decrease dose or increase dosing interval in neonatal patients.
Small mammals: 15–50 mg/kg i.m., s.c., p.o. q12h; Mice: 50 mg/kg i.m. q12h, 200 mg/kg p.o. q12h.
Birds: 50 mg/kg i.v., i.m. q8h, 75 mg/kg p.o. q8h.
Reptiles: Most species: 40–50 mg/kg i.m., s.c., p.o. q24h.

Caution: Humans exposed to chloramphenicol may have an increased risk of developing a fatal aplastic anaemia. Products should be handled with care.

Adverse effects and contraindications: Adverse effects include nausea, vomiting and diarrhoea. A dose-related reversible bone marrow suppression is seen in all species. The development of irreversible aplastic anaemia does not appear to be a significant problem. The cat, which has a reduced capacity to metabolize chloramphenicol, is more susceptible to bone marrow suppression. Topical use is not associated with such adverse effects. Patients with hepatic or renal dysfunction may need an adjustment to their dose. As chloramphenicol crosses into the milk (50% of serum levels in man), give with caution to nursing bitches or queens, especially those with neonates.

Drug interactions: Chloramphenicol is an irreversible inhibitor of a large number of hepatic cytochrome P450-dependent enzymes and so increases the plasma levels of **pentobarbital**, **phenobarbital** and **oral hypoglycaemic** agents. Recovery from the inhibitory effect of chloramphenicol requires synthesis of new liver enzymes and can take up to 3 weeks. **Rifampin** accelerates the metabolism of chloramphenicol, thus decreasing serum levels.

Chlorhexidine (Hibiscrub*; **Nolvadent**; **Savlon**; **Stomadhex** GSL; **Malaseb** POM)

Indications: Chlorhexidine is a topical antiseptic with antifungal action. It is used topically on skin and in the eye to control bacterial infections and localized dermatophytosis, and in the ear as a part of the management of resistant *Pseudomonas* infections. It is found in dental products to control oral bacterial proliferation and the development of halitosis. It is not inactivated by organic matter.

Forms:
Topical: 7.5% solution (Savlon); 2% shampoo (Malaseb).
Surgical scrub 4% solution in non-ionic detergent base (Hibiscrub).
Oral: Cleansing solution (Nolvadent); Slow release patch (Stomadhex).
Ophthalmic: 0.05% aqueous solution.

Dose: *Cats, Dogs, Small mammals:*
Apply to affected area q8h at 0.5–2.0% concentrations. 0.05% solution in water can be used as a safe wound flush. When treating dermatophytosis continue treatment for 2 weeks after apparent clinical cure and negative fungal culture results.
Otic: Dilute topical products to a 1.0% concentration and apply topically q8–12h.
Ophthalmic: Apply 1 drop q8–12h.

Adverse effects and contraindications: Chlorhexidine is highly ototoxic. If the eardrum is perforated, use only as a very dilute flushing solution under general anesthesia and rinse ear well with saline after application. Chlorhexidine is irritant to the eye in higher concentrations and povidone-iodine solution is preferred for ophthalmic use.

Chlorphenamine (Chlorpheniramine) (Piriton*) P

Indications: Chlorphenamine is an alkylamine antihistamine used in the management of allergies and anaphylactic reactions. It has been advocated for the short-term management of mild sound phobias in dogs and for control of mild anxiety conditions in dogs and cats, including anxiety related to car travel. Chlorphenamine has been used in the management of night-time activity in cats and in compulsive scratching. It has a variable but usually short duration of activity (<6 hours).

Forms:
Injectable: 10 mg/ml solution.
Oral: 4 mg tablet; 2 mg/5ml oral syrup.

Dose:
Cats: 2–4 mg/cat p.o. q8–12h.
Dogs: Small to medium size: 2–4 mg p.o. q8–12h; 2.5–5 mg i.m. q12h.
Medium to large size: 4–8 mg p.o. q8–12h; 5–10 mg i.m. q12h.
Maximum recommended dose 0.5 mg/kg q12h in both cats and dogs.

Adverse effects and contraindications: Use with caution in patients with narrow angle glaucoma, hypertension, G.I. or urinary obstruction, hyperthyroidism and cardiovascular disease. Drowsiness may occur. Injections may be irritant. Diarrhoea, vomiting and anorexia may occur. May cause paradoxical excitement in cats and palatability may be a problem.

Drug interactions: There may be enhancement of the sedative effects following concurrent administration of other **sedative drugs**. May partially counteract anti-coagulant effects of **heparin** and **warfarin**.

Chlorpheniramine – see Chlorphenamine

Chlorpropamide (Chlorpropamide*) *POM*

Indications: Chlorpropamide is a sulphonylurea that augments insulin secretion. It has been used in the management of diabetes mellitus where residual pancreatic beta cell activity is present, although it is relatively ineffective in the dog. Other sulphonylureas (glipizide) may have a greater effect. Chlorpropamide may be of use in the management of diabetes insipidus by enhancing the effect of antidiuretic hormone.

Forms: *Oral:* 100 mg, 250 mg tablets.

Dose: *Cats, Dogs:* 5–40 mg/kg p.o. q24h.

Adverse effects and contraindications: Adverse effects include hypoglycaemia, vomiting, hyponatraemia and weight gain (in patients on long-term chlorpropamide). Do not use if ketoacidosis is present. Use with caution in patients with hepatic or renal failure.

Drug interactions: Phenylbutazone and **potentiated sulphonamides** may enhance the effect of chlorpropamide. The effect of chlorpropamide may be antagonized by **loop** and **thiazide diuretics** and **cortico-steroids**. There is an increased risk of hyponatraemia if chlorpropamide is used concurrently with **potassium-sparing diuretics** and **thiazides**.

Chlortetracycline (Aureomycin) *POM*

Indications: Chlortetracycline is a bacteriostatic antibiotic that inhibits the growth of many Gram-positive and Gram-negative bacteria, ricketsiae, mycoplasmas, spirochaetes and other microbes. It inhibits protein synthesis and is selectively concentrated in bacterial cells. It is used topically to treat ocular infections.

Forms: *Topical:* 1% chlortetracycline hydrochloride ophthalmic ointment.

Dose: *Cats, Dogs:* Apply at least three times daily to the affected eye. Use a separate tube for each animal to avoid contamination.

Cholecalciferol – see Vitamin D

Cholestyramine – see Colestyramine

Chorionic gonadotrophin (Chorulon) *POM*

Indications: Chorionic gonadotrophin is a glycoprotein that has a similar effect to luteinizing hormone (LH). It is used to supplement or replace LH in cases of ovulation failure or delay, to induce lactation post-partum, or in bitches who fail to hold to mating. In males, chorionic gonadotrophin stimulates the secretion of testosterone and is used to manage reduced libido. Chorionic gonadotrophin is used in ferrets to move them out of persistent oestrus.

Forms: *Injectable:* 1500 IU powder for reconstitution.

Dose:
Cats, Dogs:
Females (delayed ovulation): 22 IU/kg i.m. q24–48h or 44 IU/kg i.m. once. Mate on behavioural oestrus.
Females (anoestrus): 500 IU i.m. followed by 20 IU/kg q24h for 10 days.
Males (deficient libido): 100–500 IU i.m. twice weekly for up to 6 weeks.
Small mammals: Ferrets: 20 IU i.m. once.

Adverse effects and contraindications: Anaphylactic reactions may occasionally occur.

Ciclosporin (Cyclosporine) (Atopica; Neoral*; Optimmune; Sandimmun*) *POM*

Indications: Ciclosporin is a fungal metabolite and potent immunosuppressant that acts as a T lymphocyte inhibitor. It is licensed for veterinary use as a topical ophthalmic preparation to treat keratoconjunctivitis sicca in dogs and as an oral preparation for treatment of atopic dermatitis in dogs. It may also be useful as an immunosuppressant in the management of chronic superficial keratoconjunctivitis (pannus), perianal fistula, sebaceous adenitis, immune-mediated disease and canine atopy.

Forms:
Topical: 0.2% ointment (Optimmune).
Oral: 10 mg, 25 mg, 50 mg, 100 mg capsules; 50 mg/ml, 100 mg/ml solution.

Dose:
Cats, Dogs:
• Ocular disease: Apply approximately 0.5 cm of ointment to the affected eye q12h. It may take 2–4 weeks for improvement to occur (occasionally up to 8 weeks). Maintenance treatment should be continued with application q12h; in cases of excessive tear production, application can be reduced to q24h but only with caution and long-term, regular monitoring of tear production.
Dogs:
• Atopic dermatitis: 5 mg/kg p.o. q24h until signs controlled, then q48h as a maintenance dose.
• Perianal fistula, sebaceous adenitis: 5 mg/kg p.o. q12–24h.
• Immunosuppression: 5 mg/kg p.o. q12–24h.

Adverse effects and contraindications: There is no evidence that systemic or ocular toxicity occurs following ocular administration. Use with caution in patients with pre-existing infections and monitor for opportunistic infections. Whilst the nephrotoxicity seen in man does not appear to be common in dogs, care should be taken in treating dogs with renal impairment, and creatinine levels should be monitored regularly. Papillomata and gingival hyperplasia may develop, but appear to resolve on cessation of treatment. Transient adverse effects of vomiting and diarrhoea may require an initial lowering of the dosage. Systemic treatment may be associated with an increased risk of malignancy.

Drug interactions: The metabolism of ciclosporin is reduced, and thus serum levels increased, by various drugs, including **diltiazem**, **doxycycline** and **imidazole** antifungal drugs. **Ketoconazole** may be used to reduce the required dose of ciclosporin. In man there is an increased risk of nephrotoxicity if ciclosporin is administered with **aminoglycosides**, **NSAIDs**, **quinolones**, **sulphonamides** and **trimethoprim**. There is an increased risk of hyperkalaemia if ciclosporin is used with **ACE inhibitors**.

Cimetidine (Cimetidine*; Tagamet*) *POM*

Indications: Cimetidine is a histamine (H_2) receptor antagonist used in the management of gastric and duodenal ulcers, uraemic gastritis, stress- or drug-related erosive gastritis, oesophagitis, hypersecretory conditions secondary to gastrinoma or mast cell neoplasia, and adjunctively to reverse metabolic alkalosis.

Forms:
Injectable: 100 mg/ml solution.
Oral: 200 mg, 400 mg, 800 mg tablets; 40 mg/ml syrup.

Dose:
Cats: 2.5–5 mg/kg i.v., i.m., p.o. q8–12h.
Dogs: 5–10 mg/kg i.v., i.m., p.o. q6–8h.

Adverse effects and contraindications: Adverse effects are rare although hepatotoxicity and nephrotoxicity have been reported. In man, cimetidine has been associated with headache, gynaecomastia and decreased libido. If used by the i.v. route, cimetidine should be administered over 30 minutes to prevent cardiac arrhythmias and hypotension.

Drug interactions: Cimetidine retards oxidative hepatic drug metabolism by binding to the microsomal cytochrome P450. Cimetidine may increase the plasma levels of **beta-blockers** (e.g. **propranolol**), **calcium-channel blockers** (e.g. **verapamil**), **diazepam**, **lidocaine**, **metronidazole**, **pethidine** and **theophylline**. Cimetidine when used with other agents that cause leucopenias may exacerbate the problem. **Sucralfate** may decrease the bioavailability of H_2 antagonists (e.g. cimetidine). Although there is little evidence to suggest that this is of clinical importance it may be a wise precaution to administer sucralfate at least 2 hours before these drugs. Stagger oral doses of cimetidine when used with **antacids**, **digoxin**, **ketoconazole** or **metoclopramide** by 2 hours.

Cinchophen (**PLT**) *POM*

Indications: Cinchophen is a quinoline NSAID with analgesic and antipyretic properties. It is used in the management of osteoarthritis in the dog.

Forms: Tablets 200 mg in combination with prednisolone (1 mg).

Dose: *Dogs:* Oral: 25 mg/kg p.o. q12h.

Adverse effects and contraindications: In man cinchophen may cause liver damage and gastric lesions. It is used in experimental animals to produce gastric ulcers at doses of 100 mg/kg. Although gastric ulceration is a risk, in the clinical setting it is very unlikely to develop. Do not use in pregnant animals, dogs with congestive heart failure, hepatic disease or those with previous adverse reactions to NSAIDs.

Ciprofloxacin (Ciloxan*) *POM*

Indications: Ciprofloxacin is a topical fluoroquinolone, a bactericidal drug (concentration-dependent mechanism) for ophthalmic use when other antibacterials are ineffective. It is active against some Gram-positive and most Gram-negative ocular pathogens, including *Pseudomonas aeruginosa* and *Staphylococcus* spp. (including beta-lactamase-producing bacteria).

Forms: *Topical:* 0.3% solution.

Dose: *Cats, Dogs:* Apply 1 drop to the affected eye q15mins for 4 doses (loading dose) then q6h.

Adverse effects and contraindications: May cause local irritation after application.

Cisatracurium (Nimbex*) *POM*

Indications: Cisatracurium is one of 10 isomers that constitute atracurium, a non-depolarizing neuromuscular blocking agent. It undergoes Hofmann elimination and so is independent of renal and hepatic function for termination of action. Laudanosine, a metabolite of both drugs, has caused hypotension and seizures in dogs. Cisatracurium has approximately 10 times the potency of atracurium; when equipotent doses are given, the risk of laudanosine toxicity is lower with the *cis* isomer. It has an intermediate (25–35 minutes) duration of action in dogs and does not appear to accumulate with repeat doses.

Forms: *Injectable:* 2 mg/ml in 2.5 ml, 5 ml ampoules; 5 mg/ml in 30 ml vials.

Dose: *Dogs:* 0.1 mg/kg i.v. to effect (prn) followed, when required, by maintenance doses of 0.02–0.04 mg/kg i.v.

Adverse effects and contraindications: Neuromuscular blocking agents **must not be used** if the provision of adequate analgesia and anaesthesia cannot be guaranteed and the means of adequate lung ventilation are unavailable. Neuromuscular blockade with cisatracurium should be antagonized with an antimuscarinic/anticholinesterase drug combination.

Drug interactions: The following agents antagonize the effects of cisatracurium: **anticholinesterases (edrophonium, neostigmine), azathioprine, potassium** and **theophylline**. The action of cisatracurium may be prolonged and intensified by **amino-glycosides, clindamycin, lincomycin, polymyxin, inhalation anaesthetics, magnesium salts** and **quinidine**.

Cisplatin (Cisplatin*) *POM*

Indications: Cisplatin is a platinum complex that binds to DNA to form intra- and interstrand cross links and DNA–protein cross links. It is used as a cell cycle non-specific antineoplastic agent against various sarcomas and carcinomas, but is used most commonly in the management of osteosarcoma.

Forms: *Injectable:* 1 mg/ml solution: 10 mg, 50 mg and 150 mg powders for reconstitution.

Dose: *Dogs:* 50–70 mg/m^2 i.v. q3–4w.
See page 293 for conversion of body weight to surface area (m^2).

Administration: The drug is irritant and must be administered via a pre-placed intravenous catheter. Do not use needles or i.v. sets containing aluminium; plastic catheters, plastic hub needles or stainless steel are compatible. Cisplatin is sensitive to daylight but is not adversely affected by normal room lighting after dilution in 0.9% saline. Do not refrigerate, as cooling of diluted solutions can lead to precipitation.

Cisplatin is a highly nephrotoxic drug; pre- and post-treatment hydration is important to ensure adequate renal clearance and reduce nephrotoxicity. Various protocols have been described:

Protocol 1: Dogs: 6 hour infusion with saline diuresis
- Pre-hydration: i.v. saline (0.9%) at 25 ml/kg/h for 3 hours
- Anti-emetic: metoclopramide 1 mg/kg 30 mins prior to cisplatin infusion
- Cisplatin 50–70 mg/m^2 in 250–500 ml 0.9% saline i.v. over 30 mins
- Diuresis: 0.9% saline continued at 15 ml/kg/h i.v. for 3 hours
- Furosemide may be administered if urine production is not adequate

Protocol 2: Dogs: Infusion with Mannitol diuresis:
- Pre-hydration: 0.9% saline at 10 ml/kg/h i.v. for 4 hours
- Anti-emetic: metoclopramide: 1 mg/kg 30 minutes prior to cisplatin infusion
- Mannitol 0.5 g/kg i.v. in saline over 20–30 minutes
- Cisplatin 50–70 mg/m^2 in 250 ml 0.9% saline given as a slow i.v. infusion over 15 minutes
- Continue saline infusion at 10 ml/kg/h for 2 hours

Caution: Cisplatin is a potent cytotoxic drug that should only be prepared and administered by trained personnel. Reconstitution or transfer to syringes or infusion bags should be carried out in designated areas, preferably a laminar flow cabinet. The fluid bag containing cisplatin should be clearly labelled so that all personnel are aware of its contents. Personnel must be protected with suitable clothing, gloves, mask and eye shield whenever the drug bottles, fluid bag, i.v. line or needle are handled.

In the event of contact with skin or eyes, the affected area should be washed with copious amounts of water or normal saline. Medical advice should be sought if the eyes are affected. Pregnant women should be excluded from handling cytotoxic agents. If urine is collected a special license is required for its disposal. Cisplatin is excreted in urine for at least 24h.

Adverse effects and contraindications: The adverse effects of cisplatin in the dog include nephrotoxicity (major concern), myelosuppression, nausea, vomiting, electrolyte abnormalities, ototoxicity, neurotoxicity, hyperuricaemia and anaphylactic reactions; patients receiving this drug should be observed carefully during administration. **Do not use in cats because of severe pulmonary reactions.**

Drug interactions: Concomitant use of **aminoglycosides** may increase the risk of nephrotoxicity and ototoxicity. Plasma concentrations of cisplatin are reduced by **anticonvulsant agents**.

Clarithromycin (Klaricid*) POM

Indications: Clarithromycin is a macrolide derived from erythromycin and has a slightly greater activity than the parent. It has bactericidal (time-dependent) or bacteriostatic properties, dependent upon the drug concentration and an organism's susceptibility. It binds to the 50S ribosome, inhibiting peptide bond formation. Clarithromycin is indicated as an alternative to penicillin in penicillin-allergic individuals, as it has a similar, although not identical, antibacterial spectrum. It is active against Gram-positive cocci (some staphylococci are resistant), Gram-positive bacilli, some Gram-negative bacilli (*Pasturella* spp.) and some spirochaetes (*Helicobacter* spp.). Some strains of *Actinomyces*, *Nocardia*, *Chlamydophila* and *Rickettsia* are also inhibited by clarithromycin. Most strains of the Enterobacteriaceae (*Pseudomonas* spp., *Escherichia coli*, *Klebsiella* spp.) are resistant. It is particularly useful in the management of respiratory tract infections, mild to moderate skin and soft tissue infections and non-tubercular mycobacterial infections. For the latter it is used in combination with enrofloxacin and rifampin (see *BSAVA Manual of Canine and Feline Infectious Diseases*).

Forms:
Oral: 250 mg, 500 mg tablets; 125 mg/ml suspension.
Injectable: 500 mg vial for reconstitution.

Dose:
Cats: 5–10 mg/kg i.v. infusion, p.o. q12h or 62.5 mg/cat p.o.
Dogs: 4–12 mg/kg i.v. infusion, p.o. q12h. Doses of 15–25 mg/kg p.o. q8–12h are recommended in the treatment of leproid granuloma syndrome. These doses are empirical and are based on a very few reports.

Adverse effects and contraindications: There is little information on the use of this drug in animals. In man similar adverse effects to those of erythromycin are seen, i.e. vomiting, cholestatic hepatitis, stomatitis and glossitis. Be cautious using it in animals with hepatic dysfunction. Reduce its dose in animals with renal impairment. Clarithromycin's activity is enhanced in an alkaline pH; administer on an empty stomach.

Drug interactions: Clarithromycin may increase serum levels of **methylprednisolone** and **theophylline**. The absorption of **digoxin** may be enhanced.

Clazuril (**Appertex**) *GSL*

Indications: Clazuril is a coccidiostat used in the treatment and control of coccidiosis caused by *Eimeria labbeana* and *E. columbarum* in homing and show pigeons. Birds should be treated following transportation to shows or races where they may have been exposed to coccidia.

Forms: *Oral:* 2.5 mg tablet.

Dose: *Birds:* Pigeons: 2.5 mg/pigeon. Treat all birds in the loft simultaneously. **Not to be used in birds intended for human consumption**; Psittacines: 7 mg/kg p.o. 3 days on, 2 days off, 3 days on.

Contraindications and adverse effects: Do not administer with drugs that may cause vomiting.

Clemastine (Tavegil*) *POM*

Indications: Clemastine is an antihistamine used in the management of allergic skin disease in the cat and dog. It is considered to act synergistically with essential fatty acids in the treatment of atopy.

Forms: *Oral:* 1 mg tablet; 0.1 mg/ml syrup.

Dose:
Cats: 0.1 mg/kg p.o. q12h.
Dogs: 0.05–0.1 mg/kg p.o. q12h.
Note: recent studies have doubted the ability of oral administration to achieve therapeutic blood levels. Until further studies are complete higher doses are not recommended.

Adverse effects and contraindications: Sedation may develop.

Clindamycin (Antirobe) *POM*

Indications: Clindamycin is a lincosamide antibiotic that binds to the 50S ribosomal subunit, inhibiting peptide bond formation. It has activity against Gram-positive cocci including penicillin-resistant staphylococci, many obligate anaerobes and against *Toxoplasma gondii*. It attains high concentrations in bone and bile. Being a weak base, it becomes ion-trapped (and therefore concentrated) in fluids that are more acidic than plasma, such as prostatic fluid, milk and intracellular fluid. Clindamycin may be bacteriostatic (time-dependent) or bactericidal depending on the organism and drug concentration. There is complete cross resistance between lincomycin and clindamycin, and partial cross resistance with erythromycin.

Forms: *Oral:* 25 mg, 75 mg, 150 mg capsules (Antirobe).

Dose: *Cats, Dogs:* 5.5–11 mg/kg p.o. q12h.
Toxoplasmosis: 12.5–25 mg/kg p.o. q12h.

Adverse effects and contraindications: Colitis and diarrhoea may develop in man. Although this is not a major problem in dogs and cats, discontinue the drug if diarrhoea develops. Lincosamides cause a potentially fatal clostridial enterotoxaemia in **rabbits, guinea pigs and hamsters**.

Drug interactions: Clindamycin may enhance the effect of **non-depolarizing muscle relaxants** (e.g. **tubocurarine**) and may antagonize the effects of **neostigmine** and **pyridostigmine**.

Clodronate (Bonefos*; Loron*) *POM*

Indications: Clodronate is a bisphosphonate that is adsorbed on to hydroxyapatite crystals, slowing their rate of growth/dissolution. It is used to treat acute moderate to severe hypercalcaemia when other therapies are ineffective, or in the long-term therapy of chronic hypercalcaemia.

Forms:
Injectable: 30 mg/ml, 60 mg/ml solution.
Oral: 400 mg capsule.

Dose: *Dogs:* 5–14 mg/kg i.v. q24h; 10–30 mg/kg p.o. q8–12h.
Note: There are few reports on the use of this drug in dogs.

Adverse effects and contraindications: Adverse effects include nausea, diarrhoea, hypocalcaemia, hypophosphataemia, hypomagnesaemia and hypersensitivity reactions.

Drug interactions: Reduced absorption is seen if administered with **antacids**, **calcium** and **iron salts**; administer 2 hours apart. Concurrent use of **aminoglycosides** may result in severe hypocalcaemia.

Clofazimine (Clofazimine*) POM

Indications: Clofazimine is a fat-soluble phenazine dye. It is a human antileprotic drug that has been used in the management of mycobacterial infections including feline leprosy.

Forms: *Oral:* 100 mg capsule.

Dose: *Cats, Dogs:* 2–12 mg/kg p.o. q24h for 2–6 months.

Adverse effects and contraindications: In man the major adverse effects are nausea, diarrhoea and renal and hepatic impairment (monitor functions during therapy). Skin discoloration has been reported in the cat.

Clomipramine (Clomicalm) *POM*

Indications: Clomipramine is a tricyclic antidepressant that blocks serotonin and noradrenaline re-uptake in the brain, thereby increasing their effects. It should be used in combination with behavioural therapy and is specifically licensed to be used in this manner for treatment of separation-related disorders manifested by destruction and inappropriate urination and defecation. It may be useful in the management of obsessive–compulsive disorders such as tail chasing, fly biting, flank sucking and licking associated with lick granuloma. Clomipramine is used for the treatment of anxiety-related urine spraying in cats and feline hyperaesthesia. In birds it is used to manage behavioural feather plucking or self-mutilation.

Forms: *Oral:* 5 mg, 20 mg, 80 mg tablets.

Dose:
Cats: 0.25–1 mg/kg p.o. q24h.
Dogs: 1–3 mg/kg p.o. q12h for a minimum of 2 months.
Birds: 1 mg/kg p.o. q24h for 6 weeks.

Adverse effects and contraindications: Do not use in male breeding dogs. It may cause sporadic vomiting, changes in appetite or lethargy. Adverse effects described in man include dry mouth, diarrhoea, excitability, arrhythmias, hypotension, syncope and, much less commonly, seizures and bone marrow disorders. Care should be used if prescribed to dogs with epilepsy, cardiovascular dysfunction, narrow angle glaucoma, reduced GI motility or urinary retention. In birds regurgitation and drowsiness have been reported.

Drug interactions: There is an increased risk of arrhythmias if clomipramine is administered concurrently with **anaesthetics** and **anti-arrhythmics**. Clomipramine antagonizes the effects of **anti-epileptic** drugs. There is enhancement of sedative effects if used with other **sedative** drugs. It may potentiate the effects of **anticholinergic drugs**, other drugs acting on the CNS and **sympathomimetics**. Do not use in conjunction with **monoamine oxidase inhibitors**. Certain drugs such as **phenytoin**, may have increased plasma levels when used simultaneously.

Clonidine (Catapres*) POM

Indications: Clonidine is an alpha-adrenergic drug used to assess the pituitary's ability to produce growth hormone (GH).

Forms: *Injectable:* 150 mg/ml solution.

Clonidine stimulation test: To assess GH production in **dogs**.
Take EDTA blood sample for GH estimation at 0 and 20 minutes. Administer 10 µg/kg clonidine i.v. (maximum 300 µg/dog) after taking the 0 sample. Separate plasma as soon as possible and store at –20°C. Send samples on dry ice to Faculty of Veterinary Medicine, University of Utrecht, Dept of Clinical Science of Companion Animals, Biochemical Lab, PO 80154, 3508 TD Utrecht, The Netherlands.
Normal baseline values 1–4 ng/ml. Following stimulation ratios of peak to basal values range from 3.4 to 111.7.
Note: Assessment of plasma insulin-like growth factor in a single sample is a useful screening test for growth hormone disorder. Low IGF is seen with growth hormone deficiency, whilst elevated IGF levels are seen with acromegaly, diabetes mellitus, hyperadrenocorticism.

Adverse effects and contraindications: Transient sedation and bradycardia may develop.

Clorazepate (Tranxene*) POM

Indications: Clorazepate is a benozodiazepine, which has been advocated by some authors for use in the treatment of anxiety-related disorders and short-term management of sound phobias.

Forms: *Oral:* 7.5 mg, 15 mg tablets.

Dose:
Cats: 0.02–0.4 mg/kg p.o. q12–24h.
Dogs: 0.55–2.2 mg/kg p.o. q4–24h.

Adverse effects and contraindications: Contraindicated in situations of renal and hepatic impairment and in patients with acute narrow-angle glaucoma. May be associated with significant levels of sedation.

Drug interactions: These are the same as for diazepam.

Clotrimazole (Canesten*; Clotrimazole*; Lotriderm*) *P*

Indications: Clotrimazole is a topical imidazole antifungal drug with a broad spectrum of activity. It has an inhibitory action on the growth of pathogenic dermatophytes, *Aspergillus* spp. and yeasts by inhibiting cytochrome P450-dependent ergosterol synthesis.

Forms: *Topical:* 1% cream and solution. Many other products are available. Some contain corticosteroids (Lotriderm).

Dose:
Cats, Dogs:
Otic: Instil 3–5 drops in ear q12h.
Topical: Apply to affected area and massage in gently q12h, if no improvement in 4 weeks re-evaluate therapy or diagnosis.
Birds: Intratracheal: 2–3 ml of a 1% solution nebulized for periods of 1 hour q24h or topically.

Cloxacillin (Orbenin) *POM*

Indications: Cloxacillin is a beta-lactamase-resistant, narrow spectrum beta-lactam antibiotic. For mode of action see ampicillin. It is used as a topical agent in the treatment of eye infections. Cloxacillin has a narrow spectrum of activity. It is less active than penicillin G or V against *Streptococcus* spp. and is indicated for the treatment of ocular infections caused by beta-lactamase-producing *Staphylococcus* spp.

Forms: *Eye ointment:* Cloxacillin benzathine ester 16.7% suspension.

Dose: *Cats, Dogs:* Apply 1/10th of a tube (0.3 g) once daily.

Adverse effects and contraindications: Do not administer penicillins to hamsters, gerbils, guinea pigs, chinchillas or rabbits.

Drug interactions: Avoid the concomitant use of bacteriostatic antibiotics (**chloramphenicol**, **erythromycin**, **tetracycline**).

Codeine (Codeine*: **Pardale–V**) *POM*

Indications: Codeine is an opioid analgesic used in veterinary medicine as a cough suppressant, and occasionally to treat diarrhoea.

Forms: *Oral:* 15 mg, 30 mg, 60 mg tablets; 3 mg/ml linctus.

Dose: *Dogs:* 0.5–2 mg/kg p.o. q12h.

Adverse effects and contraindications: Adverse effects include sedation, ataxia, respiratory depression and constipation. Use with caution in patients with severe renal insufficiency, Addisons' disease, increased intracranial pressure and hypothyroidism.

Colchicine (Colchicine*) *POM*

Indications: Colchicine inhibits collagen synthesis, may enhance collagenase activity and blocks the synthesis and secretion of serum amyloid A. It has been used, with limited success, in the management of fibrotic hepatic and pulmonary diseases and renal amyloidosis.

Forms: *Oral:* 0.5 mg tablet.

Dose: *Dogs:* 0.03 mg/kg p.o. q8–72h in conjunction with appropriate specific/dietary therapy.

Adverse effects and contraindications: The commoner adverse effects include vomiting, abdominal pain and diarrhoea. Rarely, renal damage, bone marrow suppression, myopathy and peripheral neuropathy may develop. Colchicine may cause elevated serum ALP and ALT values, decreased platelet counts and false-positive results when testing urine for RBCs and haemoglobin.

Drug interactions: Possible increased risk of nephrotoxicity and myotoxicity when colchicine given with **ciclosporin**.

Colecalciferol – see Vitamin D

Colestyramine (Cholestyramine) (Questran*) *POM*

Indications: Colestyramine is an ion exchange resin used in the rabbit for absorbing toxins produced in the GI tract following the development of overgrowth of *Clostridium* spp. It is used in dogs for the reduction of serum cholesterol in idiopathic hypercholesterolaemia.

Forms: *Oral:* 4g powder/sachet.

Dose:
Dogs: 1–2 g/dog q12h.
Small mammals: Rabbits: 2 g/rabbit given orally with 20 ml water.

Adverse effects and contraindications: Constipation may develop.

Drug interactions: It reduces the absorption of **digoxin, anti-coagulants, diuretics** and **thyroxine**.

Contrast media – see Barium sulphate contrast media and
Iodine-containing contrast media

Crisantaspase (L–Asparaginase) (Erwinase*) *POM*

Indications: Crisantaspase, the enzyme asparaginase, hydrolyses the
essential amino acid asparagine. Lymphoid tumour cells are not able
to synthesize asparagine and are dependent upon supply from the
extracellular fluid. Asparaginase deprives malignant cells of this amino
acid, which results in cessation of protein synthesis and cell death. The
main indication for asparaginase is in the treatment of lymphoproliferative disorders.

Forms: Injection, powder for reconstitution, 10,000 IU crisantaspase.

Dose: *Cats, Dogs:* 10,000–40,000 IU/m² q7 days or more; i.m. route is
recommended.
See page 293 for conversion of body weight to surface area (m²).

Adverse effects and contraindications: Anaphylaxis may follow
administration, particularly when the drug is administered i.v.
Premedication with an antihistamine is recommended if other routes
are used. Haemorrhagic pancreatitis has been reported in dogs.

Drug interactions: If crisantaspase is used in combination with
vincristine, the vincristine should be given 12–24 hours before the
enzyme. Administration of crisantaspase with or before vincristine may
reduce clearance of vincristine and increase toxicity.

Cyanocobalamin – see Vitamin B12

Cyclopentolate (Minims cyclopentolate*) *POM*

Indications: Cyclopentolate is a short-acting antimuscarinic, used for
mydriasis (dilate pupil) and cycloplegia (paralyse the ciliary body
muscle). It has a longer duration of action than tropicamide but shorter
than atropine. It is used mainly pre-operatively for intraocular surgery
to prevent intra-operative miosis.

Forms: 0.5%, 1% solutions.

Dose: *Cats, Dogs:* 1 or 2 drops as required.

Adverse effects and contraindications: Cyclopentolate should not
be used as a diagnostic aid due to its onset and duration of action. It
may cause chemosis in dogs and increased salivation in cats.

Cyclophosphamide (Cyclophosphamide*; Cytoxan (USA)*; Endoxana (UK)*) *POM*

Indications: Cyclophosphamide is an antineoplastic and immuno-suppressive alkylating agent of the nitrogen mustard group. It is used in the treatment of lymphoproliferative diseases, myeloproliferative disease and immune-mediated diseases and may have a role in the management of certain sarcomas and carcinomas.

Forms:
Injectable: 100 mg, 200 mg, 500 mg, 1000 mg powder for reconstitution.
Oral: 50 mg tablet (available in UK), 25 mg tablet (available in USA, trade name Cytoxan).

Dose: *Cats, Dogs:*
- Treatment of lymphoid neoplasms: Generally 50 mg/m^2 p.o. q48h or 4 consecutive days/week; or 200–300 mg/m^2 i.v. q3 weeks.
  See Chemotherapy protocols on pages 295–296.
- Immunosuppression: 50 mg/m^2 p.o. or 1.5 mg/kg p.o. (dogs weighing >25 kg); 2 mg/kg p.o. (dogs weighing 5–25 kg); 2.5 mg/kg p.o. (cats and dogs weighing <5 kg).
  Give for 4 consecutive days/week or q48h.
  See page 293 for conversion of body weight to surface area (m^2).

Caution: Cyclophosphamide is a potent cytotoxic drug. Intravenous preparations should only be prepared and administered by trained personnel. Reconstitution or transfer to syringes or infusion bags should be carried out in designated areas, preferably a laminar flow cabinet. Personnel must be protected with suitable clothing, gloves, mask and eye shield. In the event of contact with skin or eyes, the affected area should be washed with copious amounts of water or normal saline. Medical advice should be sought if the eyes are affected. Pregnant women should be excluded from handling cytotoxic agents.

Adverse effects and contraindications: The major adverse effect is that of myelosuppression, with the nadir usually occurring 7–14 days after the start of therapy. Regular monitoring of WBCs is recommended. A metabolite of cyclophosphamide (acrolein) may cause a sterile haemorrhagic cystitis, particularly following i.v. administration. The cystitis may be persistent. The risk may be reduced by increasing water consumption and ensuring adequate urine flow. Other effects include vomiting, diarrhoea, hepatotoxicity, nephrotoxicity and a reduction in hair growth rate. With severe renal impairment, extend the dosing interval.

Drug interactions: An increased risk of myelosuppression may occur if **thiazide diuretics** are given concomitantly with cyclophosphamide. Absorption of orally administered **digoxin** may be decreased by cyclophosphamide; this may occur several days after cyclophosphamide is administered. **Barbiturates** increase cyclophosphamide toxicity due to an increased rate of conversion to its metabolites. **Phenothiazines**, **chloramphenicol** and **corticosteroids** reduce cyclophosphamide efficacy; the latter two by interfering with metabolism to its active form. **Cisplatin** has a synergistic effect. If administered with **doxorubicin** there is an increased risk of cardiotoxicity. **Insulin** requirements are altered by concurrent cyclophosphamide therapy.

Cyclosporine – see Ciclosporin

Cyproheptadine (Periactin*) P

Indications: Cyproheptadine is an antihistamine with serotonin antagonistic effects. It provides symptomatic relief in cases of allergic skin disease, and acts as an appetite stimulant.

Forms: *Oral:* 4 mg tablet.

Dose: *Cats, Dogs:* 0.1–0.5 mg/kg p.o. q8–12h.

Adverse effects and contraindications: Cyproheptadine may cause sedation, unwanted polyphagia and weight gain.

Cytarabine (Cytarabine*) POM

Indications: Cytarabine (cytosine arabinoside) is an antimetabolite that interferes with pyrimidine synthesis. It is used as an antineoplastic agent in the management of lymphoproliferative and myeloproliferative disorders.

Forms: *Injectable:* 100 mg, 500 mg powder for reconstitution.

Dose: *Cats, Dogs:* 100 mg/m^2 i.v. q24h for 4 days, or 100 mg/m^2 by i.v. infusion over 24 hours, or 20 mg/m^2 intrathecally q1–5d.
See page 293 for conversion of body weight to surface area (m^2).

Adverse effects and contraindications: Adverse effects include vomiting, diarrhoea and leucopenia. As it is a myelosuppressant, careful haematological monitoring is required. After reconstitution store at room temperature and discard after 48 hours or if a slight haze develops.

Drug interactions: The oral absorption of **digoxin** is decreased by cytarabine. The activity of **gentamicin** may be reduced by the agent. Simultaneous administration of **methotrexate** increases the effect of cytarabine.

Dacarbazine (Dacarbazine*) *POM*

Indications: Dacarbazine is an alkylating agent that inhibits DNA and protein synthesis. Its use has been reported in the management of lymphoproliferative diseases, melanoma and soft tissue sarcomas.

Forms: *Injectable:* 100 mg, 200 mg, 500 mg powder for reconstitution.

Dose: *Cats, Dogs:* 200–250 mg/m^2 daily on days 1–5. Repeat cycle every 21–28 days.
See page 293 for conversion of body weight to surface area (m^2).

Caution: Dacarbazine is a potent cytotoxic drug. It should only be prepared and administered by trained personnel. Reconstitution or transfer to syringes or infusion bags should be carried out in designated areas, preferably a laminar flow cabinet. Personnel must be protected with suitable clothing, gloves, mask and eye shield. In the event of contact with skin or eyes, the affected area should be washed with copious amounts of water or normal saline. Medical advice should be sought if the eyes are affected. Pregnant women should be excluded from handling cytotoxic agents.

Adverse effects and contraindications: Adverse effects may be severe and include myelosuppression, intense nausea and vomiting.

Drug interactions: Phenobarbital increases the metabolic activation of dacarbazine.

Dactinomycin D (Actinomycin-D) (Cosmogen Lyvac*) *POM*

Indications: Dactinomycin is an anti-tumour antibiotic product of the *Streptomyces* species. It binds to single and double stranded DNA, resulting in inhibition of DNA synthesis and function. Inhibition of RNA and protein synthesis may contribute to its cytotoxic effects. In veterinary medicine Dactinomycin has been used in rescue protocols for canine lymphoma.

Forms: *Injectable:* 0.5 mg powder for reconstitution.

Dose: *Dogs:* 0.75–1.5 mg/m^2 slow i.v. via a pre-placed catheter.
See page 293 for conversion of body weight to surface area (m^2).

Adverse effects and contraindications: Myelosuppression is the main dose-limiting toxicity. Gastrointestinal toxicity may also occur. The drug is vesicant and tissue damage will result from extravasation.

Danazol (Danazol*) *POM*

Indications: Danazol is a synthetic androgen. It has a synergistic action with corticosteroids in the control of immune-mediated thrombo-cytopenia and immune-mediated haemolytic anaemia. This action is thought to be mediated through a reduction in macrophage cell surface immunoglobulin receptors and a decrease in the amount of antibody on target cells. The onset of action may be slow, with the effects taking several weeks to become apparent.

Forms: *Oral:* 100 mg, 200 mg capsules.

Dose:
Cats: 5 mg/kg p.o. q8h.
Dogs: 4–10 mg/kg p.o. q8–12h, although an initial dose of 5 mg/kg p.o. q8h is suggested.

Adverse effects and contraindications: Danazol is teratogenic and must not be used in pregnant animals. It is principally metabolized in the liver and may cause hepatotoxicity. Avoid use in patients with cardiac, renal or hepatic impairment. Other effects result from androgen actions: virilization in females, increased muscle mass, testicular atrophy and alopecia.

Drug interactions: Danazol inhibits the metabolism of **ciclosporin**.

Danthron – see Dantron

Dantrolene (Dantrium*) *POM*

Indications: Dantrolene inhibits calcium release from the sarcoplasmic reticulum of skeletal muscle, and diminishes the strength of evoked muscle contraction. It is used in the management of muscle spasms, e.g. urethral spasm and tetanus, and for the prevention (oral preparation), or treatment (i.v. preparation) of malignant hyperthermia.

Forms:
Injectable: 20 mg powder for reconstitution.
Oral: 25 mg, 100 mg capsules.

Dose: *Cats, Dogs:* 2–5 mg/kg i.v. (for malignant hyperthermia), and 0.5–2 mg/kg p.o. q12h (other indications).

Adverse effects and contraindications: Increase the dose slowly. Avoid in animals with hepatic impairment and use with caution if cardiac and pulmonary function is impaired. Monitor liver function during therapy.

Dantron (Codanthramer*; Codanthrusate*) POM

Indications: A faecal softener/stimulant used to treat constipation.

Forms: *Oral:* 5 mg/ml dantron and 40 mg/ml poloxamer '188' solution (codanthramer); 50 mg dantron plus 60 mg docusate capsule (codanthrusate).

Dose: *Cats, Dogs:* 2.5–5ml p.o. q12h.

Adverse effects and contraindications: Do not use if GI obstruction present.

Dapsone (Dapsone*) POM

Indications: Dapsone is an anti-inflammatory, antibacterial agent with immunomodulatory properties, including inhibition of neutrophil chemotaxis and stabilization of mast cells. In dogs dapsone has been used to treat subcorneal pustular dermatitis and vasculitis.

Forms: *Oral:* 50 mg tablets.

Dose: *Dogs:* 1 mg/kg p.o. q24h.

Adverse effects and contraindications: Serious blood dyscrasias, thrombocytopenia and hepatotoxicity have been reported, albeit very rarely. Haematology and serum biochemistry should be monitored regularly in treated dogs.

Deferoxamine (Desferrioxamine) (Desferal*) POM

Indications: Deferoxamine chelates iron, and the complex is excreted in the urine. It is used to remove iron from the body following poisoning. It may be useful in the management of reperfusion injury. If administered prior to reperfusion, it limits the availability of iron for free radical production.

Forms: *Injectable:* 500 mg vial for reconstitution.

Dose: *Cats, Dogs:* 12.5–20 mg/kg diluted in 10–20 ml of water for injection, i.v., i.m. q2h for 2 doses then 10 mg/kg i.v., i.m. q8h for 24h or 15 mg/kg/hour i.v. infusion. Maximum 80 mg/kg or 6 g in 24h. If used to manage reperfusion injury, continuous infusion recommended.

Adverse effects and contraindications: Intramuscular administration is painful. Anaphylactic reactions and hypotension may develop if administered rapidly i.v.

Delmadinone acetate (Tardak) *POM*

Indications: Delmadinone is a progestin with antiandrogen and antioestrogen effects. It is used in the treatment of hypersexuality (male dog and cat), prostatic hypertrophy, anal adenomas and hormonally driven canine aggression. The use of this drug as an indicator of the effect of surgical castration on behavioural problems is limited by its central calming effect and this should be taken into consideration when assessing the response to treatment with this drug. Dogs that show a reduced level of aggression when treated with delmadinone will not automatically show the same behavioural response to surgical castration. In situations of fear- or anxiety-related aggressive behaviour, the surgical approach can exacerbate the behaviour. In birds it may be useful for behavioural regurgitation or behaviour associated with sexual frustration.

Forms: *Injectable:* 10 mg/ml suspension.

Dose: *Cats, Dogs:* <10 kg 1.5–2 mg/kg; 10–20 kg 1–1.5 mg/kg; >20 kg 1 mg/kg i.m., s.c. repeated after 8 days if not response. Animals that respond to treatment may need further treatment after 3–4 weeks.
Birds: 1 mg/kg i.m. once.

Adverse effects and contraindications: Possible adverse effects include a transient reduction in fertility and libido, polyuria and polydipsia, an increased appetite and hair colour change at the site of injection.

Desferrioxamine – see Deferoxamine

Desmopressin (DDAVP*; Desmospray*; Desmotabs*; Nocutol*) *POM*

Indications: Desmopressin, a vasopressin analogue, has a longer duration of action than vasopressin and, unlike vasopressin, has no vasoconstrictor activity. It is used in the diagnosis and treatment of central diabetes insipidus, and to boost plasma levels of factor VIII and von Willebrand's factor in patients with mild to moderate haemophilia A or von Willebrand's disease.

Forms:
Intranasal: 100 µg/ml solution (DDAVP), 10 µg metered spray (Desmospray, Nocutol).
Injectable: 4 µg/ml solution (DDAVP).
Oral: 100 µg, 200 µg tablets (DDAVP, Desmotabs).

Dose:
Cats: 5 µg/cat or 0.05 ml (1–2 drops) intranasally or on to the conjunctiva q8–24h, or 5 µg/cat p.o. q8–24h initially. The dose and frequency of dosing can be increased or decreased according to response.
Dogs:
* Coagulopathies: 1–4 µg/kg i.v. once. Dilute in 20 ml saline and administer over 10 minutes.
* Diabetes insipidus diagnosis: 1–4 µg/dog i.v. once (*see Modified water deprivation test, below*)
* Diabetes insipidus treatment: 1–4 µg/dog i.v., i.m. or 5–20 µg/dog or 0.05–0.2 ml/dog intranasally or on to the conjunctiva q8–24h, or 5 µg/kg p.o. q8–24h initially (maximum dose 400 µg p.o. q8h). The dose and frequency of dosing can be increased or decreased according to response.

Modified water deprivation test: To assess the ability of the kidney to concentrate urine in patients with suspect diabetes insipidus. **Do not perform this test in patients with renal disease, dehydration or hypercalcaemia. Assess renal and adrenocortical function first.** Starve patient overnight for 12 hours. Weigh patient, obtain urine sample and record specific gravity. Remove water. Every 2–4 hours weigh the patient, empty bladder and check urine specific gravity. Once urine specific gravity has reached 1.030 (dogs) or 1.035 (cats), or the animal has lost 5% of its body weight, then stop test. If urine is still dilute once a 5% weight loss has occurred then empty the bladder, administer **desmopressin** (2 µg i.v., i.m. or 20 µg intranasally) and check urine specific gravity 2 hours later. An increase in urine specific gravity is consistent with central diabetes insipidus. If the urine specific gravity remains low, nephrogenic diabetes insipidus or medullary washout should be considered.

Dexamethasone (Colvasone; **Dexadreson**; **Dexafort**; **Duphacort Q**; Maxidex*; Maxitrol*; **Opticorten**; **Voren**) *POM*

Indications: Dexamethasone is a corticosteroid with high glucocorticoid but low mineralocorticoid activities. This makes it suitable for high-dose therapy in conditions where water retention would be a disadvantage. Its anti-inflammatory potency is 7.5 times greater than prednisolone. On a dose basis 0.15 mg dexamethasone is equivalent to 1 mg prednisolone. Dexamethasone has a long duration of action and is therefore unsuitable for long-term daily or alternate-day use. It is used as an anti-inflammatory drug or in the management of shock and in the assessment of adrenal function in suspect cases of hyperadrenocorticism (HAC).

Forms:
Ophthalmic: 0.1% solution (Maxitrol, Maxidex). Maxitrol also contains 6000 IU/ml polymyxin B, 3500 IU/ml neomycin.

Injectable: 2 mg/ml solution; 1 mg/ml, 3 mg/ml suspension; 2.5 mg/ml suspension with 7.5 mg/ml prednisolone.
Oral: 0.25 mg tablet.

Dose:
Cats, Dogs:
- Ophthalmic: Apply small amount of ointment to affected eye(s) q6–24h or 1 drop of solution in affected eye(s) q6–12h.
- Cerebral oedema or spinal cord trauma: 2–3 mg/kg i.v., then 1 mg/kg s.c. q6–8h; taper off.
- Inflammation: 0.01–0.16 mg/kg i.m., s.c., p.o. q24h for 3–5 days maximum.
- Immunosuppression: 0.3–0.64 mg/kg i.m., s.c., p.o. q24h for up to 5 days.
- Shock: 5 mg/kg i.v. using sodium phosphate salt.

Small mammals: Anti-inflammatory: 0.05–0.2 mg/kg i.m., s.c. q12–24h.
Birds: 1.2–5 mg/kg i.v., 2–4 mg/kg i.m. q12–24h. Use higher doses for shock/trauma.
Reptiles: 2–4 mg/kg i.v., i.m. q24h.

Dexamethasone 1 mg $\equiv$ dexamethasone acetate 1.1 mg $\equiv$ dexamethasone isonicotinate 1.3 mg $\equiv$ dexamethasone sodium phosphate 1.3 mg $\equiv$ dexamethasone trioxa-undecanoate 1.4 mg.

Dexamethasone suppression tests:

Low-dose dexamethasone screening test: Used to diagnose HAC. Assess blood cortisol levels at 0, 3 and 8 hours. Give 0.01–0.015 mg/kg dexamethasone i.v. after the 0 hour sample.
Interpretation:
- Normal: Cortisol suppressed to < 50% of the basal level after 3 hours and <40 nmol/l after 8 hours.
- HAC: Fail to suppress at 3 and 8 hours, although some cases show partial suppression at 3 hours.

High-dose dexamethasone suppression test: Differentiates between pituitary-dependent and adrenal-dependent HAC (largely superseded by ACTH assay).
Protocol as for the low-dose test except administer 1.0 mg/kg dexamethasone i.v. (**dogs** and **cats**).
Interpretation:
- PDH: Most cases will suppress to <50% of the basal level after 3 hours and to <40 nmol/l after 8 hours.
- Adrenal tumours: Most fail to suppress or show partial suppression at 3 hours.

Adverse effects and contraindications: Prolonged use of glucocorticoids suppresses the hypothalamic–pituitary axis (HPA), causing adrenal atrophy. Animals on chronic therapy should be tapered off steroids when discontinuing the drug. A single dose of dexamethasone or dexamethasone sodium phosphate suppresses adrenal gland function for up to 32 hours. Adverse effects include elevated liver enzymes, cutaneous atrophy, weight loss, PU/PD, vomiting and diarrhoea. GI ulceration may develop. Hyperglycaemia and decreased serum T4 values may be seen in patients receiving dexamethasone. Do not use in pregnant animals. Systemic corticosteroids are generally contraindicated in patients with renal disease and diabetes mellitus. Impaired wound healing and delayed recovery from infections may be seen. Topical corticosteroids are contraindicated in ulcerative keratitis.

Drug interactions: There is an increased risk of GI ulceration if used concurrently with **NSAIDs**. The risk of developing hypokalaemia is increased if corticosteroids are administered concomitantly with **amphotericin B** or **potassium-depleting diuretics** (**furosemide**, **thiazides**). Dexamethasone antagonizes the effect of **insulin**. **Phenobarbital** or **phenytoin** may accelerate the metabolism of glucocorticoids.

Dexamfetamine sulphate (Dexedrine*) *POM*

Indications: Dexamfetamine is a CNS stimulant used in the diagnosis of the rare condition of canine hyperkinesis.

Forms: *Oral:* 5 mg tablets.

Dose: *Dogs:* Test for hyperkinesis: 0.2–0.5 mg/kg p.o. and then monitor respiratory rate, heart rate and activity levels every 30 minutes for 1–2 hours. Dogs suffering from hyperkinesis show a paradoxical decrease in all of these parameters.

Adverse effects and contraindications: Contraindicated in patients with epilepsy, hypertension, cardiovascular disease and glaucoma. Adverse effects include convulsions and elevated blood pressure. In animals unaffected by canine hyperkinesis there is an increase in heart rate and respiratory rate and the risk of anorexia, tremors, aggression, insomnia and hyperthermia.

Dextrans (Dextran 40*; Dextran 70*) *POM*

Indications: Dextrans are slowly metabolized macromolecular substances, which are used in the short term to expand and maintain blood volume in various forms of shock including hypovolaemic, traumatic, haemorrhagic and septic shock. They may be used as an immediate short-term measure to manage haemorrhage until blood is available. They are rarely required when shock is due to water and sodium depletion. Dextran 40 increases plasma volume by 50% at 1 hour and 110% at 2 hours. Dextran 70 increases plasma volume by 38%. Dextran 70 is indicated for volume expansion, whilst dextran 40 is used to improve peripheral blood flow in ischaemic and thromboembolic diseases.

Forms: *Intravenous infusion:* Dextran 40 and dextran 70 solutions.

Dose: *Cats, Dogs:* 10–20 ml/kg/day i.v. infusion.

Adverse effects and contraindications: Use with caution in animals with congestive heart failure and renal insufficiency as they will increase the risk of circulatory overload. Dextrans may interfere with some serum biochemistry assays and blood cross-matching. Thus, blood samples should be obtained prior to infusion. Dextrans should not be used where bleeding disorders due to thrombocytopenia or hypofibrinogenaemia are present. Increased bleeding times and acute renal failure are unusual adverse effects. Anaphylactic reactions may develop.

Diazepam (Diazepam*) *POM*

Indications: Diazepam is a benzodiazepine compound, used as an anticonvulsant, an anxiolytic, a skeletal muscle relaxant (e.g. urethral muscle spasm, tetanus) and in cats also as an appetite stimulant. It may be used with ketamine to offset the muscle hypertonicity associated with 'dissociative anaesthesia', and with opioids and/or acepromazine, for pre-anaesthetic medication in the critically ill. Diazepam is used in behavioural medicine for the short-term control of canine sound phobias and for short management of anxiety-related disorders. Used in birds for the short-term management of feather plucking.

Forms:
Injectable: 5 mg/ml solution.
Oral: 2 mg, 5 mg, 10 mg tablets, 2 mg/5 ml oral solution.

Dose:
Cats, Dogs:
- Status epilepticus: 0.5 mg/kg i.v. repeated every 10 min up to 3 times as required.
- Pre-ictal treatment of seizures: 2–15 mg p.o. q8h.
- Control of generalized cluster seizures: 2–15 mg p.o. q8h starting after first seizure or 0.5 mg/kg of injectable solution per rectum after the first seizure and when a second or third seizure occurs.
- Anaesthetic premedicant/sedative: 0.1–0.25 mg/kg i.v. It is unreliable as a sedative as it may cause excitement and is thus often used in combination with other drugs.

Cats:
- Anxiolytic: 0.2–0.4 mg/kg p.o. q8h.
- Appetite stimulant: 0.5–1 mg/kg i.v.
- Spraying/muscle relaxant: 1.25–5 mg/cat p.o. q8h.

Dogs:
- Anxiolytic: 0.55–2.2 mg/kg p.o. as required.
- Scottie cramp: 0.5–2 mg/kg i.v. until effect, then p.o. q8h.
- Skeletal muscle relaxation: 2–10 mg/dog p.o. q8h.

Small mammals: 2–5 mg/kg i.m. (1 mg/kg i.m. or 2.5 mg/kg i.p. if used in conjunction with ketamine or fentanyl.)

Birds: 0.5–1.0 mg/kg i.m., i.v. (0.5 mg/kg if given in conjunction with ketamine).

See Sedation protocols, pages 297–301.

Adverse effects and contraindications: Fulminant hepatic necrosis in cats has been associated with repeated oral administration of diazepam. Rapid i.v. injection may cause marked excitation and elicit signs of pain in normal dogs; i.v. injections should be made slowly (over at least 1 minute for each 5 mg). Intramuscular injection is painful, and results in erratic drug absorption. Chronic dosing leads to a shortened half-life due to activation of the hepatic microsomal enzyme system, and tolerance to anticonvulsant effects in dogs may develop. Conversely the duration of action may be prolonged after repeated doses, in older animals, those with liver dysfunction, and those receiving beta$_1$ antagonists. Diazepam is contraindicated in the long-term treatment of canine and feline behavioural disorders due to risks of disinhibition and interference with memory and learning. A paradoxical increase in activity is possible following oral administration.

Drug interactions: Do not dilute or mix with other agents. If injecting through infusion tubing, do it as close to the vein as possible. Up to 80% of diazepam in a solution is adsorbed on to plastic infusion systems and thus the use of i.v. infusions of diazepam cannot be recommended. Due to extensive metabolism by the hepatic microsomal enzyme system, interactions with other drugs metabolized in this way are common. **Cimetidine** and **omeprazole** inhibit metabolism of diazepam and may prolong clearance. Concurrent use of **phenobarbital** may lead to a decrease in the half-life of diazepam. Hypotension may be enhanced if **propranolol** is given with diazepam. An enhanced sedative effect may be seen if **anti-histamines** or **opioid analgesics** are administered with diazepam. When given with diazepam, the effects of **digoxin** may be increased.

Diazoxide (Eudemine*) *POM*

Indications: Diazoxide is a benzothiadiazide diuretic that causes vasodilation and inhibits insulin secretion by blocking calcium mobilization. It is used to manage hypoglycaemia caused by hyperinsulinism. In man it is also used in the short-term management of acute hypertension.

Forms:
Injectable: 15 mg/ml solution.
Oral: 50 mg tablet.

Dose: *Dogs:*
- Hypertension: 1–3 mg/kg rapid i.v. injection (less than 30 seconds); maximum single dose of 150 mg.
- Hypoglycaemia: 3.3 mg/kg p.o. q8h initially, increasing to 20 mg/kg p.o. q8h.

Adverse effects and contraindications: The commonest adverse effects are anorexia, vomiting and diarrhoea. Hypotension, tachy-cardia, bone marrow suppression, pancreatitis, cataracts and electrolyte and fluid retention may occur. Its efficacy may diminish over a period of months.

Drug interactions: Phenothiazines and **thiazide diuretics** may increase the hyperglycaemic activity of diazoxide, whilst alpha-adrenergic blocking agents (e.g. **phenoxybenzamine**) may antagonize the effects of diazoxide.

Dichlorophen (Dichlorophen) *GSL*

Indications: Dichlorophen is a cestocide used in the control of tapeworm infections in dogs and cats over 6 months of age.

Forms: *Oral:* 500 mg tablet.

Dose: *Cats, Dogs:* 500 mg/2.5 kg p.o. Give only 250 mg if less than 2.5 kg. Give a maximum of 6 tablets at one time, and give the rest 3 hours later if no vomiting. Administer whole or crushed in food.

Adverse effects and contraindications: Vomiting may be seen.

Diclofenac (Voltarol Ophtha*) *POM*

Indications: Diclofenac is an NSAID used in cataract surgery to prevent intra-operative miosis and reflex (axonal) miosis caused by ulcerative keratitis. It is used to control pain and inflammation associated with corneal surgery and in ulcerative keratitis when topical corticosteroid use is contraindicated.

Forms: *Topical:* 0.1% solution in single-use vial.

Dose: *Cats, Dogs:* 1 drop q30min for 2h prior to cataract surgery (there is a wide variation in protocols for cataract surgery).

Adverse effects and contraindications: Diclofenac may cause local irritation. Topical NSAIDs can be used in ulcerative keratitis but with caution. They can delay epithelial healing and have been associated with an increased risk of corneal melting. Regular monitoring is advised.

Digitoxin (Digitoxin*) *POM*

Indications: See digoxin for mode of action and indications. There is little reason to use this drug over digoxin. Digitoxin is metabolized in the liver and may be of value in patients with renal failure.

Forms: *Oral:* 100 µg tablet.

Dose: *Dogs:* 14–33 µg/kg p.o. q8h.

Adverse effects and contraindications: Signs of toxicity include anorexia, vomiting, diarrhoea, depression or arrhythmias (e.g. heart block, bigeminy, paroxysmal ventricular or atrial tachycardias with block and multifocal ventricular premature contractions). **Do not use in cats.**

Drug interactions: Antacids, chemotherapy agents (e.g. **cyclophosphamide, cytarabine, vincristine**), **cimetidine** and **metoclopramide** may decrease digitoxin absorption from the GI tract. The following may increase the serum level, decrease the elimination rate or enhance the toxic effects of digitoxin: **acetazolamide, antimuscarinics, diazepam, erythromycin, loop** and **thiazide diuretics** (hypokalaemia), **quinidine** and **verapamil. Spironolactone** may enhance or decrease the toxic effects of digitoxin.

Digoxin (Digoxin*) *POM*

Indications: Digoxin, a cardiac glycoside, inhibits Na^+–K^+ ATPase, leading to an increase in intracellular sodium. Sodium is exchanged for calcium, resulting in an increase in intracellular calcium. This results in an increase in the force of myocardial contraction. Digoxin acts on specialized conducting tissue and the SA node, increasing the refractory period, while decreasing conduction velocity, thereby slowing the heart. The combination of a slower heart and increased force of contraction increases cardiac output. Digoxin normalizes baroreceptor reflexes that are impaired in heart failure. Digoxin is used in the management of heart failure and supraventricular tachycardias.

Forms:
Injectable: 100 μg/ml, 250 μg/ml for i.v. use.
Oral: 62.5 μg, 125 μg, 250 μg tablets; 50 μg/ml elixir.

Dose:
Cats: 1–1.6 μg/kg i.v. q12h, 10 μg/kg p.o. q24–48h, $^1/_4$ of a 125 μg tablet q24–48h.
Dogs: 2.2–4.4 μg/kg i.v. q12h, 5.5–11μg/kg p.o. q12h (tablets), 5–8 μg/kg p.o. q12h (elixir). For larger dogs (>22 kg) a more accurate dosing regimen is 0.22 mg/m². *See page 293 for conversion of body weight to surface area (m²).* Dosing should be based on lean body weight.

Use of the i.v. route is rarely indicated. Administer i.v. slowly with extreme care, as it may cause vasoconstriction.
The bioavailability of digoxin varies between the different dosage routes: i.v. = 100%, tablets = 60% and elixir = 75%.

Adverse effects and contraindications: Cats are more sensitive to the toxic effects of digoxin than dogs. Signs of toxicity include anorexia, vomiting, diarrhoea, depression or arrhythmias (e.g. heart block, bigeminy, paroxysmal ventricular or atrial tachycardias with block, and multifocal ventricular premature contractions). If these are seen or the drug is ineffective, serum levels of digoxin should be assessed; the ideal therapeutic serum level is in the region of 1 ng/ml to optimize beneficial effects and minimize toxic side-effects.
Lidocaine, **phenytoin** and **procainamide** may be used to control digitalis-associated arrhythmias. Decreased dosages or an increase in dosing intervals may be required in geriatric patients, obese animals or those with significant renal dysfunction (digoxin is predominantly excreted by the kidneys).

Drug interactions: Antacids, chemotherapy agents (e.g. **cyclophosphamide, cytarabine, doxorubicin, vincristine**), **cimetidine** and **metoclopramide** may decrease digoxin absorption from the GI tract. The following may increase the serum level, decrease the elimination rate or enhance the toxic effects of digoxin: **antimuscarinics, diazepam, erythromycin, loop** and **thiazide diuretics** (hypokalaemia), **quinidine, oxytetracycline** and **verapamil**. **Spironolactone** may enhance or decrease the toxic effects of digoxin.

Diltiazem (Diltiazem*; **Hypercard**) *POM*

Indications: Diltiazem is a calcium-channel blocker. It interferes with the inward movement of calcium ions through slow channels in myocardial cells and cells within the specialized conduction system in the heart and vascular smooth muscle; vascular smooth muscle is more sensitive to diltiazem than myocardial tissues (relative activity of 7:1). Systemic resistance vessels and large arteries respond to calcium-channel blockers more readily than venous capacitance vessels and pulmonary vasculature. Diltiazem causes a reduction in myocardial contractility (negative inotrope, although less effective than verapamil), depressed electrical activity (retarded AV conduction) and decreases vascular resistance (vasodilation of cardiac vessels and peripheral arteries and arterioles). It is primarily used to control supraventricular tachyarrhythmias, and to slow the heart rate in dogs with atrial fibrillation as an adjunct to digoxin. Diltiazem is preferred to verapamil by many because it has effective anti-arrhythmic properties with minimal negative inotropy. Calcium-channel blockers are preferred to propranolol for the management of feline hypertrophic cardiomyopathy by some because they improve myocardial relaxation, increase ventricular filling and dilate coronary vasculature. Diltiazem is less effective than amlodipine in the management of hypertension.

Forms: *Oral:* 10 mg (Hypercard), 60 mg (generic) tablets.

Dose:
Cats: 1.5–2.5 mg/kg p.o. q8h or 7.5–15 mg/cat p.o. q8h.
Dogs: 0.5–2.0 mg/kg p.o. q8h.

Adverse effects and contraindications: Diltiazem is contraindicated in patients with 2nd or 3rd degree heart block, hypotension, sick sinus syndrome, or with severe left ventricular dysfunction. Reduce the dose of diltiazem if hepatic or renal impairment exists. In dogs, bradycardia is the commonest adverse effect, whilst in cats it is vomiting.

Drug interactions: If diltiazem is administered concurrently with **beta-adrenergic blockers** (e.g. **propranolol**), there may be additive negative inotropic and chronotropic effects. Diltiazem's activity may be adversely affected by **calcium salts** or **vitamin D**. Plasma digoxin values are increased by diltiazem. Monitoring of **digoxin** serum levels is recommended if used concurrently with diltiazem. **Cimetidine** inhibits the metabolism of diltiazem, thereby increasing plasma concentrations. Diltiazem enhances the effect of **theophylline** which may lead to toxicity. It may affect **quinidine** and **ciclosporin** concentrations. Diltiazem may displace highly protein-bound agents from plasma proteins. Diltiazem may increase intracellular **vincristine** levels by inhibiting the drug's outflow from the cell.

Dimercaprol (British anti-lewisite) (Dimercaprol*) *POM*

Indications: Dimercaprol chelates heavy metals. It is used in the treatment of acute toxicity caused by arsenic, gold, bismuth and mercury, and as an adjunct (with edetate calcium disodium) in lead poisoning.

Forms: *Injectable:* 50 mg/ml solution in peanut oil.

Dose: *Cats, Dogs:* 2.5–5 mg/kg i.m. q4h for 2 days, then q8h for 10 days or until recovery. (Note: The 5 mg/kg dose should only be used on the first day when severe acute intoxication occurs). Alternatively, for arsenic poisoning when gastroenteritis is present 6–7 mg/kg i.m. q8h or 3–4 mg/kg i.m. q6h. Increase intervals between doses on 3rd day and q12h dosing at the lower dosage levels may begin on day 4; continue to day 10. Aggressive supportive therapy should be maintained throughout the treatment period.

Adverse effects and contraindications: Intramuscular injections are painful. Dimercaprol–metal complexes are nephrotoxic. This is particularly so with iron, selenium or cadmium; do not use for these metals. Alkalinization of urine during therapy may have protective effects for the kidney. The use of dimercaprol is contraindicated if severe hepatic failure is present.

Drug interactions: Iron salts should not be administered during therapy.

Dimethylsulfoxide (Dimethylsulphoxide; DMSO)
(Rimso–50*) *POM*

Indications: DMSO has various pharmacological actions, including free radical scavenging, membrane stabilization, analgesia, enhancement of local blood flow, amyloid resorption, anti-inflammatory effect, and it may affect immune responses at the local level. It is used topically to control otitis externa, and in the management of haemorrhagic cystitis induced by cyclophosphamide, as well as i.v. to decrease intracranial pressure following CNS trauma (efficacy is controversial) and in the treatment of renal amyloidosis (efficacy unproven). DMSO's free radical scavenging ability may be useful in the management of reperfusion injury; administer prior to reperfusion to be effective.

Forms: 50%, 90% liquid. DMSO should be kept in a tightly closed container as it is very hygroscopic. Medical grade only available as a 50% solution from Brittania (Rimso–50).

Dose: *Dogs:*
- Otic: 4–6 drops of a 60% solution in affected ear q12h for up to 14 days.
- CNS trauma: 1 g DMSO/kg i.v. over 45 minutes. Use a 10% solution, prepared by diluting 32 ml of a 90% solution in 250 ml of sterile water for injection. Caution: the LD_{50} for DMSO in dogs is 2.5 g/kg.
- Renal amyloidosis: 80 mg/kg s.c. 3 times/wk; 125–300 mg/kg p.o. q24h.
- Topically: Apply 90% solution to affected areas q8–12h; total daily dose should not exceed 20 ml. Do not apply for longer than 14 days.

Caution: DMSO is rapidly absorbed through the skin; handle product with care and wear gloves.

Adverse effects and contraindications: DMSO should not be mixed with potentially toxic ingredients and applied to the skin because of profound enhancement of systemic absorption. Adverse effects include local irritation, erythema, an oily garlic-like odour from the site and on the breath. Following i.v. administration with concentrations in excess of 20%, haemolysis may occur and a diuretic effect is seen. Chronic use may cause lens refractive index changes in the eye which are slowly reversible upon discontinuation of the drug.

Dinoprost tromethamine (Enzaprost*; Lutalyse*) *POM*

Indications: Dinoprost (prostaglandin $F_{2\alpha}$) is a luteolytic agent used in the termination of pregnancy at any stage of gestation and to stimulate uterine contractions in the treatment of open pyometra. Dinoprost may be used to manage egg binding in birds, where it relaxes the vagina and increases uterine tone.

Forms: *Injectable:* 5 mg dinoprost/ml solution.

Dose:
Cats: Abortifacient: 0.025 mg/kg s.c. q24h for up to 5 days, after day 40 of pregnancy.
Dogs:
• Abortifacient: First half of gestation: 0.05–0.25 mg/kg s.c. q12h for 4 days starting at least 5 days after the onset of cytological dioestrus. Second half of gestation: 0.05–0.25 mg/kg s.c. q12h until abortion is complete; monitor radiographically or ultrasonographically. Use low doses initially (0.05–0.1 mg/kg) to assess the severity of any adverse effects. Assess serum progesterone concentration at the end of treatment to ensure that complete luteolysis has occurred.
• Open pyometra: 0.1–0.25 mg/kg s.c. q12h until the uterus is empty; usually 3–5 days treatment required.
Birds: 0.02–0.1 mg/kg i.m. or directly into the cloacal mucosa.

Caution: Pregnant woman and asthmatics should avoid handling this agent.

Adverse effects and contraindications: Hypersalivation, panting, tachycardia, vomiting, urination, defecation, transient hyperthermia, locomotor incoordination and mild CNS signs have been reported. Such effects usually diminish within 30 minutes of drug administration. There is no adverse effect on future fertility. Do not use for the treatment of closed pyometra as there is a risk of uterine rupture.

Dinoprostone (Prostaglandin E₂) (Prostin E2*) *POM*

Indications: Prostaglandin E_2 is used to relax the vagina and induce uterine contractions in egg-bound birds.

Forms: *Topical:* 0.4 mg/ml gel.

Dose: *Birds:* Apply to cloacal mucosa.

Adverse effects and contraindications: Uterine rupture may occur.

Diphenhydramine (Dreemon*; Medinex*; Nightcalm*; Nytol*) *P*

Indications: Diphenhydramine is an antihistamine of the ethanolamine class. It has pronounced sedative, antimuscarinic and anti-emetic properties. It is a component of some cough suppressants and is used in the management of coughing. Its antihistaminergic (H_1) effects are used to reduce pruritus and prevent motion sickness. It has been advocated for the control of mild anxiety conditions in dogs and cats, including anxiety related to car travel. It has been used in the management of night-time activity in cats and in compulsive scratching. In birds it is used in the management of allergic rhinitis and hypersensitivity reactions. In ferrets it is used prevaccination if a previous vaccine reaction has been encountered.

Forms: *Oral:* Dreemon, Medinex 2 mg/ml solution; Dreemon, Nightcalm, Nytol 25 mg tablet. Liquid is very distasteful. Other products are available of various concentrations and most contain other active ingredients.

Dose:
Dogs:
• Cough suppression and anti-emesis: 2–4 mg/kg p.o. q6–8h.
• Suppression of pruritus: 1–2 mg/kg p.o. q8–12h.
Small mammals: Ferrets: 0.5–2 mg/kg p.o. q8–12h.
Birds: 2–4 mg/kg p.o. q8–12h.

Adverse effects and contraindications: Use is contraindicated in cases of urine retention, glaucoma and hyperthyroidism. Paradoxical excitement may be seen in cats.

Drug interactions: An increased sedative effect may occur if used with **benzodiazepines** or other **anxiolytics/hypnotics**. Avoid the concomitant use of other **sedative agents**. It may enhance the effect of adrenaline and partially counteract anticoagulant effects of heparin and warfarin.

Diphenoxylate with atropine (Lomotil*) POM

Indications: Diphenoxylate is a non-analgesic opiate that increases segmental smooth muscle tone, decreases the propulsive activity of intestinal smooth muscle, and decreases electrolyte and water secretion into the intestinal lumen. It is used in the management of diarrhoea and irritable bowel syndrome. Atropine is added in a sub-therapeutic dose to discourage abuse of diphenoxylate.

Forms: *Oral:* 2.5 mg diphenoxylate, 0.025 mg atropine tablet.

Dose: *Dogs:* 0.05–0.1 mg/kg diphenoxylate p.o. q6–8h.

Adverse effects and contraindications: Adverse effects include sedation, constipation and ileus. Do not use in animals with liver disease, intestinal obstruction, neoplastic or toxic bowel disease.

Drug interactions: Diphenoxylate may potentiate the sedative effects of **barbiturates** and other **tranquillizers**.

Dipyrone – see Butylscopolamine/Metamizole

Disopyramide (Disopyramide*; Rythmodan*) *POM*

Indications: Disopyramide is an oral anti-arrhythmic (class 1A) that has pharmacological properties similar to procainamide and quinidine (membrane stabilizing). It is used in patients with ventricular/supraventricular arrhythmias.

Forms:
Injectable: 10 mg/ml solution.
Oral: 100 mg, 150 mg capsule.

Dose: *Dogs:* 2 mg/kg i.v. over at least 5 minutes; 7–30 mg/kg p.o. q2–4h.

Adverse effects and contraindications: Adverse effects include antimuscarinic effects (dry mouth, urinary retention), AV block and hypotension. As disopyramide impairs myocardial contractility, its use should be avoided in patients with congestive failure. Do not use in patients with glaucoma, or hepatic or renal impairment.

Drug interactions: The toxicity of disopyramide may be increased if hypokalaemia develops with **acetazolamide**, **loop diuretics** and **thiazides**. Do not use within 48 hours of **verapamil**. Widening of QRS complexes or QT interval may occur when used with other **anti-arrhythmic agents**; use with caution. Additive anticholinergic effects if used with **atropine** or **glycopyrrolate**. May need to increase dose if used with **phenobarbital**. May need to adjust **warfarin** dose if used with disopyramide.

Dobutamine (Posiject*) *POM*

Indications: Dobutamine is a dopamine analogue acting principally as a beta$_1$ agonist, with lesser degrees of alpha$_1$ and beta$_2$ agonistic effects. It increases cardiac contractility with little effect on heart rate at normal doses. Dobutamine is indicated for short-term inotropic support in patients with cardiac failure due to decreased contractility (e.g. dilated cardiomyopathy), and septic and cardiogenic shock. Its mild beta$_2$ and alpha$_1$ actions on the peripheral vasculature offset one another, thereby minimizing effects on blood pressure. Although chemically related to dopamine it does not cause the release of endogenous noradrenaline. Dobutamine is preferred over dopamine by many in the management of cardiac failure.

Forms: *Injectable:* 50 mg/ml solution. Dilute to a 0.025% (25 µg/ml) solution in 5% dextrose or normal saline (if not sodium-restricted).

Dose:
Cats: 2–5 µg/kg/min constant rate of i.v. infusion.
Dogs: 5–20 µg/kg/min constant rate of i.v. infusion.

Start at the bottom of the dose range and increase gradually over several hours with continuous ECG monitoring, if possible. Frequently evaluate heart rate, rhythm, arterial pulse quality, mucous membranes, CRT and respiratory rate.
Administer with an i.v. infusion pump or other i.v. flow controlling device.

Adverse effects and contraindications: Dobutamine should only be used in an intensive care unit. Adverse effects include tachycardia and a marked increase in systolic blood pressure. Monitor the ECG for ventricular arrhythmias. In cases of atrial fibrillation pretreat with digoxin prior to administering dobutamine and even then use it with great caution. A synergistic effect on the improvement of cardiac output has been recorded when nitroprusside and dobutamine were used concomitantly. Diabetic patients treated with dobutamine may experience increased insulin requirements. The reconstituted i.v. solution is stable for 24 hours although a slight colour change may occur during this period.

Drug interactions: Increase in systemic vascular resistance may develop if dobutamine administered with **beta-blocking drugs** (e.g. **propranolol**), **doxapram** or MAOI's (e.g. **selegiline**). Concomitent use with **halothane** may result in an increased incidence of ventricular arrythmias.

Docusate sodium (Codanthrusate*; Dioctyl*; Docusol*; Fletchers Enemette*; Waxsol*) *P*

Indications: Docusate is a surfactant and detergent used as a faecal softener and laxative and as a ceruminolytic.

Forms:
Oral: 100 mg tablets; 12.5 mg/5 ml, 50 mg/5 ml syrup; 50 mg dantron plus 60 mg docusate/5 ml (codanthrusate; Docusol).
Enema: 90 mg docusate, 3.8 g glycerol/5 ml solution (Fletchers enemette).

Topical: 0.5% docusate solution (Waxsol).
Docusate is also a component of many mixed topical preparations.

Dose:
Cats: 50 mg p.o. q12–24h, or 2 ml of a 5% solution mixed with 50 ml
of water instilled per rectum prn, or a few drops in the affected ear
q8–12h or 5–15 minutes prior to flushing.
Dogs: 50–100 mg p.o. q12–24h, or 10–15 ml of 5% solution mixed
with 100 ml of water instilled per rectum prn or a few drops in the
affected ear q8–12h or 5–15 minutes prior to flushing.

Drug interactions: Avoid the concurrent use of docusate and **mineral oil**.

Domperidone (Motilium*) *POM*

Indications: Domperidone is a potent anti-emetic with a similar
mechanism of action to metoclopramide, but with fewer adverse CNS
effects, although it may not be a prokinetic in dogs.

Forms: 10 mg tablet, 1 mg/ml suspension.

Dose: *Cats, Dogs:* 2–5 mg per animal q8h.

Adverse effects and contraindications: There is little information on
the use of this drug in veterinary medicine, but it may cause
gastroparesis in dogs.

Dopamine (Dopamine*) *POM*

Indications: Dopamine is an endogenous catecholamine and the
precursor of noradrenaline. Dopamine acts directly and indirectly (by
releasing noradrenaline) on $alpha_1$ and $beta_1$ receptors, and has
dopaminergic effects. It is used to manage haemodynamic imbalances
present in shock and to treat oliguric renal failure. At low doses
(≤ 10 µg/kg/min) dopamine acts on dopaminergic and $beta_1$ receptors
causing vasodilation, resulting in increases in organ perfusion, renal
blood flow, urine production and cardiac output; systemic vascular
resistance remains largely unchanged. At higher doses (>10 µg/kg/min)
dopaminergic effects are over-ridden by the alpha and beta effects,
resulting in an increase in systemic peripheral resistance, heart rate and
force of contraction, but reduced renal and peripheral blood flow.

Forms: *Injectable:* 40 mg/ml, 160 mg/ml solutions.
To prepare a solution: add contents of a vial to 1 litre of either normal
saline, 5% dextrose, or lactated Ringer's. The resultant solution will
contain a concentration of 200 µg/ml (if 40 mg/ml vial used) or 800 µg/ml
(if 160 mg/ml vial used). In small dogs and cats it may be necessary to
use less dopamine so that the final concentration will be lower.

Dose:
Cats: 1–5 µg/kg/min as a constant i.v. infusion.
Dogs: 2–10 µg/kg/min as a constant i.v. infusion; occasionally doses
up to 50 µg/kg/min may be required for cases of cardiogenic shock.
See above under **Indications** to determine initial dose rate.
Use an i.v. pump or other flow controlling device to increase precision
in dosing. Constant monitoring is required.

Adverse effects and contraindications: Nausea, vomiting, ectopic
beats, tachycardia, palpatation, hypo/hyper tension, dyspnoea,
headache and vasoconstriction may be seen. Dopamine should only
be used in an intensive care unit. Extravasation injuries can be very
serious with dopamine (necrosis and sloughing of surrounding tissue).
Should extravasation occur, infiltrate the site (ischaemic areas) with a
solution of 5–10 mg phentolamine in 10–15 ml of normal saline. A
syringe with a fine needle should be used. Monitor parameters such as
urine flow, cardiac rate and rhythm, and blood pressure. If overdosage
occurs, systemic blood pressure will rise. Discontinue the drug or
reduce the dosage if arrhythmias develop.

Drug interactions: Risk of severe hypertension when **MAOIs,
doxapram** and **oxytocin** are used with dopamine. **Halothane** may
increase myocardial sensitivity to catecholamines. **Propranolol** can be
used to treat dopamine-induced ventricular arrythmias.

Dorzolamide (Trusopt*) *POM*

Indications: Dorzolamide is a topical carbonic anhydrase inhibitor
used in the control of glaucoma. It can be used alone or in combination
with other topical glaucoma drugs.

Forms: *Topical:* 2% solution.

Dose:
Cats: 1 drop/eye q12h.
Dogs: 1 drop/eye q6–8h.

Adverse effects and contraindications: Do not use where severe
hepatic impairment or renal impairment is present. In man ocular
irritation and irreversible corneal oedema have been reported. In dogs,
irritation and blepharitis may be seen.

Doxapram (Dopram-V) *POM*

Indications: Normal doses of doxapram stimulate respiration by
increasing the sensitivity of aortic and carotid bodies (chemoreceptors)
to arterial gas tensions, increasing the tidal volume. Doxapram
stimulates respiration in certain types of perioperative respiratory
depression, and in neonates. Doxapram is preferred to naloxone in

animals that require opioid-induced analgesia. In these circumstances doxapram activity is short lived and may be followed by profound depression unless repeated doses or an infusion are given.

Forms:
Injectable: 20 mg/ml solution.
Oral: 20 mg/ml solution.

Dose:
Cats, Dogs: 5–10 mg/kg i.v.; may repeat prn (duration of effect generally does not exceed 15–20 min).
Neonates: 1–2 drops under tongue (oral solution) or 0.1 ml i.v. in umbilical vein; *see below.*
Small mammals: 5 mg/kg i.v., s.c. q15min.
Birds: 10 mg/kg i.m.; 0.5 mg on tongue.
Reptiles: 5–10 mg/kg i.v.

Adverse effects and contraindications: Doxapram must not be used indiscriminately, e.g. when the airway is occluded. Its use may aggravate dyspnoea. Severe respiratory depression should be controlled by (1) tracheal intubation, followed by (2) intermittent positive pressure ventilation of the lungs, and then (3) resolution of the inciting cause. Doxapram may be useful in single-handed resuscitation attempts for 'buying time' in animals whose airway is unprotected. Use with caution in neonates as the injection contains benzyl alcohol which is toxic. Doxapram is irritant and may cause a thrombophlebitis; avoid extravasation or repeated i.v. dosing in same vein. Overdosage symptoms include hypertension, skeletal muscle hyperactivity, tachycardia and generalized CNS excitation, including seizures. Treatment is supportive using short-acting i.v. barbiturates and oxygen. Its effects in pregnant/lactating animals are not known.

Drug interactions: Hypertension may occur with **sympathomimetics**. The use of **theophylline** concurrently with doxapram may cause increased CNS stimulation. As doxapram may stimulate the release of adrenaline, its use within 10 minutes of the administration of anaesthetic agents that sensitize the myocardium to catecholamines (e.g. **halothane**) should be avoided. Doxapram is compatible with **5% dextrose** or **normal saline**, but is incompatible with **sodium bicarbonate** and **thiopental**.

Doxepin (Sinequan*) POM

Indications: Doxepin is a tricyclic antidepressant with potent antihistaminic (H_1), anticholinergic and alpha$_1$-adrenergic blocking properties. It has been advocated to be of use in the management of pruritus and psychogenic dermatoses where there is a component of anxiety, including canine acral lick dermatitis and compulsive disorders. Data are lacking as to its efficacy at the suggested doses. It is used in birds for the management of feather plucking.

Forms: *Oral:* 10 mg, 25 mg, 50 mg, 75 mg tablets.

Dose:
Cats: 0.5–1.0 mg/kg p.o. q12–24h.
Dogs: 3–5 mg/kg p.o. q12h, maximum dose 150 mg q12h.
Birds: 0.5–1 mg/kg p.o. q12h.

Adverse effects and contraindications: Adverse effects reported in man include sedation, dry mouth, diarrhoea, vomiting, excitability, arrhythmias, hypotension, syncope, weight gain and, less commonly, seizures and bone marrow disorders. Doxepin is less cardiotoxic than other tricyclics. Do not use in animals with glaucoma or urinary retention.

Drug interactions: There is an increased risk of arrhythmias if doxepin is administered concurrently with **anaesthetics** and **anti-arrhythmics**. Tricyclics antagonize the effects of **anti-epileptics**. There is enhancement of sedative effects if used with other **sedative** drugs. Do not use in combination with **monoamine oxidase inhibitors**.

Doxorubicin (Doxorubicin*) POM

Indications: Doxorubicin is a cytotoxic anthracycline glycoside antibiotic that binds to DNA and inhibits nucleic acid synthesis. It is used in the treatment of lymphoma, soft tissue sarcomas, osteosarcoma and haemangiosarcoma, and may have a role in the management of carcinomas in the dog and soft tissue sarcomas in the cat. It may be used alone or in combination with other antineoplastic therapies.

Forms: *Injectable:* 10 mg, 50 mg powder for reconstitution; 10 mg, 50 mg/vial solutions.
After reconstitution the drug is stable for at least 48 hours at 4°C. A 1.5% loss of potency may occur after 1 month at 4°C but there is no loss of potency when frozen at −20°C. Filtering through a 0.22 μm filter will ensure adequate sterility of the thawed solution.

Dose: The usual doses are:
Cats: 20–25 mg/m^2 i.v. q3–5 weeks.
Dogs: 30 mg/m^2 i.v. q3 weeks, or 10 mg/m^2 on days 1, 2, 3 q4 weeks maximum total dose not to exceed 240 mg/m^2.
The drug is highly irritant and must be administered via a preplaced intravenous catheter.
The reconstituted drug should be administered over a minimum period of 10 minutes into the side port of a freely running i.v. infusion of 0.9% NaCl. *See page 293 for conversion of body weight to surface area (m^2).*

Caution: Doxorubicin is a potent cytotoxic drug that should only be prepared and administered by trained personnel. Reconstitution or transfer to syringes or infusion bags should be carried out in designated areas, preferably a laminar flow cabinet. Personnel must be protected with suitable clothing, gloves, mask and eye shield. In the event of contact with skin or eyes, the affected area should be washed with copious amounts of water or normal saline. Medical advice should be sought if the eyes are affected. Pregnant women should not come into contact with the drug.

Adverse effects and contraindications: Allergic reactions to the drug have been reported. Premedication with i.v. diphenhydramine, chlorphenamine or dexamethasone prior to therapy is recommended. When antihistamines are used, give 10 mg to dogs up to 10 kg, 20 mg to dogs 10–30 kg, and 30 mg to dogs >30 kg, or give 0.5 mg/kg dexamethasone. Acute anaphylactic reactions should be treated with adrenaline, steroids and fluids. Doxorubicin is known to cause a dose-dependent cumulative cardiotoxicity in dogs (dilated cardiomyopathy and congestive heart failure). This rarely develops in dogs given a total dose of < 240 mg/m^2. It may also cause a tachycardia and arrhythmias on administration; monitor with ECGs and/or echocardiograms. Anorexia, vomiting, severe leucopenia, thrombocytopenia, haemorrhagic gastroenteritis and nephrotoxicity (in cats if dosages exceed 100 mg/m^2) are the major adverse effects. A CBC and platelet count should be monitored whenever therapy is given. If the neutrophil count drops below 2 x 10^9/l or if the platelet count drops below 50 x 10^9/l, treatment should be suspended. Once the counts have stabilized, doxorubicin can then be restarted at the same dose. If haematological toxicity occurs again, or if GI toxicity is recurrent the dose should be reduced to 20 mg/m^2.

Drug interactions: Barbiturates increase plasma clearance of doxorubicin. Concurrent administration with **cyclophosphamide** increases the risk of nephrotoxicity in cats. The agent causes a reduction in serum **digoxin** levels. Do not mix doxorubicin with other drugs.

Doxycycline (Doxirobe gel; Doxyseptin 300; **Ornicure**; **Ronaxan**) *POM*

Indications: Doxycycline is a lipid-soluble tetracycline with antibacterial (including spirochaetes such as *Helicobacter* spp. and *Campylobacter* spp.), anti-rickettsial (e.g. *Haemobartonella*), anti-mycoplasmal and anti-chlamydial activity. It is the drug of choice to treat avian chlamydiosis. Bacteriostatic agent inhibiting protein synthesis at the initiation step by interacting with the small ribosomal subunit. It is not affected by and does not affect renal function as it is excreted in faeces and is therefore recommended when tetracyclines are indicated in animals with renal impairment. It is preferred by some to oxytetracycline for use in birds. Being extremely lipid-soluble, it penetrates well into prostatic fluid and bronchial secretions.

Forms: *Oral:* 20 mg, 100 mg capsules (Ronaxan); 300 mg tablets (Doxyseptin); 260 mg/sachet powder (Ornicure); 8.5% gel (Doxirobe).

Dose:
Cats, Dogs: 10 mg/kg p.o. q24h with food. Oral gel (dogs) – apply to periodontal pockets.
Birds: Except psittacines: 15–50 mg/kg p.o. q12–24h, 130 mg/l drinking water; Psittacines: Amazons 50 mg/kg p.o. q24h; Macaws/Cockatoos 35 mg/kg p.o. q24h.
Reptiles: 10 mg/kg p.o. q24h.

Adverse effects and contraindications: Do not administer Doxyseptin to dogs <15 kg. Adverse effects include nausea, vomiting and diarrhoea. Oesophagitis and oesophageal ulceration may develop; administer with food to reduce this risk.

Drug interactions: Absorption of doxycycline is reduced by **antacids**, **calcium**, **magnesium** and **iron salts**, and **sucralfate**, although the effect is less marked than seen with water-soluble tetracyclines. **Phenobarbital**, **phenytoin** and **primidone** may increase its metabolism, thus decreasing plasma levels. Do not use **zinc**-containing products (e.g. **chlorhexidine** solutions formulated with **zinc gluconate**) when using the oral gel formation of doxycycline to fill periodontal pockets.

Edetate calcium disodium (CaEDTA): (Ledclair*; **Sodium calcium edetate**) *POM*

Indications: Edetate calcium disodium is a heavy metal chelating agent used to treat lead and zinc poisoning.

Forms: *Injectable:* 200 mg/ml solution.

Dose:
Cats, Dogs: 25 mg/kg s.c. q6h for 2–5 days. Dilute strong solution to a concentration of 10 mg/ml in 5% dextrose before use. The total daily dose should not exceed 2 g. Dogs that respond slowly or have an initial (pre-treatment) blood lead level of >4.5 μmol/l may need another 5-day course of treatment after a rest period of 5 days. Blood lead levels may be confusing, therefore monitor clinical signs during therapy. Measure blood lead levels 2–3 weeks after completion of treatment in order to determine whether a second course is required or if the animal is still being exposed to lead.
Small mammals: Rabbits: 27.5 mg/kg s.c. q6h for 5 days.
Birds: 20–35 mg/kg i.m., s.c. q8–12h for 5 days followed by 2–5 days of no treatment, or until metal particles are no longer visible on radiographs.

Adverse effects and contraindications: The most serious adverse effect noted with CaEDTA therapy is a reversible nephrotoxicity. This is usually preceded by other symptoms of toxicity (e.g. depression, vomiting, diarrhoea). Dogs showing GI effects may benefit from zinc supplementation. Injections are painful.

Edrophonium chloride (Edrophonium*) POM

Indications: Edrophonium is a rapid- and short-acting anticholinesterase prolonging the action of acetylcholine. It is used in the diagnosis of myasthenia gravis, to treat atrial tachycardia (vagal effects) and to antagonize non–depolarizing neuromuscular blockade.

Forms: *Injectable:* 10 mg/ml solution.

Dose:
Cats:
- Diagnosis of myasthenia gravis: 2.5 mg/cat i.v. Improvement should be noted within 30 seconds, with the effects dissipating within 5 minutes, for a positive test. Atropine should be available (0.04 mg/kg) to control cholinergic side-effects (e.g. salivation, urination).
- Atrial tachycardia after failure of vagal manoeuvres: 1.5 mg i.v. **(Note: This step is not advised in cases of heart failure.)**
Dogs:
- Diagnosis of myasthenia gravis: 0.11–0.22 mg/kg i.v. (maximum of 5 mg). Improvement should be noted within 30 seconds, with the effects dissipating within 5 minutes, for a positive test. Atropine should be available (0.05 mg/kg) to control cholinergic side-effects (e.g. salivation, urination).
- Atrial tachycardia after failure of vagal manoeuvres: 1.5 mg i.v. **(Note: This procedure is ill advised in cases of heart failure.)**
- To antagonize non-depolarizing neuromuscular blockade: edrophonium (0.5–1.0 mg/kg) is mixed with atropine (0.04 mg/kg) and injected i.v. over 2 minutes once signs of spontaneous recovery from 'block', e.g. diaphragmatic 'twitching' are present. Continued ventilatory support should be provided until full respiratory muscle activity is restored.

Adverse effects and contraindications: These include nausea, vomiting, increased salivation and diarrhoea. Overdosage may lead to muscle fasciculations and paralysis. Severe bradyarrythmias, even asystole, may occur if edrophonium is used to antagonize neuromuscular block without the co-injection of atropine.

Enalapril (Enacard) POM

Indications: Enalapril is an ACE inhibitor that inhibits conversion of angiotensin I to angiotensin II. Angiotensin II is a potent vasopressor, stimulates release of aldosterone and vasopressin, facilitates the central and peripheral effects of the sympathetic nervous system and preserves glomerular filtration when renal blood flow is reduced. Blocking angiotensin II production results in veno- and arteriodilation and decreased salt and water retention (reduced aldosterone production). It is indicated for the treatment of CHF and hypertension. Enalapril reduces proteinuria seen in patients with diabetes mellitus, hypertension and protein-losing nephropathy (PLN). This has been attributed to efferent arteriolar dilation, resulting in a reduced glomerular filtration pressure.

Forms: *Oral:* 1 mg, 2.5 mg, 5 mg, 10 mg, 20 mg tablets.

Dose:
Cats: Cardiac disease, PLN: 0.25 mg/kg p.o. q12–24h.
Dogs:
• Cardiac disease, PLN: 0.25–1 mg/kg p.o. q12–24h.
• Hypertension: Doses up to 3 mg/kg are recommended by some.

Adverse effects and contraindications: Hypotension, renal impairment, hyperkalaemia, anorexia, vomiting and diarrhoea are the main adverse effects. Hypotension is the main concern if an overdose is given. Treat with normal saline to expand blood volume and support the blood pressure. The dose of enalapril may need to be reduced in patients with renal dysfunction; monitor renal function after starting treatment. Hypersensitivity reactions, e.g. angioneurotic oedema, have been reported in man. Serum biochemical abnormalities reported in man include hyperkalaemia, hyponatraemia, and increased liver enzymes and bilirubin.

Drug interactions: Concomitant treatment with **NSAIDs, potassium-sparing diuretics**, and **potassium** supplementation may increase the risk of hyperkalaemia developing. The concurrent use of **diuretics** or **vasodilators** with enalapril may cause hypotension; normal saline is recommended to correct blood pressure.

Enilconazole (Imaverol) *P*

Indications: Enilconazole is an imidazole antifungal agent used to treat fungal infections of the skin and nasal aspergillosis. It inhibits cytochrome P450-dependent synthesis of ergosterol in fungal cells.

Forms: *Topical:* 100 mg/ml (10%) liquid.

Dose: *Cats, Dogs, Small mammals:*
• Dermatological indications: Dilute 1 volume enilconazole in 50 volumes of water to produce a 0.2 mg/ml (0.2%) solution. Apply every 3 days for 3–4 applications.

- Nasal aspergillosis: 10 mg/kg q12h instilled into the nasal cavities and sinuses through indwelling tubes for 7–10 days. Dilute the solution of enilconazole (100 mg/ml) 50:50 with water. The instilled volume should be kept low (<10 ml) to reduce the risk of inhalation and the tubes flushed with an equivalent volume of air. Make up a fresh solution as required. **Note: This is not an authorized use of enilconazole.**

Adverse effects and contraindications: Enilconazole is hepatotoxic if swallowed.

Enrofloxacin (Baytril) *POM*

Indications: Enrofloxacin, a fluoroquinolone class antimicrobial agent, has a broad spectrum of activity. It is bactericidal inhibiting bacterial DNA gyrase, and is active against *Mycoplasma* spp and many Gram-positive and Gram-negative organisms including *Pasteurella* spp., *Staphylococcus* spp., *Pseudomonas aeruginosa*, *Klebsiella* spp., *Escherichia coli*, *Mycobacterium* spp., *Proteus* spp. and *Salmonella* spp. Enrofloxacin is effective against many beta-lactamase-producing bacteria, but is ineffective in treating obligate anaerobic infections. The bactericidal action is concentration-dependent, meaning that 'pulse' dosing regimens may be effective particularly against Gram-negative bacteria. The fluoroquinolones are highly lipophilic drugs that attain high concentrations within cells in many tissues and are particularly effective in the management of soft tissue, urogenital (including prostatic) and skin infections.

Forms:
Injectable: 25 mg/ml, 50 mg/ml, 100 mg/ml solutions.
Oral: 15 mg, 50 mg, 150 mg tablets; 25 mg/ml solution.

Dose:
Cats, Dogs: 5 mg/kg s.c. q24h; 2.5 mg/kg p.o. q12h, or 5 mg/kg p.o. q24h. Some isolates of *Pseudomonas aeruginosa* may require higher doses – contact the manufacturer to discuss individual cases.
Notes:
- For the treatment of non-tubercular mycobacterial disease, enrofloxacin can be combined with clarithromycin and rifampin.
- I.v. administration is not licensed but has been used in cases of severe sepsis. If this route is used, administer slowly as the carrier contains potassium.
Small mammals: 5–10 mg/kg s.c., p.o. q12h or 20 mg/kg s.c., p.o. q24h.
Birds: 10 mg/kg i.m., p.o. q12h or 20 mg/kg i.m., p.o. q24h.
Reptiles: 5–10 mg/kg i.m., p.o. q24–48h.

Adverse effects and contraindications: Fluoroquinolones are relatively contraindicated in growing dogs, as cartilage abnormalities have been reported in young dogs (but not cats). A similar warning exists for children but the risk is considered small and fluoroquinolones are used 'off-label' in children. Enrofloxacin is not licensed in cats <8 weeks of age. In birds, joint lesions have been induced in nestling pigeons with high doses of enrofloxacin, and muscle necrosis may be seen following i.m. administration. Enrofloxacin should be used with caution in epileptics until further information is available, as in man they potentiate CNS adverse effects when administered concurrently with NSAIDs. In cats retinal blindness has occurred and the higher the dose the greater the risk of this being irreversible.

Drug interactions: Adsorbents and **antacids** containing cations (Mg^{2+}, Al^{3+}) may bind to fluoroquinolones and prevent their absorption from the GI tract. The absorption of fluoroquinolones may also be inhibited by **sucralfate** and **zinc salts**; separate doses of these drugs by at least 2 hours. Fluoroquinolones increases plasma **theophylline** concentrations. **Cimetidine** may reduce the clearance of fluoroquinolones and so should be used with caution in combination with these drugs.

Epinephrine – see Adrenaline

Epirubicin (4'–Epi–doxorubicin) (Pharmorubicin*) *POM*

Indications: Epirubicin is a cytotoxic anthracycline glycoside antibiotic that has cytotoxic properties. It is a stereoisomer of doxorubicin. Intracellularly its metabolism results in production of free radicals that are cytotoxic. It also binds irreversibly to DNA, thereby preventing replication and it alters membrane functions. Epirubicin has demonstrated efficacy against human breast, ovarian, pancreatic, lung, gastric, bladder, thyroid, hepatic, colorectal and cervical neoplasms. In the dog the drug has only been assessed against lymphoma (similar efficacy to doxorubicin). It may be used alone or in combination with other antineoplastic therapies.

Forms: Injectable: 10 mg, 20 mg, 50 mg powder for reconstitution; 2 mg/ml solution. After reconstitution the drug is stable for 24 hours at room temperature (protect from light).

Dose: *Dogs:* 30 mg/m² i.v. q3 weeks; maximum total dose not to exceed 240 mg/m² The drug must be given i.v. As extravasation of the drug is likely to result in severe tissue necrosis, use of an indwelling catheter taped in place is recommended for administration. The reconstituted drug should be administered over a minimum period of 10 minutes into the side port of a freely running i.v. infusion of 0.9% NaCl.
See page 293 for conversion of body weight to surface area (m²).

Caution: Epirubicin is a potent cytotoxic drug that should only be prepared and administered by trained personnel. Reconstitution or transfer to syringes or infusion bags should be carried out in designated areas, preferably a laminar flow cabinet. Personnel must be protected with suitable clothing, gloves, mask and eye shield. In the event of contact with skin or eyes, the affected area should be washed with copious amounts of water or normal saline. Medical advice should be sought if the eyes are affected. Pregnant women should be excluded from handling cytotoxic agents.

Adverse effects and contraindications: Allergic reactions to the drug may develop, therefore premedication with i.v. diphenhydramine, chlorphenamine or dexamethasone prior to therapy is recommended. When antihistamines are used, give 10 mg to dogs up to 10kg, 20 mg to dogs 10–30 kg and 30 mg to dogs >30 kg, or give 0.5 mg/kg dexamethasone. Acute anaphylactic reactions should be treated with adrenaline, steroids and fluids. Epirubicin causes a dose-dependent cumulative cardiotoxicity in dogs (dilated cardiomyopathy and congestive heart failure) but possibly at a lower incidence than that of doxorubicin. This rarely develops in dogs given a total dose of <240 mg/m^2. It may also cause a tachycardia and arrhythmias on administration. Dogs with pre-existing cardiac disease should be routinely monitored with ECGs and/or echocardiograms. Anorexia, vomiting, pancreatitis, severe leucopenia, thrombocytopenia, haemorrhagic gastroenteritis and nephrotoxicity are major adverse effects. A complete CBC and platelet count should be monitored whenever therapy is given. If the neutrophil count drops below 2 x 10^9/l or if the platelet count drops below 50 x 10^9/l, treatment should be suspended. Once the counts have stabilized, epirubicin can then be restarted at the same dose. If haematological toxicity occurs again, or if GI toxicity is recurrent the dose should be reduced to 20 mg/m^2.

Epoetin alfa and beta (r–Human erythropoietin)
(Eprex*; Neorecormon*) *POM*

Indications: Erythropoietin is a key regulator of erythropoiesis. Recombinant human erythropoietin (r-HuEPO) is predominantly used to treat anaemia associated with chronic renal failure, although it is also used to treat anaemic human patients with cancer and rheumatoid arthritis, and cats with FeLV-associated anaemia. Erythropoietin is not indicated in conditions where high serum concentrations of the hormone already exist (e.g. haemolytic anaemia, anaemia due to blood loss), where the anaemia is due to iron deficiency or where systemic hypertension is present.

Forms: *Injectable:* 1000 IU, 2000 IU, 5000 IU powders for reconstitution; 2000 IU/ml, 4000 IU/ml, 10,000 IU/ml, 40,000 IU/ml solutions. Neorecormon is epoetin beta. Eprex is epoetin alfa.

Dose: *Cats, Dogs:* Epoetin beta: 50–100 IU/kg s.c. 3 times/week until PCV is normal. Then gradually reduce frequency of dosing to maintain PCV at lower end of normal.
Epoetin alfa: 50 IU/kg i.v. over 1–5 mins 3 times/week. Once anaemia resolved, maintenance dose 75–300 IU/kg i.v. once weekly or divided doses.

Adverse effects and contraindications: Do not administer epoetin alfa subcutaneously. Local and systemic allergic reactions may rarely develop (skin rash at the injection site, pyrexia, arthralgia and mucocutaneous ulcers). The production of cross-reacting antibodies to r–HuEPO occurs in 20% of treated dogs and 30% of treated cats 4 weeks or more after treatment. These antibodies reduce the efficacy of the drug leading to a reappearance of the anaemia. The drug should be discontinued if this develops.

Erythromycin (Erythrocin*; Erythromycin*; Erythroped*) *POM*

Indications: Erythromycin is a macrolide antibiotic that may be bactericidal (time-dependent) or bacteriostatic, depending upon drug concentration and bacterial susceptibility. It binds to the 50S ribosome, inhibiting peptide bond formation. Erythromycin has a similar antibacterial spectrum to penicillins. It is active against Gram-positive cocci (some staphylococci are resistant), Gram-positive bacilli and some Gram-negative bacilli (*Pasturella* spp.). Some strains of *Actinomyces*, *Nocardia*, *Chlamydia* and *Rickettsia* are also inhibited by erythromycin. Most of the Enterobacteriaceae (*Pseudomonas* spp., *Escherichia coli*, *Klebsiella* spp.) are resistant. It is used in hamsters to treat proliferative ileitis (*Lawsonia intracellularis*). Being a lipophilic weak base, it is concentrated in fluids that are more acidic than plasma, including milk, prostatic fluid and intracellular fluid. Resistance to erythromycin can be quite high, particularly in staphylococcal organisms. Erythromycin may act as a GI prokinetic by stimulating motilin receptors. Different esters of erythromycin are available. It is likely that the kinetics and possibly the toxicity will differ, depending on the ester used.

Forms:
Injectable: 200 mg/ml solution; 1g/vial powder.
Oral: 250 mg, 500 mg tablets capsules; 25 mg/ml suspension.

Dose:
Cats, Dogs: 10–20 mg/kg p.o. q8–12h.
As a gastrointestinal prokinetic: 0.5–1 mg/kg p.o. q8h.
Small mammals: Hamsters: 20 mg/kg p.o., 0.13 mg/ml drinking water.
Birds: 20 mg/kg i.m., s.c. q8h; 60 mg/kg p.o. q12h, 125 mg/ml of drinking water; 200 mg/kg soft feed.

Adverse effects and contraindications: The commonest adverse effect is vomiting. This can be avoided by using enteric coated products. In man the erythromycin estolate salt has been implicated in causing cholestatic hepatitis. Although not demonstrated in veterinary medicine, this salt should be avoided in animals with hepatic dysfunction. Erythromycin's activity is enhanced in an alkaline pH (pK_a of erythromycin = 8.6). As the base is acid-labile it should be administered on an empty stomach. It can cause enterotoxaemia in rodents.

Drug interactions: Erythromycin may enhance the absorption of **digoxin** from the GI tract and increase serum levels of **methylprednisolone, theophylline,** and **terfenadine**. The interaction with **terfenadine** proved particularly significant in human medicine leading to fatal arrhythmias in some patients receiving both drugs.

Erythropoietin – see Epoetin

Esmolol (Brevibloc*) *POM*

Indications: Esmolol is an ultra-short-acting beta-blocker, used to treat supraventricular tachycardias (including atrial fibrillation, atrial flutter and atrial tachycardia). It is relatively cardioselective.

Forms: *Injectable:* 10 mg/ml solution.

Dose: *Cats, Dogs:* 0.05–0.1 mg/kg slow i.v. bolus q5min to a total cumulative dose of 0.5 mg/kg; 50–200 µg/kg/min constant rate infusion.

Adverse effects and contraindications: Adverse effects are most frequently seen in geriatric patients with chronic heart disease or in patients with rapidly decompensating cardiac failure. They include bradycardia, impaired AV conduction, myocardial depression, heart failure, syncope, glucose intolerance, bronchospasm, diarrhoea and peripheral vasoconstriction. The use of esmolol is contraindicated in patients with supraventricular bradycardia and AV block and relatively contraindicated in animals with congestive heart failure. Depression and lethargy are occasionally seen and are a result of esmolol's high lipid solubility and its penetration into the CNS. Esmolol may reduce the glomerular filtration rate and therefore exacerbate any pre-existing renal impairment.

Drug interactions: As the beta effects of **sympathomimetics** (e.g. **adrenaline, phenylpropanolamine, terbutaline**) may be blocked by esmolol, the unopposed alpha effects may result in severe hypertension and a decreased heart rate. The hypotensive effect of esmolol is enhanced by **anaesthetic agents** that depress myocardial activity, **phenothiazines, antihypertensive** drugs (e.g. **hydralazine, prazosin**),

diazepam, **diuretics** and other **anti-arrhythmics**. There is an increased risk of bradycardia, severe hypotension, heart failure and AV block if esmolol is used concurrently with **calcium-channel blockers**. Concurrent **digoxin** administration potentiates bradycardia. Esmolol may increase serum **digoxin** levels by up to 20%. **Cimetidine** may decrease the metabolism of esmolol, thereby increasing its blood levels. **Morphine** may increase esmolol serum concentration by up to 50%. Esmolol may enhance the effects of **muscle relaxants** (e.g. **suxamethonium**, **tubocurarine**). Hepatic enzyme induction by **phenobarbital** may increase the rate of metabolism of esmolol. The bronchodilatory effects of **theophylline** may be blocked by esmolol.

Estradiol benzoate (Oestradiol benzoate) (Mesalin) POM

Indications: Estradiol is indicated for the management of misalliance.

Forms: *Injectable:* 0.2 mg/ml solution.

Dose: *Dogs:* Misalliance: 0.01 mg/kg i.m., s.c. on day 3 and day 5 after mating. Administer a third dose on day 7 after mating where the exact date of mating is unclear or if the bitch was mated several times.

Adverse effects: Oestrogens may be toxic to bone marrow. The incidence of bone marrow aplasia is increased with higher doses, or chronic or repeated therapy. **Do not use in cats.**

Estriol (Incurin) POM

Indications: Estriol is a synthetic, short-acting oestrogen with a high affinity for oestrogen receptors in the lower urogenital tract. It increases muscle tone, improving urodynamic function, and is indicated in the management of urethral sphincter mechanism incompetence that develops in spayed bitches.

Forms: *Oral:* 1 mg tablet.

Dose: *Dogs:* The dose has to be determined for each animal individually. Start at a dose of 1 mg/dog p.o. q24h. If treatment is successful reduce the dose to 0.5 mg/dog p.o. q24h. If treatment is unsuccessful increase to 2 mg/dog p.o. q24h. Alternate-day dosing can be considered once a response has been seen. The minimum effective dose is 0.5 mg/dog q24–48h. The maximum dose is 2 mg/dog q24h.

Adverse effects and contraindications: Do not use in intact bitches. Oestrogenic effects are seen in 5–9% of bitches receiving 2 mg q24h. Do not use if PU/PD present.

Drug interactions: No specific drug interactions have been reported.

Etamiphylline camsilate (Millophylline V) *POM*

Indications: Etamiphylline is a phosphodiesterase inhibitor used to treat bronchial constriction and pulmonary oedema. It also has a mild diuretic action and is a mild cardiac and respiratory stimulant.

Forms:
Injectable: 140 mg/ml solution.
Oral: 100 mg, 200 mg, 300 mg tablets.

Dose:
Cats: 70–140 mg i.m., s.c. or 100 mg p.o. q8h.
Dogs: BW <10 kg: 70–140 mg i.m., s.c. or 100 mg p.o. q8h; 10–30 kg: 140–420 mg i.m., s.c. or 100–300 mg p.o. q8h; >30 kg: 420–700 mg i.m., s.c. or 300–400 mg p.o. q8h.

Adverse effects and contraindications: Occasional CNS stimulation may develop; treat with a sedative (e.g. diazepam). It is recommended that the drug should not be used in animals <3 kg.

Drug interactions: Phenobarbital may decrease the effects of etamyphylline. **Allopurinol**, **cimetidine** and **erythromycin** may increase the effects of etamyphylline. Etamiphylline may reduce the effects of **pancuronium**. Etamiphylline and **beta-adrenergic blockers** (**propranolol**) may antagonize each other's effect. There is an increased risk of cardiac dysrhythmias if used with **halothane** and an increased risk of seizures if used with **ketamine**.

Ethanol (Alcohol*; Ethanol*) *POM*

Indications: Ethanol is used to prevent the metabolization of ethylene glycol (*See also Fomepizole*) or methanol to toxic metabolites and to cleanse skin.

Forms: Injectable: 95% solution. To prepare a solution for i.v. use, dilute to 20% in sterile water and administer through a 22 μm filter.

Dose:
Cats: 5 ml of 20% ethanol solution/kg i.v. q6h for 5 treatments, then q8h for 4 additional treatments.
Dogs: 5.5 ml of 20% ethanol solution/kg given i.v. q4h for 5 treatments, then q6h i.v. for 4 additional treatments. Alternatively, give an i.v. loading dose (rapidly infused over 15 minutes) of 1.4 ml/kg of 20% solution, then begin a constant infusion of 0.62 ml/kg/h, maintain for 48–56 hours.

Adverse effects and contraindications: Adjust dose to maintain blood ethanol levels above 35 mg/dl in dogs. Ethanol may cause additive depression and mask CNS symptoms of ethylene glycol toxicity, and cause diuresis. Monitor fluid and electrolyte balance during ethanol therapy.

Etherified starch (eloHAES*; HAES–steril*; Hemohes*) *POM*

Indications: Etherified starch comprises >90% amylopectin that has been etherified with hydroxyethyl groups. Hetastarch has a higher degree of etherification than pentastarch. They are slowly metabolized macromolecular substances, used in the short term to expand and maintain blood volume in all forms of shock, and may be used as an immediate short-term measure to manage haemorrhage until blood is available. They are rarely required when shock is due to water and sodium depletion.

Forms: *Injectable:* Hetastarch (eloHAES) 6% solutions; Pentastarch (HAES–steril, Hemohes) 6% solution.

Dose: *Cats, Dogs:*
Hetastarch: 10–20 ml/kg/day i.v. infusion; maximum daily dose 1500 ml.
Pentastarch: 10–40 ml/kg/day i.v. infusion; maximum daily dose 2000 ml.

Adverse effects and contraindications: Etherified starches should be used with caution in animals with congestive heart failure and renal impairment. They may interfere with some serum biochemistry assays; obtain blood samples prior to their use. Etherified starch should not be used where bleeding disorders due to thrombocytopenia (due to its effects on platelets) or hypofibrinogenaemia are present. Anaphylactic reactions may occasionally develop. No oxygen-carrying capacity, and so it is not a replacement for whole blood or red cells.

Ethinylestradiol (Ethinyloestradiol) – see Methyltestosterone

Ethylestrenol (Ethyloestrenol) (Nandoral) *POM*

Indications: Ethylestrenol is a potent anabolic drug, derived from nandrolone. It is used wherever excessive tissue breakdown or extensive repair processes are present.

Forms: *Oral:* 0.5 mg tablet.

Dose: *Cats, Dogs:* 0.05 mg/kg p.o. q24h.

Adverse effects and contraindications: Adverse effects include virilism if unduly prolonged dosage or overdosages are administered. Monitor CBC to determine the efficacy of treatment and liver enzymes.

Drug interactions: Anabolic steroids may enhance the effects of **warfarin**. The **insulin** requirements of diabetics may need to be decreased following the administration of anabolic steroids. The concurrent use of anabolic steroids with **adrenal steroids** may potentiate the development of oedema.

Etidronate (Didronel*) *POM*

Indications: Etidronate is a bisphosphonate that is adsorbed on to hydroxyapatite crystals, slowing their rate of growth and dissolution. It is used to treat acute moderate to severe hypercalcaemia when other therapeutic regimens are ineffective, or for long-term therapy of chronic hypercalcaemia.

Forms:
Injectable: 50 mg/ml solution.
Oral: 200 mg tablet.

Dose: *Dogs:* 7.5 mg/kg q24h i.v. for 3 days; 20 mg/kg p.o. q24h. Note: There are few reports on the use of this drug in dogs. The oral route appears to be relatively ineffective in comparison to other bisphosphonates (pamidronate, clodronate).

Adverse effects and contraindications: Adverse effects may include nausea, diarrhoea, hypocalcaemia, hypophosphataemia, hypomagnasaemia and hypersensitivity reactions.

Drug interactions: Concurrent use of **aminoglycosides** may result in severe hypocalcaemia.

Famotidine (Famotidine*; Pepcid*) *POM*

Indications: Famotidine is a potent H_2 receptor antagonist that reduces gastric acid secretion. It is used to treat gastroduodenal ulceration and severe reflux oesophagitis.

Forms: *Oral:* 20, 40 mg tablets.

Dose: *Cats, Dogs:* 0.5–1.0 mg/kg p.o. q12–24h.

Adverse effects and contraindications: There is little information on the use of this drug in veterinary medicine. No adverse effects reported yet. They may be similar to those for cimetidine.

Fat/Triglyceride preparations (Intralipid*; MCT oil*; MCT pepdite) *POM*

Indications: Fat is an essential component of the diet. Lipid emulsions (Intralipid) are used parenterally in animals receiving nutritional support, to provide fat for energy production and essential fatty acids for cellular metabolism. Seek specialist advice prior to using parenteral nutrition. *See also Amino acid solutions and Glucose.* Medium chain triglycerides (MCT oil) were thought to be absorbed directly into the portal system and were used as energy sources in animals requiring low-fat diets, e.g. hyperlipidaemia, lymphangiectasia. However, recent work indicates significant lymphatic transport.

Forms:
Injectable (Intralipid)*:* 20% soybean emulsion for i.v. use only. Contains 2 kcal/ml (8.4 kJ/ml), 268 mOsm/l. Do not use if separation of the emulsion occurs. There are several other human products available.
Oral: Medium chain triglycerides (MCT oil): Several products are available. Several human licensed products are available that also contain peptides and simple sugars.

Dose: *Cats, Dogs:*
- Parenteral use: The amount required will be governed by the animal's physiological status and its tolerance of the fat. Generally fat is used to supply 40–60% of energy requirements in dogs and cats.
- MCT oil: Each ml provides 8 kcal and the total given should not exceed 20% of the animal's daily energy intake. A dose of 1–2 ml/kg can be used in dogs. A gradual introduction is necessary as initial tolerance is poor. A more palatable 50% emulsion is available (Liquigen) although the volume given must be doubled.

Adverse effects and contraindications: Intralipid is isotonic with blood and may be administered through a peripheral vein. Be aware that hyperlipidaemia, liver failure and pancreatitis may develop in some patients. The use of MCTs is contraindicated in cats as they may cause hepatoencephalopathy and possibly hepatic lipidosis. In dogs they should be started gradually to allow tolerance to build up; poor palatability and diarrhoea are common complications. As MCTs are unpalatable their use may result in reduced food intake. Unabsorbed MCTs induce abdominal pain and diarrhoea, and they should therefore be used with caution in animals with fat maldigestion/malabsorption.

Febantel (Drontal plus; Drontal puppy suspension) *PML*

Indications: Febantel is an antiparasitic drug that interferes with carbohydrate metabolism in the different developmental stages of helminths, including larvae in eggs.

Forms: *Oral:* 150 mg febantel with praziquantel and pyrantel (Drontal plus);15 mg/ml febantel with pyrantel suspension (Drontal puppy suspension).

Dose: *Dogs:* 15 mg/kg p.o.

Adverse effects and contraindications: Do not use Drontal puppy suspension in pregnant or lactating bitches as studies have not been carried out in these animals.

Drug interactions: It has a synergistic effect when used in combination with **pyrantel**. Do not use simultaneously with **piperazine** as this reduces efficacy.

Fenbendazole (Granofen; Panacur; Zerofen) PML

Indications: Fenbendazole is an oral anthelmintic active against ascarids (including larval stages), hookworms, whipworms, tapeworms (*Taenia* spp.), *Oslerus osleri, Aelurostrongylus abstrusus, Angiostrongylus vasorum, Capillaria aerophila, Ollulanus tricuspis, Physaloptera rara* and *Paragonimus kellicotti* infections. It shows a 60–70% efficacy against *Dipylidium caninum*. Fenbendazole has a 100% efficacy in clearing *Giardia* cysts. It is used in rabbits for the treatment of *Encephalitozoon cuniculi*.

Forms: *Oral:* 222 mg/g granules (22%); 25 mg/ml (2.5%), 100 mg/ml (10%) suspension, 0.187g/g paste in a syringe; 500 mg and 1000 mg chewable tablets; 8 mg capsule (for pigeons).

Dose:
Cats, Dogs:
- Roundworms, Tapeworms: Animals <6 months 50 mg/kg p.o. q24h for 3 consecutive days or 20 mg/kg p.o. q24h for 5 days (cats); animals >6 months 100 mg/kg as a single dose p.o. Treatment of *Capillaria* may need to be extended to 10 days. Repeat q3 months. For pregnant bitches 25 mg/kg p.o. q24h from day 40 until 2 days post-whelping (approximately 25 days).
- *Aelurostrongylus abstrusus:* 50 mg/kg p.o. q24h for 3 days or 20 mg/kg p.o. q24h for 5 days; *Angiostrongylus vasorum, Oslerus osleri* : 50 mg/kg p.o. q24h for 7 days.
- Giardiasis: 50 mg/kg p.o. q24h for 3 days or 20 mg/kg p.o. for 5 days (cats).
Small mammals: 50 mg/kg p.o. q24h for 5 consecutive days.
Rabbits: *E. cuniculi*: 20 mg/kg p.o. q24h for 28 days.
Birds:
- Nematodes: 10–50 mg/kg p.o. – administer 2 doses separated by 10 days.
- Microfilariae and trematodes: 10–50 mg/kg p.o. q24h for 3 consecutive days.
- Capillariasis: 10–50 mg/kg p.o. q24h for 5 consecutive days.
- Pigeons: 16 mg/kg p.o. once only; repeat after 10 days if necessary.
Reptiles: 100 mg/kg p.o. q24h for 5 consecutive days.

Adverse effects and contraindications: Pigeons and doves are susceptible to fenbendazole intoxication. Mortality of 50% has occurred at doses of 20 mg/kg p.o. given on 3 consecutive days. Fenbendazole appears to affect intestinal function and may be hepatotoxic. Vomiting, depression and death within 96 hours are recorded.

Fentanyl (Duragesic*: Fentanyl*: Sublimaze*) POM Scheduled 2 Controlled Drug

Indications: Fentanyl is a pure OP3 (mu) agonist of the phenylpiperidine series. Its high lipid solubility confers a rapid onset (1–2 minutes) with peak effects apparent 2–5 minutes after injection. It has a short, dose-dependent duration of action (10–20 minutes). It shows moderate cumulative properties when infused for longer than one hour. It is given intravenously by repeated doses in dogs to provide profound intra-operative analgesia and post-operative 'rescue' analgesia when pain proves difficult to control. It can be used with benzodiazepines to provide profound sedation in unhealthy dogs. Fentanyl patches are used in the prolonged management of pain associated with surgery, trauma or neoplastic disease. Following patch application, fentanyl plasma levels peak in 3 to 6 hours in cats but may require 12–24 hours in dogs to reach full effect. Plasma drug levels are sustained for 24–72 hours, but fall rapidly once the patches are removed. It is a potent respiratory depressant and a means of supporting ventilation should be available whenever fentanyl is used in unconscious animals.

Forms: 0.05 mg/ml solution in 2 ml and 10 ml ampoules (Fentanyl, Sublimaze): 0.025, 0.050, 0.075 and 0.1 mg/hour skin patches (Duragesic).

Dose:
Cats:
- Topical: A 0.025 mg/hour patch is suitable for 3–5 kg cats. In smaller cats, only half the protective liner should be removed. The chest wall should be clipped and then shaved, and dried before the patch is applied. The patch should be covered with a light dressing. A single patch should suppress pain for about 24 to 72 hours so will need to be substituted every two to three days if 'troughs' in analgesia are to be avoided. After removal, fentanyl blood levels drop rapidly within 24 hours because of the drug's brief elimination half-life.

Dogs:
- Intravenous: 0.001–0.005 mg/kg i.v. for intra-operative analgesia. Repeated injections may be required at 10–20 minute intervals. Infusion rates of 0.0025–0.010 mg/kg/h are required to produce profound sustained analgesia.
- Topical: In 20 kg dogs, a single 0.050 or 0.075 mg/h patch is applied 24 hours before the anticipated time that analgesia will be required.

Adverse effects and contraindications: Rapid injection can cause severe bradycardia, even asystole. This may be prevented by slow injection or the prior/co-injection of atropine (0.04 mg/kg) or glycopyrronium (0.010 mg/kg). Fentanyl is a potent respiratory depressant; IPPV must be imposed whenever fentanyl is used. In respect of the fentanyl patches, high individual variability in plasma fentanyl concentrations after patch application mandates that animals be observed for the adequacy of analgesia and adverse effects. The latter includes sedation, respiratory depression, bradycardia, ataxia and appetite suppression, although occasionally euphoria and appetite stimulation may be seen. Overdose is possible if the patch becomes inadvertently hot, i.e., following contact with a heater blanket. Patches must be removed if signs of overdose arise. Parenteral analgesics may be required for 'rescue' analgesia if 'peaks' in postoperative pain are refractory to fentanyl. Patches should be removed if skin irritation arises, and a topical corticosteroid ointment applied. Fentanyl patches may be toxic if swallowed by the subject, children or other animals.

Drug interactions: The intravenous dose requirement for fentanyl will be reduced by drugs with central nervous depressant effects. Similarly any drug causing CNS depression, including **sedatives**, **antihistamine** preparations and **opioid** analgesics are likely to produce a disproportionately greater effect in animals being treated with fentanyl patches. Fentanyl will reduce the dose requirements of concurrently administered anaesthetics, including inhaled anaesthetics, by at least 50%.

Filgrastim (G–CSF) (Neupogen*) *POM*

Indications: Filgrastim is recombinant human granulocyte colony stimu-lating factor (rhG-CSF). G-CSF is a cytokine produced by bone marrow stromal cells, monocytes/macrophages, fibroblasts and endothelial cells. In man it stimulates granulocyte production and is indicated in the management of neutropenia, especially in patients receiving high-dose chemotherapy. Neutrophil counts rise within 24 hours. Following discontinuation of therapy, neutrophil counts drop to normal after 5 days. There are few reports on the use of G-CSF in dogs or cats. It is most likely to be used in the management of febrile patients, particularly those receiving cytotoxic drugs with neutrophil counts $< 1 \times 10^9/l$.

Forms: *Injectable:* 30 million IU (300 µg)/ml solution.

Dose: *Cats, Dogs:* 500,000 IU (5 µg)/kg/day i.v. infusion, s.c., for 3–5 days.

Adverse effects and contraindications: Normal dogs produce neutralizing antibodies to rhG-CSF. This limits repeated use and may result in neutropenia. This does not appear to be the case in canine chemotherapy patients. A variety of adverse effects have been reported in man, including musculoskeletal pain, transient hypotension, dysuria, allergic reactions, proteinuria, haematuria and increased liver enzymes. Reported adverse effects are bone pain at high doses and irritation at the injection site.

Finasteride (Proscar*) *POM*

Indications: Finasteride is a 5-alpha-reductase inhibitor that inhibits dihydrotestosterone (DHT) production within the prostate. DHT is the main hormonal stimulus for the development of benign prostatic hyperplasia. Finasteride is used in the management of this disorder as an alternative to castration.

Forms: *Oral:* 5 mg tablet.

Dose: *Dogs:* 5 mg per dog p.o. q24h.

Caution: Women of child-bearing potential should avoid handling crushed or broken tablets.

Adverse effects and contraindications: Finasteride is secreted into semen and as it causes fetal anomalies must not be used in breeding dogs. It is potentially teratogenic.

Fipronil (**Frontline**; **Frontline Combo**) *POM*

Indications: Fipronil is a phenylpyrazoline drug used in the treatment and prevention of flea, biting lice and tick infestations. It can help in the control of dermatoses caused by harvest mites (*Neotrombicula autumnalis*). It blocks GABA receptors to kill the parasite on contact. It is a non-systemic ectoparasiticide.

Forms: *Topical:* Spot-on: 10% w/v: 50 mg, 67 mg, 134 mg, 268 mg, 402 mg pipettes; Pump spray: 0.25% w/v.
In combination with s-methoprene (Frontline Combo).

Dose: *Cats, Dogs, Ferrets:* 7.5–15 mg/kg.
Regular local treatment of feet and legs may be necessary to control harvest mites.

Adverse reactions and contraindications: Do not use on rabbits.

Flucloxacillin (Flucloxacillin*; Magna pen*) *POM*

Indications: Flucloxacillin is a beta-lactamase-resistant, narrow spectrum beta-lactam antibiotic. It binds to penicillin-binding proteins, decreasing bacterial cell wall strength and rigidity, and affecting cell division, growth and septum formation. It is bactericidal with a time-dependent mechanism. As animal cells lack a cell wall it is safe. Flucloxacillin is stable in gastric acid so can be given orally but food significantly reduces its bioavailability. It is less active than penicillin G or V against *Streptococcus* spp. and obligate anaerobic bacteria and is indicated for the treatment of infections caused by beta-lactamase-producing *Staphylococcus* spp. Formulations of flucloxacillin with ampicillin are available (Magna pen cofluampicil).

Forms:
Injectable: Flucloxacillin sodium: 250 mg, 500 mg, 1 g powders for reconstitution.
Oral: Flucloxacillin sodium capsules – 250 or 500 mg; oral suspension (as sodium salt) – 125 mg, 250 mg powder for reconstitution with water.

Dose: *Cats, Dogs:* Flucloxacillin sodium 15 mg/kg i.v., i.m., p.o., q6h. As flucloxacillin kills in a time-dependent fashion, dosing regimens should be designed to maintain tissue concentrations above the MIC value throughout the interdosing interval.

Adverse effects and contraindications: 250 mg of flucloxacillin sodium contains 0.57 mEq of sodium. This may be clinically important for patients on restricted sodium intakes. Patients with significant renal or hepatic dysfunction may need dosage adjustment. **Do not administer penicillins to hamsters, gerbils, guinea pigs, chinchillas or rabbits.**

Drug interactions: Avoid the concomitant use of bacteriostatic antibiotics. The **aminoglycosides** (e.g. **gentamicin**) may inactivate penicillins when mixed together in parenteral solutions. Although flucloxacillin is absorbed from the GI tract, food has a significant inhibitory effect on its bioavailabilty – doses must be given on an empty stomach.

Fluconazole (Diflucan*; Fluconazole*; **Itrafungol**) *POM*

Indications: Fluconazole is a triazole antifungal agent effective against *Blastomyces*, *Candida*, *Cryptococcus*, *Coccidioides*, *Histoplasma* and *Microsporum canis* infections and variably effective against *Aspergillus* and *Penicillium* infections. Fluconazole is licensed in the form of an oral solution for the treatment of dermatophytosis in cats caused by *M. canis*. It acts by inhibiting the synthesis of ergosterol in fungal cell membranes, thus causing increased cell wall permeability and allowing leakage of cellular contents. It attains therapeutic concentrations in the CNS and respiratory tract. It is excreted by the kidney, producing high concentrations in urine.

Forms:
Injectable: 2 mg/ml solution.
Oral: 50 mg, 150 mg, 200 mg capsules; 10 mg/ml, 40 mg/ml suspensions.

Dose:
Cats: Ocular/CNS cryptococcosis: 50 mg/cat i.v. infusion, p.o. q24h; Dermatophytosis, nasal cryptococcosis: 5 mg/kg p.o. q24h. For dermatophytosis administer for three periods of 7 days, with 7 days without treatment in between.
Dogs: 2.5–5 mg/kg p.o. q12h.
Birds: 15 mg/kg p.o. q12h.

Adverse effects and contraindications: Reduce the dose if renal impairment is present. Adverse effects may include nausea and diarrhoea. Do not use in cats with impaired liver function. Do not use in pregnant/lactating queens.

Drug interactions: Fluconazole (due to inhibition of cytochrome P450-dependent liver enzymes) may increase plasma **theophylline** concentrations. In man, fluconazole has led to **terfenadine** toxicity when the two drugs were administered together. It may increase **ciclosporin** blood levels.

Flucytosine (Ancotil*) *POM*

Indications: Flucytosine (5-FC) is a fluorinated pyrimidine antifungal agent, used to treat cryptococcosis (often in conjunction with amphotericin B or ketoconazole), systemic and urinary yeast infections (e.g. candidiasis). It has a narrow spectrum of antifungal activity – most strains of *Aspergillus* and dermatophytes, other filamentous fungi and dimorphic fungi are not susceptible. The drug is almost exclusively excreted by the kidney and thus attains high concentrations in urine. Fungal cells convert 5-FC into 5-fluorouracil (5-FU) which inhibits DNA and RNA synthesis in the cell. Mammalian cells are spared. Resistance to 5-FC develops readily.

Forms: *Injectable:* 10 mg/ml solution for i.v. infusion.

Dose:
Cats: 25–35 mg/kg i.v. q8h.
Dogs: 25–50 mg/kg i.v. q6h.

Adverse effects and contraindications: Use flucytosine with caution in patients with hepatic or renal impairment; reduce the dose and monitor haematological, renal and hepatic parameters. Vomiting and diarrhoea may develop; alleviate by dosing over 15 minutes. Flucytosine may be teratogenic.

Drug interactions: Synergy with **amphotericin B** has been demonstrated, although there is an increased risk of nephrotoxicity.

Fludrocortisone acetate (Florinef*) *POM*

Indications: Fludrocortisone is a mineralocorticoid used to treat adrenocortical insufficiency (Addison's disease).

Forms: *Oral:* 0.1 mg tablet.

Dose: *Cats, Dogs:* Start at 0.01 mg/kg p.o. q24h depending on size of animal. Monitor sodium and potassium levels q1–2 weeks and adjust dose by 0.05–0.1 mg accordingly. Following stabilization, monitor serum sodium and potassium, blood urea and creatinine q4–5 months. Most patients once stabilized will require approximately 0.1 mg/5 kg p.o. q24h. Supplemental doses may be required during times of stress.

Adverse effects and contraindications: Adverse effects include hypertension, oedema (including cerebral oedema) and hypokalaemia with overdosages.

Drug interactions: Hypokalaemia may develop if fludrocortisone is administered concomitantly with **amphotericin B** or **potassium-depleting diuretics (furosemide, thiazides)**.

Flunixin meglumine (Finadyne) *POM*

Indications: Flunixin is a potent NSAID, inhibiting COX-1 enzyme, thereby limiting prostaglandin production. NSAIDs have antipyretic, analgesic, anti-inflammatory and anti-platelet effects. Flunixin controls moderate to severe visceral and somatic pain and is used to minimize the effects of endotoxaemia.

Forms:
Injectable: 10 mg/ml.
Oral: 5 mg, 20 mg tablets.

Dose:
Cats: 1 mg/kg i.v., i.m., p.o. q24h for a maximum of 3 days, although one dose only is preferable.
Dogs: 1.1 mg/kg s.c. or slowly i.v. q24h, or 1 mg/kg p.o. q24h; not to exceed 3 days of therapy; one dose only is preferable.
Small mammals: Rabbits: 1.1 mg/kg i.m., s.c. q12h; Rodents: 2.5 mg/kg i.m., s.c. q12h; not to exceed 3 days of therapy; one dose only is preferable.

Adverse effects and contraindications: Adverse effects are dose-related and reflect the pathophysiological changes expected with reduced prostaglandin synthesis. GI irritation and ulceration and renal papillary necrosis (renal failure) are the most common adverse effects, particularly if hypotension, dehydration or other nephrotoxic drugs are present. Blood dyscrasias, hepatotoxicity and exacerbation of heart failure may be seen rarely. Do not use if gastric or duodenal ulceration is suspected, in haemorrhagic syndromes or in cases of cardiac or renal failure. Severe toxicity (usually with an acute overdose) may present with vomiting, pyrexia, metabolic acidosis, depression, coma, seizures and GI bleeding. Treatment of acute toxic ingestion includes emptying the gut, treating the acidosis, alkalinizing urine with sodium bicarbonate and supportive therapy.

Drug interactions: Do not use with **corticosteroids** or other **NSAIDs** (increased risk of GI ulceration). In man there is an increased risk of convulsions if NSAIDs are administered with **fluoroquinolones**. NSAIDs may antagonize the hypotensive effects of **anti-hypertensives** (e.g. **beta-blockers**). The concomitant use of **diuretics** may increase the risk of nephrotoxicity.

Fluorometholone (FML*) *POM*

Indications: Fluorometholone is a topical corticosteroid used for superficial ocular inflammation or anterior uveitis. It is most commonly used when there is concern about raised intraocular pressure.

Forms: *Topical:* 0.1% drops.

Dose: *Cats, Dogs:* 1 drop topically to affected eye q6–8h, although dose frequency is dependent on the severity of inflammation and response to therapy.

Adverse effects and contraindications: Topical corticosteroids can cause cataract and glaucoma in man. They are contraindicated in cases of suspected infectious aetiology and corneal ulceration. Systemic effects may be apparent with prolonged use.

Fluorouracil (Fluorouracil*: Efudix*) *POM*

Indications: 1,5-Fluorouracil (5-FU) is an antineoplastic pyrimidine analogue. It has been used in the treatment of basal cell and squamous cell carcinoma (topically), intestinal carcinoma, transitional carcinoma of the bladder and mammary carcinoma.

Forms:
Injectable: 250 mg/vial, 500 mg/vial, 2500 mg/vial solutions.
Topical: 5% cream (Efudix).

Dose: *Dogs:* 75 mg/m^2 i.v. q24h for 5 days every 4–5 weeks, or 150–200 mg/m^2 i.v. once weekly for 6 weeks. In patients that have liver, renal or bone marrow impairment, reduce dose by half
Topical use: Apply to affected area q24h.
See specific protocols prior to use.
See page 293 for conversion of body weight to surface area (m^2).

Adverse effects and contraindications: Adverse effects include anorexia, vomiting, stomatitis, diarrhoea, leucopenia with a nadir between 7 and 14 days, thrombocytopenia, anaemia, alopecia, hyperpigmentation, dermatitis, cerebellar ataxia and seizures. **Do not use in the cat as it causes seizures.**

Drug interactions: Cimetidine inhibits the metabolism of 5-FU. There is synergism between 5-FU and **cisplatin** as well as an increased risk of neurotoxicity. **Methotrexate** is synergistic if administered before 5-FU but is antagonistic if administered afterwards. **Vincristine** increases the cytotoxicity of 5-FU.

Fluoxetine (Fluoxetine*) *POM*

Indications: Fluoxetine is a selective serotonin re-uptake inhibitor (SSRI). It is an antidepressant with little sedative effect compared to tricyclic antidepressants. Fluoxetine has been used in animals to treat aberrant compulsive behaviours, e.g. lick granulomas, self-mutilation and psychogenic pruritus/alopecia. It is also advocated in the management of generalized and recurrent anxieties and problems of impulse control. In birds it may be used to manage feather plucking.

Forms: *Oral:* 20 mg, 60 mg capsules; 4 mg/ml syrup.

Dose:
Cats: 0.5–1.0 mg/kg p.o. q24h.
Dogs: 0.5–1 mg/kg p.o. q24h up to a maximum of 20 mg.
Birds: 0.4 mg/kg p.o. q24h.

Adverse effects and contraindications: Fluoxetine should not be used in patients with epilepsy, cardiovascular disease, renal or hepatic compromise or in pregnant and lactating animals. Use in cases involving aggression should be undertaken with care due to the risk of disinhibition. In man fluoxetine has been reported to cause aplastic anaemia, ecchymoses, GI haemorrhage, eosinophilic pneumonia, haemolytic anaemia, pancreatitis, thrombocytopenia, tachycardia and bradycardia. As it has been little used in veterinary medicine the incidence of these effects in cats or dogs is unknown.

Drug interactions: Do not use in combination with **MAOIs, anti-epileptics**, **anti-arrhythmic drugs**, **propranolol** or **benzodiazepines**.

Flurbiprofen (Ocufen*) *POM*

Indications: Flurbiprofen is a topical NSAID for ophthalmic use. It is most commonly used for cataract surgery. It is also useful for anterior uveitis and ulcerative keratitis when topical corticosteroids are contraindicated.

Forms: *Topical:* 0.3% solution in single use vials.

Dose: *Cats, Dogs:* 1 drop/eye q6–12h depending on severity of inflammation. 1 drop q30min for 4 doses preoperatively (pre-surgery protocols vary widely).

Adverse effects and contraindications: As with other topical NSAIDs, flurbiprofen may cause local irritation (stinging). Topical NSAIDs can be used in ulcerative keratitis, but with caution. They can delay epithelial healing and have been associated with an increased risk of corneal melting. Regular monitoring is advised.

Fluvoxamine (Fluvoxamine*) *POM*

Indications: Fluvoxamine is a selective serotonin (5-hydroxytryptamine) reuptake inhibitor used in the treatment of canine compulsive disorders, phobias and panic attacks, especially when involving signs of impulsiveness and aggression.

Forms: *Oral:* 50 mg, 100 mg tablet.

Dose: *Dogs:* 1–2 mg/kg p.o. q12h.

Adverse effects and contraindications: Fluvoxamine should not be used in pregnant and lactating animals or those with epilepsy, cardiovascular disease, diabetes mellitus, a history of bleeding disorder, or renal or hepatic compromise. Tachycardia or bradycardia may develop. Use in cases involving aggression should be undertaken with care due to the risk of disinhibition.

Drug interactions: Not to be used in combination with **MAOIs, anti-epileptics, anti-arrhythmia** drugs or **propranolol**.

Fomepizole (Antizole*) *POM*

Indications: Fomepizole inhibits alcohol dehydrogenase and is used in the treatment of ethylene glycol (antifreeze) toxicity in dogs. It inhibits the metabolism of ethylene glycol to oxalate, thereby preventing precipitation of calcium oxalate in the kidney. Fomepizole is not effective in the cat. Fomepizole is extremely expensive and only available from poisons information centres on a named patient basis.

Forms: *Injectable:* 1g/ml solution.

Dose: *Dogs:* 20 mg/kg i.v. infusion of 30 minutes initially, then 15 mg/kg i.v. slowly over 15–30 minutes 12 and 24 hours later, then 5 mg/kg i.v. q12h until ethylene glycol concentration is negligible or the dog has recovered. Make required dose up in 100 ml normal saline for infusion.

Framycetin (**Canaural**; Soframycin*) *POM*

Indications: Framycetin is an aminoglycoside antibiotic used in the treatment of ocular infections causing conjunctivitis or blepharitis, and aural infections. It has a broad spectrum of activity but is particularly effective against Gram-negative bacteria.

Forms: *Topical:* 0.5% solution/ointment (Soframycin); 5 mg/g suspension (Canaural).

Dose: *Cats, Dogs:* 1–2 drops in the affected eye q8h (Soframycin), although dosing frequency may vary depending on the severity of the condition. 5–10 drops/ear q12h (Canaural)

Frusemide – see Furosemide

Furosemide (Frusemide) (**Dimazon**; **Frusecare**; **Frusedale**; **Frusemide**; Lasilactone*) *POM*

Indications: Furosemide is a loop diuretic, inhibiting the reabsorption of chloride and sodium in the thick ascending limb of the loop of Henlé. As a consequence it promotes natriuresis and reduces water reabsorption. It acts within 1 hour following oral dosing and within 5–30 minutes if given i.v. The diuresis is completed within 2–6 hours so that, if necessary, it can be given twice a day without interfering with sleep. Furosemide is used in the management of congestive cardiac failure, pulmonary oedema, non-cardiogenic ascites, hypercalcuric nephropathy, acute renal failure, uraemia, hyperkalaemia and hypertension. The use of chronic diuretic monotherapy in the management of cardiac failure should be avoided, as patients receiving diuretics alone may deteriorate more rapidly than those receiving other treatment modalities concurrently.

Forms:
Injectable: 50 mg/ml solution.
Oral: 20 mg, 40 mg, 1 g tablets.
Lasilactone: Furosemide 20 mg, Spironolactone 50 mg capsule.

Dose:
Cats, Dogs:
- Cardiogenic or pulmonary oedema: 1–2 mg/kg (may increase up to 8 mg/kg for acute short-term situations) i.v., i.m. q4–6h; start on oral therapy once stabilized, at 2 mg/kg p.o. q8–12h.
- Hypercalcuric nephropathy: Hydrate before therapy. Give 5 mg/kg bolus i.v., then begin 5 mg/kg/h infusion. Maintain hydration status and electrolyte balance with normal saline and added KCl. Furosemide generally reduces serum calcium levels by 0.5–1.5 mmol/l.
- Acute renal failure/uraemia: After replacing fluid deficit give furosemide at 2 mg/kg i.v. If no diuresis within 1 hour repeat dose at 4 mg/kg i.v. If no response within 1 hour give another dose at 6 mg/kg i.v. The use of low dose dopamine as adjunctive therapy is often recommended.
- To promote diuresis in hyperkalaemic states: 2 mg/kg i.v.

Small mammals: 1–2.5 mg/kg i.m., s.c., p.o. q8–12h.
Birds: 7.5 mg/kg i.m., s.c.

Adverse effects and contraindications: As furosemide affects fluid and electrolyte balance, monitor patients for hydration status and electrolyte imbalances (hypokalaemia, hypocalcaemia, hypomagnesaemia and hyponatraemia); dehydration occurs readily. Lasilactone helps to restrict potassium excretion so protecting against hypokalaemia. The reduction in ventricular filling pressures associated with furosemide may be beneficial in patients whose cardiac performance is operating on the flat portion of the ventricular function curve. However, in patients whose cardiac performance operates on the ascending limb of the curve, a marked reduction in filling pressure may result in a precipitous decline in cardiac output; this effect may be seen in normal animals with pulmonary disease, those with hypertrophic cardio-myopathy, left ventricular hypertrophy, pericardial and myocardial disorders, tamponade and severe hypertension. Other adverse effects include ototoxicity, GI disturbances, leucopenia, anaemia, weakness and restlessness.

Drug interactions: Nephrotoxicity/ototoxicity associated with **aminoglycosides** may be potentiated when furosemide is also used. Furosemide may induce hypokalaemia, thereby increasing the risk of **digoxin** toxicity. Increased risk of hypokalaemia if furosemide given with **acetazolamide, corticosteroids, thiazides** and **theophylline**. The excretion of **aspirin** and furosemide may be reduced as they both compete for renal excretory sites; dose reduction may be required. Furosemide may inhibit the muscle relaxation qualities of **tubocurarine**, but increase the effects of **suxamethonium**.

Fusidic acid (Canaural; Fuciderm; Fucithalmic Vet) *POM*

Indications: Fusidic acid is an antibacterial agent active against Gram-positive bacteria, particularly *Staphylococcus intermedius*. It is used topically in the management of staphylococcal infections of the conjunctiva, skin or ear. Fusidic acid is able to penetrate skin and into the cornea and anterior chamber of the eye. The carbomer gel vehicle in the ocular preparation may also be efficacious as it has a surface lubricative effect.

Forms: *Topical:* Canaural: 5 mg/g fusidate suspension (also contains framycetin, nystatin and prednisolone). Fuciderm: 0.5% fusidic acid and 0.1% betamethasone. Fucithalmic Vet: 1% fusidic acid.

Dose:
Cats, Dogs: Canaural: 5–10 drops/affected ear q12h.
Fucithalmic Vet: 1 drop/eye q12–24h.
Dogs: Fuciderm: Apply to affected area q12h for 5 days.
Small mammals: Rabbits: Fucithalmic Vet: 1 drop/eye q12–24h.

Adverse effects and contraindications: Do not use compounds containing corticosteroids in pregnant animals.

Gelatine (Gelofusine; Haemaccel) *POM*

Indications: Gelatine is an artificial colloid used as a plasma substitute to restore circulating blood volume in cases of shock. It mimics the oncotic action of plasma proteins, expanding plasma volume by an amount equivalent to twice the administered dose. Because of the strong shift of fluid from the interstitium, a crystalloid should be administered at the same time. With severe haemorrhage, blood transfusion should be considered as gelatin has no oxygen-carrying capacity.

Forms:
Gelofusine: 40 g/l succinylated gelatine in saline.
Haemaccel: 35 g/l degraded gelatine with NaCl, KCl and $CaCl_2$.

Dose: *Cats, Dogs:* Infuse a volume equivalent to the estimated blood loss.

Gentamicin (Clinagel Vet; Genticin*; Pangram; Tiacil) *POM*

Indications: Gentamicin is an aminoglycoside bactericidal antibiotic. It binds to the bacterial 30S ribosome, causing misreading of the genetic code. Aminoglycosides produce concentration-dependent killing, leading to a marked post-antibiotic effect that allows pulse-dosing regimens to be used effectively. The aminoglycosides as a class are more active against Gram-negative bacteria, but some staphylococcal and streptococcal (*S. faecalis*) species are sensitive. All obligate anaerobic bacteria and many haemolytic streptococci are resistant. Aminoglycosides require an oxygen rich environment to be effective, thus they are ineffective in sites with low oxygen (abscesses, exudates). When used for 'blind' therapy of undiagnosed serious infections gentamicin is usually given in conjunction with a penicillin and/or metronidazole. Aminoglycosides are more active in an alkaline environment. Their use in domestic animals is limited by nephrotoxicity and, more rarely, ototoxicity and neuromuscular blockade. Microbial resistance is a concern, although many bacteria resistant to gentamicin may be susceptible to amikacin.

Forms:
Injectable: 40 mg/ml solution for i.v., i.m., s.c. injection, 50 mg/ml solution for i.m., s.c. injection.
Ophthalmic/aural solution: 0.3% solution (Tiacil); 0.3% gel (Clinagel).
Topical ointment: 0.3% ointment.
Note: Gentamicin is a component of many topical ear preparations.

Dose:
Cats, Dogs:
Otic: 2–4 drops in affected ear or apply ointment to affected area q6–8h.
Ophthalmic: 1 drop/eye q6–8h. Severe ocular infections may require dosing q1–2h. A fortified topical solution (100 mg gentamicin in 5 ml of 0.3% solution making 14.3 mg/ml) can be used.
Systemic: 2–4 mg/kg i.v. (over 30 min), i.m. or s.c. q6–8h; 6-hourly dosing is recommended by some for serious systemic infections. Alternatively 5–10 mg/kg i.v., i.m., s.c. q24h may be less nephrotoxic.
Small mammals: 2 mg/kg i.m. q12h; topically q6–8h. Rabbits: 2–4 mg/kg i.v. (over 30 min), i.m., s.c. q6–8h; topically q6–8h.
Birds: 2.5–10 mg/kg i.v., i.m. q24h; topically q6–8h.
Reptiles: Snakes: 2.5 mg/kg s.c. q72h. Chelonians: 3–6 mg/kg s.c. q72h.

Adverse effects and contraindications: Geriatric animals or those with reduced renal function should only be given this drug systemically when absolutely necessary and then the interdosing interval should be 12 hours or longer. Monitoring serum gentamicin levels is recommended for those with pre-existing renal dysfunction if the use of this drug is considered essential. The trough serum level should be allowed to fall below 2 μg/ml. Cellular casts in urine sediment are an early sign of impending nephrotoxicity; serum creatinine levels rise later. Gentamicin delays epithelial healing in corneal ulcers and may cause local irritation. Use with caution in birds as it is toxic. Monitor uric acid levels in birds and reptiles.

Drug interactions: Avoid the concurrent use of other nephrotoxic, ototoxic or neurotoxic agents (e.g. **amphotericin B**, **cisplatin**, **furosemide**). Increase monitoring and adjust dosages when these drugs must be used together. Aminoglycosides may be chemically inactivated by **beta-lactam antibiotics** (e.g. **penicillins**, **cephalosporins**) or **heparin** when mixed *in vitro*. The effect of non-depolarizing muscle relaxants (e.g. **atracurium**, **pancuronium**, **vecuronium**) may be enhanced by aminoglycosides. Synergism may occur when aminoglycosides are used with **penicillins** or **cephalosporin.**

Glibenclamide (Glibenclamide*) POM

Indications: Glibenclamide is a sulphonylurea that augments insulin secretion. It is indicated in the management of diabetes mellitus only where some residual pancreatic beta-cell activity is present.

Forms: *Oral:* 2.5 mg, 5 mg tablets.

Dose: *Dogs:* 0.2 mg/kg p.o. q24h. Adjust the dose until normoglycaemia is attained.

Adverse effects and contraindications: Hypoglycaemia and vomiting may develop. Its use is relatively contraindicated in cases of hepatic or renal impairment.

Glipizide (Glipizide*; Minodiab*) POM

Indications: Glipizide is a sulphonylurea that exerts hypoglycaemic effects by stimulating insulin secretion by the beta-cells of the pancreas and by improving tissue sensitivity to circulating insulin. It is used in the management of type II non-insulin-dependent diabetes mellitus, where there is some residual insulin production (beta-cell dysfunction). In these cases it may be effective alone or administered with insulin to reduce insulin requirements. It is ineffective when there is an absolute insulin deficiency or when insulin resistance is present.

Forms: *Oral:* 2.5 mg, 5 mg tablets.

Dose: *Cats:* 0.25–0.5 mg/kg p.o. q12h. Start at the lower end of the dose range, increasing the dose as required if no adverse effects are reported after 2 weeks. An effect on blood glucose may not be seen for 4–8 weeks. Administer with food.

Adverse effects and contraindications: Glipizide may cause GI disturbances, e.g. vomiting, and sensitivity reactions, e.g. jaundice, rashes, fever. Do not use if ketoacidosis present.

Drug interactions: The effects of glipizide may be enhanced by **ACE inhibitors**, **NSAIDs**, **chloramphenicol**, **potentiated sulphonamides** and **fluoroquinolones**.

Glucose (**Aqupharm No. 3, No. 18**; Dextrose monohydrate*; **Duphalyte**; Glucose*) *POM*

Indications: Dilute glucose solutions are used for fluid replacement (primarily where intracellular and interstitial losses have occurred). Concentrated glucose solutions are used parenterally as an energy source or in the treatment of hypoglycaemia. Patients requiring parenteral nutritional support will require mixtures comprising combinations of amino acid, glucose solutions and fat. *See also Amino acid solutions and Fat/Triglyceride preparations.*

Forms: *Injectable:* 4–50% sterile solutions in water or mixed with sodium chloride; 50% solutions contain 2 kcal/ml (8.4 kJ/ml) and are hypertonic (2525 mOsm/l).

Dose: *Cats, Dogs:*
- Fluid therapy: Fluid requirements depend upon the degree of dehydration and ongoing losses. In uncomplicated cases 5% dextrose, 5.5% dextrose/0.9% NaCl, or 4% dextrose/0.18% NaCl solutions should be administered at a dose of 50–60 ml/kg/day i.v. Higher doses may be required in dehydrated animals. *See Parenteral fluids table on page 294 for further details.*
- Parenteral nutrition: The amount required will be governed by the animal's physiological status and its ability to tolerate high blood glucose levels. Generally glucose is used to supply 40–60% of the energy requirement. Seek specialist advice before giving parenteral nutrition.
- Hypoglycaemia: 1–5 ml 50% dextrose i.v. slowly over 10 min.

Adverse effects and contraindications: 10–50% solutions are irritant; administer through a jugular catheter.

Glycerol (Glycerol*) *POM*

Indications: Glycerol acts as an osmotic diuretic and lowers intraocular pressure. It can be used in the management of acute glaucoma and is helpful for emergency home use although its use has been superceded by topical agents. Maximal reduction in pressure is seen approx 1 hour after dosing and will last for approx 5 hours. Glycerol is also used as a topical emollient and solvent, and as a laxative when given rectally in cats.

Forms:
Oral solution: 50% glycerol in 180 ml bottle.
Reagent grade 100% solution.

Dose:
Cats, Dogs: Acute glaucoma: 1–2 ml/kg p.o. as a single dose.
Cats: Laxative: 3 ml (100% solution) per rectum.

Adverse effects and contraindications: Adverse effects include vomiting and dehydration. Oral glycerol is contraindicated in diabetes mellitus, dehydration and suspected renal dysfunction. Renal function should be assessed before treatment as prerenal azotaemia or renal failure can result.

Glyceryl trinitrate (Glyceryl trinitrate*; Nitrocine*; Percutol*)
POM

Indications: Glyceryl trinitrate is a systemic vasodilator. Although a potent coronary vasodilator, its major benefit follows from a reduction in venous return as a consequence of venodilation. A decrease in venous return reduces left ventricular work. It is used in the short-term management of oedema (particularly acute pulmonary oedema) and to reduce ventricular filling pressures in animals with congestive cardiac failure.

Forms:
Topical: 2% ointment to be applied to skin (Percutol).
Oral: 2.6 mg, 6.4 mg, 10 mg modified-release tablets – longer acting tablets (Sustac).
Injectable: 500 μg/ml, 1 mg/ml, 5 mg/ml solutions (Glyceryl trinitrate, Nitrocine).

Dose:
Cats: 3–6 mm ($^1/_8$–$^1/_4$ inches) topically to the skin q6–8h; 5 μg/min i.v. infusion increasing in increments of 10–20 μg/min until an effect is reached; 2.6 mg p.o. q8–12h (modified-release tablets).
Dogs: 6–50 mm ($^1/_4$–2 inches) applied topically to the skin q6–8h; 5 μg/min i.v. infusion increasing in increments of 10–20 μg/min until an effect is reached; 2.6–6.4 mg p.o. q8–12h (modified-release tablets). Where it is used chronically for the management of heart failure (e.g. nocturnal dyspnoea) use q24h to avoid tolerance.

Caution: Owners should be cautioned to avoid contact with areas where the ointment has been applied and to wear non-permeable gloves when applying.

Adverse effects and contraindications: These include orthostatic hypotension (reduce dose), tachycardia and a rash at the site of application (rotate application sites). Suggested sites include the thorax, groin, or inside the ears. Rub ointment well into the skin. Tachyphylaxis can occur. Headaches are common in humans and may be an adverse effect in animals also.

Drug interactions: Concurrent use of **ACE inhibitors**, **anaesthetics**, **beta-blockers**, **calcium-channel blockers**, **corticosteroids** and **diuretics** may enhance the hypotensive effect. **NSAIDs** may antagonize its hypotensive effects.

Glycopyrronium bromide (Robinul*) *POM*

Indications: Glycopyrronium is a long-acting antimuscarinic (parasympatholytic) drug used pre-operatively to decrease oral and bronchial secretions and to inhibit vagal efferent activity. Its routine use for pre-anaesthetic medication is controversial. Glycopyrronium is used with long-acting anticholinesterase drugs, e.g. neostigmine, pyridostigmine, during antagonism of neuromuscular block. Glycopyrronium is longer acting than atropine and, being a quaternary ammonium compound, does not readily cross the blood–brain or placental barriers. This, in theory, limits the risk of adverse reactions in overdose.

Forms: *Injectable:* 200 μg/ml solution.

Dose:
Cats, Dogs:
- Premedication: 2–10 μg/kg i.v., i.m. 10–15 min prior to anaesthetic induction.
- Neuromuscular blockade antagonism: Glycopyrronium (10 μg/kg) with neostigmine (50 μg/kg).

Small mammals: Rabbits: 11 μg/kg i.v., i.m.

Adverse effects and contraindications: Adverse effects include sinus tachycardia, ventricular arrythmias, ileus, urinary retention and drying of bronchial secretions. The incidence of adverse effects is lower than that seen with atropine. Low doses may produce paradoxical bradycardia before the desired response supervenes.

Drug interactions: Glycopyrronium is physically compatible with the following: **atropine**, **5% dextrose**, **fentanyl**, **lidocaine**, **morphine**, **neostigmine**, **pethidine**, **pyridostigmine**, **Ringer's solution** and **0.9% sodium chloride**. When mixed with alkaline drugs (e.g. **barbiturates**) a precipitate may form. The adverse effects of antimuscarinics may be increased by **antihistamines**, **benzo-diazepines**, prolonged **corticosteroid** use (may increase intraocular pressure), **pethidine**, **phenothiazines**, **procainamide** and **quinidine**. Antimuscarinics may enhance the actions of **sympathomimetics** and **thiazide diuretics**. Antimuscarinics may antagonize the actions of **metoclopramide**.

Gonadotrophin releasing hormone (GnRH) – see Buserelin

Griseofulvin (Grisovin*) POM

Indications: Griseofulvin is a fungistatic antibiotic produced by *Penicillium* spp. It acts on susceptible fungi by disrupting the mitotic spindle, thereby arresting cell division in metaphase. Griseofulvin is active against *Trichophyton* spp., *Microsporum* spp. and *Epidermophyton* spp.

Forms: *Oral:* 125 mg, 500 mg tablets.

Dose:
Cats, Dogs: 15–30 mg/kg p.o. q24h.
Some texts recommend higher doses for cats and dogs (40–50 mg/kg daily). The duration required is usually 3–4 weeks but can be up to 12 weeks. To enhance absorption administer with 2.5–5 ml of corn oil or after a meal high in fat.
Small mammals: 25–30 mg/kg p.o. q24h.

Caution: Personnel should wear gloves when handling this product; women of child-bearing age should take particular care.

Adverse effects and contraindications: Adverse effects include GI distress, hypersensitivity reactions, decreased spermatogenesis, hepatotoxicity and, in cats, a leucopenia. Griseofulvin is teratogenic in cats and may be a teratogen in other animals; if possible avoid its use in pregnant animals. Tumours have developed in laboratory animals given griseofulvin long term.

Drug interactions: Barbiturates may accelerate the metabolism of griseofulvin.

Growth hormone – see Somatotropin

Haemoglobin glutamer-200 (bovine) (Oxyglobin) POM

Indications: This is an ultrapurified, polymerized haemoglobin of bovine origin in modified Ringer's lactate solution. It is isosmotic to blood and has a lower viscosity. It is indicated for the provision of oxygen carrying capacity and has been shown to be of benefit in anaemic dogs regardless of cause (e.g. haemorrhage, haemolysis etc.). It has an intravascular half-life of 30–40 hours in healthy dogs. Because there is no red cell membrane, pre-treatment compatibility testing is not required. The effect of repeated dosing is unknown. It has a long shelf life (>2 years). The product is not licensed for use in cats.

Forms: *Injectable:* 130 mg/ml solution in a 125 ml oxygen-impermeable delivery bag. Discard after 24 hours even if stored in a fridge as it has no preservative and slow oxygenation results in methaemoglobin formation.

Dose:
Cats: 5–10 ml/kg i.v. at a rate of 0.5–1ml/kg/h.
Dogs: 30 ml/kg i.v. at a rate of 0.5–3 ml/kg/h.

Adverse effects and contraindications: Rapid administration to normovolaemic animals could result in hypervolaemia. The solution causes a discoloration of plasma (red, brown) and mucous membranes, sclera, urine and skin (yellow, brown or red). Vomiting, diarrhoea and fever have been reported. There is an increase in plasma total protein and haemoglobin that can artefactually change derived red cell indices on blood screens. Increased liver enzymes have been noted in toxicity trials in Beagles. Haemoglobinuria is expected and significant urine discoloration can interfere with other colorimetric changes on dipsticks. The package insert contains notes of known interferences with clinical chemistry analysers. Ideally obtain all diagnostic blood and urine samples before administration. The product is not licensed for use in cats. Use with caution in animals with advanced heart disease or renal impairment (oliguria/anuria) as it can cause volume overload. The main complication in cats is volume overload, leading to pulmonary oedema and pleural effusions; partly due to its potent colloid osmotic effects (slightly better than those of hetastarch) but probably also due to its nitric oxide-scavenging properties leading to vasoconstriction.

Drug interactions: Avoid concomitant administration with other **plasma-volume expanders**. The manufacturer states that no other medications should be added to the infusion line whilst oxyglobin is being administered. No specific interactions are yet reported.

Halothane (Fluothane; Halothane) *POM*

Indications: Halothane is a volatile halogenated hydrocarbon, suitable for the induction and maintenance of anaesthesia for all types of surgery and in all species, irrespective of age. Halothane is potent and highly volatile, and so should only be delivered from a suitable, calibrated vaporizer.

Forms: 250 ml bottle.

Dose: *Cats, Dogs, Small mammals, Reptiles:* The *expired* concentration of halothane required to maintain surgical anaesthesia in 50% of recipients is about 0.8–1.0% in animals, but does depend on other drugs used (*see **Drug interactions,** below*). Even though halothane is more soluble in blood compared with isoflurane, changes in vaporizer setting rapidly alters the 'level of anaesthesia' and the cessation of administration results in rapid recovery.

Adverse effects and contraindications: Halothane causes dose-dependent hypotension through depression of heart rate and myocardial contractility, although these adverse effects wane with time. Respiratory depression is also dose-dependent. Halothane facilitates the generation of ventricular arrhythmias in the presence of other arrhythmogenic factors, e.g. catecholamines, hypoxia, hypercapnia. Halothane crosses the placental barrier and will affect neonates delivered by caesarean operation.

Drug interactions: Opioid agonists, **benzodiazepines** and **N$_2$O** reduce the concentration of halothane required to achieve surgical anaesthesia.

Hartmann's solution – see Lactated Ringer's solution

Heparin (Heparin*) POM

Indications: Heparin is an anticoagulant that exerts its effects primarily by enhancing the binding of anti-thrombin III (AT III) to factors IIa, IXa, Xa, XIa and XIIa; it is only effective if adequate AT III is present. The AT III/clotting factor complex is subsequently removed by the liver. Heparin inactivates thrombin and blocks the conversion of fibrinogen to fibrin. The inhibition of factor XII activation prevents the formation of stable fibrin clots. Heparin does not significantly change the concentrations of clotting factors, nor does it lyse pre-existing clots. Heparin's uses in small animal medicine include the treatment of DIC and thromboembolic disease, and the maintenance of i.v. catheter patency. Its use in DIC is controversial. Uncontrolled case series in man claim success whereas a benificial effect has not been shown in controlled clinical trials.

Forms: Heparin sodium 1,000–25,000 IU/ml solutions.

Dose: *Cats, Dogs:*
• Treatment of DIC: 100–200 IU/kg i.v. initially; may repeat in 4 hours, then adjust dose prn and repeat s.c. q8h. It is only effective if sufficient AT III is present; provision of fresh or frozen plasma is required in AT III-deficient animals for heparin to be effective. For the successful treatment of DIC, heparin therapy is only one aspect. Addressing the precipitating cause, administration of fluids, fresh whole blood, aspirin and diligent monitoring of coagulation tests (APTT, OSPT), fibrin degradation products and fibrinogen are all important factors.

- Treatment of thromboembolic disease: 100–200 IU/kg i.v. as a loading dose, followed by 200–300 IU/kg s.c. q6–8h; adjust dosage so that the APTT is 1.5–2.5 times normal.
  Note: The doses of heparin are controversial, with some texts recommending lower or higher doses or the use of constant i.v. infusions.
- For maintaining catheter patency: 1250 IU in 100 ml water for injection.

Adverse effects and contraindications: If an overdosage occurs protamine can be used as an antidote *(see Protamine sulphate)*. Heparin should not be administered i.m. as it may result in haematoma formation. Its use in DIC may worsen haemorrhage and some texts indicate it is contraindicated where DIC is due to sepsis. Heparin-induced thrombocytopenia is a concern.

Drug interactions: Use with caution with other drugs that can cause changes in coagulation status (e.g. **aspirin**, **NSAIDs**, **warfarin**). Heparin may antagonize **ACTH**, **corticosteroids** or **insulin**. Heparin may increase plasma levels of **diazepam**. The actions of heparin may be partially counteracted by **antihistamines**, **digoxin** and **tetracyclines**. Do not mix other drugs in the same syringe as heparin.

Hetastarch – see Etherified starch

Hexamine hippurate – see Methenamine hippurate

Hyaluronate (VisLube*) *POM*

Indications: Sodium hyaluronate is a viscoelastic fluid with mucomimetic properties. It is used as a tear replacement and is beneficial for the management of keratoconjunctivitis sicca. It has longer corneal contact time than the aqueous tear substitutes.

Forms: *Topical:* 0.18% solution in single use vials.

Dose: *Cats, Dogs:* 1 drop/eye q4–6h, although it can be used hourly if required.

Adverse effects and contraindications: It is tolerated well and ocular irritation is unusual.

Hydralazine (Hydralazine*) *POM*

Indications: Hydralazine acts directly on arteriolar smooth muscle causing vasodilation; it is able to decrease systemic vascular resistance to about 50% of the baseline value. Thus the effects of hydralazine are to reduce afterload, and increase heart rate, stroke volume and cardiac output. It is particularly used to treat congestive heart failure in dogs secondary to mitral value insufficiency. It can be used to treat systemic hypertension, although not typically as a first-line drug.

Forms: 25 mg, 50 mg tablets.

Dose:
Cats: 2.5–10 mg/cat p.o. q12h.
Dogs: 0.5–3 mg/kg p.o. q8–12h.

Start at low doses and titrate upwards.

Adverse effects and contraindications: Adverse effects include reflex tachycardia, severe hypotension (monitor and adjust doses as necessary), anorexia and vomiting (the latter two effects commonly seen in cats). As hydralazine may activate the renin–angiotensin–aldosterone system, concomitant use of diuretic therapy, ACE inhibitors and/or salt restriction is often necessary. Caution in hypovolaemic and hypotensive patients or those with renal impairment or intracerebral bleeding.

Drug interactions: The hypotensive effects of hydralazine may be enhanced by **ACE inhibitors** (e.g. **enalapril**), **anaesthetics**, **beta-blockers** (e.g. **propranolol**), **calcium-channel blockers** (e.g. **diltiazem**, **verapamil**), **corticosteroids**, **diuretics** and **NSAIDs**. **Sympathomimetics** (e.g. **phenylpropanolamine**) may cause an additive tachycardia.

Hydrochlorothiazide (Co-amilozide*) *POM*

Indications: Hydrochlorothiazide is a thiazide diuretic that acts on the proximal portion of the distal convoluted tubule to inhibit resorption of sodium and cause secretion of potassium. It has an onset of action of 2 hours, peak activity after 4 hours and a duration of 12 hours. Hydrochlorothiazide is indicated in the management of ascites, pleural effusion, oedema and hypertension. It is formulated with a potassium-sparing diuretic (amiloride) and may be useful where compliance is a problem.

Forms: *Oral:* 25 mg hydrochlorothiazide with 2.5 mg amiloride and 50 mg hydrochlorothiazide with 5 mg amiloride tablets.

Dose:
Cats: 12.5 mg i.m. or 2–4 mg/kg p.o. q12h with a salt-restricted diet.
Dogs: 12.5–25 mg i.m. or 1–5 mg/kg p.o. q12h with a salt-restricted diet.

Adverse effects and contraindications: Adverse effects include hyperglycaemia, hypokalaemia, hyponatraemia and volume contraction. It enhances the effects of the renin–angiotensin–aldosterone system in heart failure. The use of hydrochlorothiazide is contraindicated in animals with renal impairment as it tends to reduce renal blood flow.

Drug interactions: There is an increased possibility of hypokalaemia developing if thiazides are used concomitantly with **corticosteroids** or loop diuretics (**furosemide**). Thiazide-induced hypokalaemia may increase the risk of **digoxin** toxicity. Thus, potassium therapy may be necessary during prolonged administration. The concurrent administration of **Vitamin D** or **calcium salts** with thiazides may exacerbate hypercalcaemia.

Hydrocortisone (Hydrocortisone*; **Hydrocortisone and Neomycin**; Hydrocortone*; Solu-cortef*; **Vetodale**) *POM*

Indications: Hydrocortisone is a corticosteroid used in veterinary medicine as an anti-inflammatory drug, in the management of hypoadrenocorticism and in the treatment of shock. It has only 1/4 the glucocorticoid potency of prednisolone and 1/30 that of dexamethasone. On a dose basis 4 mg of hydrocortisone is equivalent to 1 mg prednisolone.

Forms:
Topical: 0.5%, 1% cream and 1% solution (Hydrocortisone). It is also a constituent of many veterinary licensed mixed topical preparations.
Injectable: 25 mg/ml solution; 100 mg, 500 mg powder for reconstitution (Solu-cortef).
Oral: 10 mg, 20 mg tablets (Hydrocortone).

Dose: *Cats, Dogs:*
• Topically: Apply to affected area q6–12h.
• Hypoadrenocorticism: 2–4 mg/kg i.v., i.m. in acute Addisonian crisis and 0.125 mg/kg p.o. q12h for maintenance.
• Anti-inflammatory, shock: 1–10 mg/kg i.v., 5–10 mg/kg i.m., 0.5 mg/kg p.o. q12h.

Caution: Wear gloves when applying topically as the cream is absorbed through skin.

Adverse effects and contraindications: Prolonged use of glucocorticoids suppresses the hypothalamic–pituitary axis (HPA) and cause adrenal atrophy. Animals on chronic therapy should be tapered off steroids when discontinuing the drug (even following topical administration). Catabolic effects of glucocorticoids leads to weight loss and cutaneous atrophy. Iatrogenic hyperadrenocorticism may develop (PU/PD, elevated liver enzymes). Vomiting and diarrhoea, or GI ulceration may develop. Glucocorticoids may increase urine glucose levels and decrease serum T3 and T4 values. Do not use in pregnant animals. Systemic corticosteroids are generally contraindicated in patients with renal disease and diabetes mellitus. Impaired wound healing and delayed recovery from infections may be seen.

Drug interactions: There is an increased risk of GI ulceration if used concurrently with **NSAIDs**. Glucocorticoids antagonize the effect of **insulin**. **Anti-epileptic** drugs (**phenobarbital, primidone**) may accelerate the metabolism of corticosteroids. There is an increased risk of hypokalaemia when corticosteroids are used with **acetazolamide, amphotericin** and **potassium depleting diuretics** (**furosemide, thiazides**).

Hydroxocobalamin – see Vitamin B12

Hydroxycarbamide (Hydroxyurea) (Hydrea*) POM

Indications: Hydroxycarbamide, a ribonucleotide reductase inhibitor, is used in the treatment of polycythaemia vera and chronic granulocytic leukaemia.

Forms: *Oral:* 500 mg tablet.

Dose:
Cats: 10 mg/kg p.o. q12h for 3 days per week until haematology is normal.
Dogs: 50 mg/kg p.o. q24h for 1–2 weeks then q48h, or 80 mg/kg p.o. q3d or 1 g/m² p.o. q24h until haematology is normal.

Once in remission, reduce dosage frequency as required to maintain remission.

Adverse effects and contraindications: Adverse effects include myelosuppression, nausea and skin reactions. Monitor haematological parameters at regular intervals.

Hydroxyzine (Atarax*; Ucerax*) POM

Indications: Hydroxyzine is a piperazine H_1 antihistamine that has a central depressant activity. It is used to manage animals with pruritus or psychogenic dermatoses, including feather plucking in birds.

Forms: *Oral:* 10 mg, 25 mg tablets.

Dose:
Cats, Dogs: 2.2 mg/kg p.o. q8h.
Birds: 2.2 mg/kg p.o. q8h.

Adverse effects and contraindications: Sedation may occasionally be seen. Occasional idiopathic polydipsia may occur.

Hyoscine – see Butylscopolamine

Hypromellose (Hypromellose*; Isopto alkaline*; Isopto plain*) *P*

Indications: Hypromellose is a cellulose tear substitute (lacromimetic) used for lubrication of dry eyes. In cases of KCS (dry eye) it will improve ocular surface lubrication, tear retention and patient comfort while lacrostimulation therapy (e.g. topical ciclosporin) is initiated. It may also be used as a vehicle base for compounding ophthalmic drugs.

Forms: *Ocular:* 0.3%, 0.5%, 1% solutions in 10 ml dropper bottle.

Dose: *Cats, Dogs, Small mammals, Birds:* 1 drop/eye q60min. Note: Patient compliance is poor if >q4h, consider using a longer acting tear replacement.

Ibafloxacin (Ibaflin) *POM*

Indications: Ibafloxacin is a fluoroquinolone antimicrobial agent with a broad spectrum of activity. It is bactericidal by inhibiting DNA gyrase. Its action is concentration-dependent, particularly against Gram-negative bacteria; pulse dosing regimens may be effective. It is active against mycoplasmas, many Gram-negative organisms and some Gram-positive organisms including *Pasteurella* spp., *Staphylococcus* spp., *Pseudomonas aeruginosa*, *Klebsiella* spp., *Escherichia coli*, *Proteus* spp. and *Salmonella* spp. It is effective against beta-lactamase-producing bacteria but ineffective against obligate anaerobes. It is highly lipophilic, attaining high concentrations within cells in many tissues and is particularly effective in the management of soft tissue, urogenital (including prostatic) and skin infections. Ibafloxacin is specifically authorized for the treatment of acute uncomplicated bacterial cystitis due to susceptible strains of *E. coli* and *Proteus spp., Enterobacter spp.* and *Klebsiella spp.*, for the treatment of pyoderma caused by susceptible strains of *Staphylococcus*, *E. coli* and *Proteus*, for the management of soft tissue infections and of upper respiratory tract infections.

Forms: *Oral:* 15 mg, 300 mg tablets.

Dose: *Dogs:* 15 mg/kg p.o. q 24h.

Adverse effects and contraindications: Cartilage abnormalities have been reported following the use of other fluoroquinolones in growing animals. Such abnormalities have not been specifically reported following the use of ibafloxacin. Some animals may show GI signs following use of fluoroquinolones (nausea, vomiting, diarrhoea or soft faeces). It should be used with caution in epileptics until further information is available from dogs, as fluoroquinolones potentiate CNS adverse effects when administered concurrently with NSAIDs in man. Ibafloxacin is specifically contraindicated for use in combination with NSAIDs. Caution should be exercised before using dose rates above those recommended by the manufacturer. The potential adverse effects of ibafloxacin on the canine retina have not been studied (*see enrofloxacin*).

Drug interactions: Absorbents and **antacids** containing cations (**Mg^{2+}**, **Al^{3+}**) may bind fluoroquinolones, preventing their absorption from the GI tract. The absorption of fluoroquinolones may be inhibited by **sucralfate** and **zinc salts**; separate doses of these drugs by at least 2 hours. **Cimetidine** may reduce the clearance of fluoroquinolones and so should be used with caution with these drugs. Antagonism may be observed with **nitrofurantoin**. As stated above, the use of **NSAIDs** in combination with ibafloxacin is contraindicated.

Imidacloprid (**Advantage**; **Advantix**) *POM*

Indications: Imidacloprid is used in the management of flea infestations. Regular treatment reduces the incidence of flea allergy dermatitis.

Forms: 40 mg, 80 mg solutions for cats; 40 mg, 100 mg, 250 mg and 400 mg pipettes for dogs.

Dose:
Cats, Rabbits: <4 kg 40 mg/animal; >4 kg 80 mg/animal.
Dogs: <4 kg 40 mg/dog; 4–10 kg 100 mg/dog; 10–<25 kg 250 mg/dog; 25–<40 kg 400 mg/dog; ≥40 kg 800 mg/dog.
Part hair and apply directly to bare undamaged skin at the base of the skull in cats and rabbits, and between the shoulder blades in dogs. Where 2 pipettes are required apply contents of both pipettes evenly in 3 or 4 different sites along the spine. Do not rub in.

Adverse effects and contraindications: The product is bitter tasting and salivation will be seen if the product is licked or ingested. Do not use on animals <8 weeks old.

Imidapril (Prilium) *POM*

Indications: Imidapril is a pro-drug, which is hydrolysed to form an active metabolite imidoprilat. Imidoprilat inhibits angiotensin-converting enzymes, thereby inhibiting conversion of angiotensin I to angiotenisn II. Angiotensin II, a potent vasopressor, stimulates release of aldosterone and vasopressin, facilitates the central and peripheral effects of the sympathetic nervous system and preserves the glomerular filtration rate. Inhibiting angiotensin II production results in veno- and arteriodilation, which leads to decreased preload and afterload, and lowered blood pressure. Imidapril reduces salt and water retention. It is used in the management of CHF and hypertension. The liquid formulation may make it easier to administer to cats than enalapril, although it is not licensed for use in this species.

Forms: *Oral:* 150 mg, 300 mg powder for reconstitution as oral solution. Tap water can be used to reconstitute the solution.

Dose: *Cats, Dogs:* 0.25 mg/kg p.o. q24h with or without food.

Adverse effects and contraindications: Hypotension, renal impairment, hyperkalaemia, diarrhoea, fatigue, anorexia and hypotension are potential adverse effects. Do not use imidapril in animals with acute renal failure, congenital heart disease, haemodynamically relevant stenoses (e.g. aortic stenosis), obstructive hypertrophic cardiomyopathy or hypovolaemia. If hypotension should develop administer normal saline.

Drug interactions: There is a risk of hyperkalaemia developing if imidapril is used with **NSAIDs**, **potassium sparing diuretics** and **potassium** supplementation. The concurrent use of **diuretics**, **vasodilators** or **low sodium** diets with imidapril may result in hypotension.

Imidocarb dipropionate (Imizol*) *POM*

Indications: Imidocarb dipropionate is used in the treatment of *Babesia canis* infection in dogs.

Forms: *Injectable:* 85 mg/ml solution.

Dose: *Dogs:* 6.6 mg/kg i.m., s.c. once, repeated in 2–3 weeks.

Adverse effects and contraindications: Do not administer i.v. The safety and effectiveness of imidocarb have not been determined in puppies or in breeding, lactating or pregnant animals. Cholinergic signs (e.g. salivation, vomiting and occasionally diarrhoea, panting, restlessness) may develop after dosing. These may be alleviated by **atropine**. Mild injection site inflammation lasting one to several days and which may ulcerate has been reported. Anaphylactoid reactions have been reported in cattle but not in dogs.

Immunoglobulins – see Antibacterial immunoglobulin, Antivenom, Tetanus antitoxin

Insulin (**Caninsulin**; Humulin*; Hypurin*; Insulatard*; **Insuvet**; Monotard*; Semitard*) POM

Indications: Insulin is used to treat insulin-dependent diabetes mellitus (IDDM) and as adjunctive therapy in the management of hyperkalaemia. There are various types of insulin. Neutral (soluble) insulin is the normal crystalline form. Isophane (NPH) contains protamine, which increases the duration of activity. The lente insulins rely on different concentrations of zinc and sizes of zinc–insulin crystals to provide different durations of activity. Of the lente type insulins, semilente (amorphous insulin zinc suspension) is the shortest acting, whilst ultralente (crystalline insulin zinc suspension) is longer acting. Lente insulin comprises a mixture of semilente and ultralente insulins.

Forms: *Injectable:* 40 IU/ml, 100 IU/ml suspensions (for s.c. injection) or 100 IU/ml soluble (for i.v. or i.m. injection).
When using in animals preference should be given to veterinary licensed products. There are many more products licensed for use in man than those listed above. Where a veterinary licensed product proves unsuitable, a human product can be considered. The tables below list the various forms.

Type		Onset	Max effect		Duration	
			Dog (hours)	Cat (hours)	Dog (hours)	Cat (hours)
Soluble (neutral)	i.v.	Immediate	0.5–2	0.5–2	1–4	1–4
	i.m.	10–30 min	1–4	1–4	3–8	3–8
	s.c.	10–30 min	1–5	1–5	4–8	4–8
Semilente (amorphous IZS)	s.c.	30–60 min	1–5	1–5	4–10	4–10
Isophane (NPH)	s.c.	0.5–3 h	2–10	2–8	6–24	4–12
Lente (mixed IZS)	s.c.	30–60 min	2–10	2–8	8–24	6–14
Ultralente (crystalline IZS)	s.c.	2–8 h	4–16	4–16	8–28	8–24
PZI	s.c.	1–4 h	4–14	3–12	6–28	6–24

IZS = insulin zinc suspension
NPH = neutral protamine Hagedorn
PZI = protamine zinc insulin

Insulin	Species of insulin	Types available
Caninsulin	Porcine	Lente
Insuvet	Bovine	Neutral, Lente, PZI
Humulin	Human	Neutral, Isophane, Lente, Ultralente
Hypurin	Bovine	Neutral, Isophane, Lente, Ultralente, PZI
Semitard	Porcine	Semilente
Insulatard	Human or porcine	Isophane
Ultratard	Human	Ultralente

Dose:
Cats: IDDM: Initially 0.25 IU/kg of PZI s.c. q12–24h. Adjust dose by monitoring blood glucose and/or fructosamine levels.
Dogs: IDDM: Initially 0.25–0.5 IU/kg (dogs >25 kg) or 0.5–1 IU/kg (dogs <25 kg) of lente, isophane or PZI insulin s.c. q24h. If the insulin does not give 24 hour coverage, either administer q12h or use a longer acting type of insulin. Adjust dose by monitoring blood glucose and/or fructosamine.
Cats, Dogs:
- Diabetic ketoacidosis: Infuse 0.025–0.06 IU/kg/h of soluble insulin. Run approximately 50 ml of i.v. solution through tubing as insulin adheres to glass and plastic; change insulin/saline solution q6h, or 0.2 IU/kg soluble insulin i.m. initially followed by 0.1 IU/kg i.m. q1h. Monitor blood glucose and ketones q2h if possible.
- Hyperkalaemic myocardial toxicity: Give a bolus of 0.5 IU/kg of soluble insulin i.v. followed by 2–3 g of dextrose/unit of insulin. Half the dextrose should be given as a bolus and the remainder administered i.v. over 4–6 h. Avoid hypoglycaemia. Patients with adrenocortical insufficiency may be susceptible to the hypoglycaemic effects of insulin.

Adverse effects and contraindications: Overdosage results in hypoglycaemia.

Drug interactions: Corticosteroids, thiazide diuretics and **thyroid hormones** may antagonize the hypoglycaemic effects of insulin. **Anabolic steroids, beta-adrenergic blockers** (e.g. **propranolol**), **ethanol, phenylbutazone, salicylates** and **tetracycline** may increase insulin's effect. Insulin can affect serum potassium levels. Therefore, administer with caution and monitor patients closely if **digoxin** is given concurrently.

Interferon alfa (Intron A*; Roferon A*; Viraferon*) *POM*

Indications: Interferon alfa has been used in the management of herpes keratitis and dendritic keratitis in the cat. Interferons are proteins that have a complex effect on immunity and cell function.

Forms: *Injectable:* 10 million units vial of powder for reconstitution; 6–36 million units/ml solution.

Dose: *Cats:* Ophthalmic: 1 drop/eye q6–8h of a 200–50,000 units/ml solution. Reconstitute vial or use solution and dilute in hypromellose to obtain a 3000 units/ml solution (take vial containing 3×10^6 units powder and reconstitute in 0.5 ml sterile saline. Dilute 50 μl (microlitres) of the resulting solution in 5 ml hypromellose). This can be stored for up to 14 days. If products with different concentrations are used the dilutions will be different. Apply 1 drop four times a day to the affected eye until resolution is seen.

Adverse effects and contraindications: If ocular irritation occurs, use a lower concentration.

Interferon omega (Virbagen omega) *POM*

Indications: The exact mechanism of action of interferon omega is not known but it is thought to enhance the non-specific defence of the body. It has been shown to reduce mortality and clinical signs of the enteric form of parvovirus in dogs. Interferon omega has been used topically in the management of ocular herpes keratitis in cats. Although used frequently with beneficial results, there is limited clinical data as to its efficacy in treating ocular disease.

Forms: *Injectable:* 5×10^6 IU, 10×10^6 units/vial powder and solvent for suspension and injection.

Dose:
Cats: (ophthalmic use): 1 drop/eye q6h of a 200–50,000 units/ml solution. Doses, protocols and storage information are anecdotal and vary widely.
Dogs: 2.5×10^6 units/kg body weight i.v. once daily for 3 consecutive days.

Adverse effects and contraindications: Hyperthermia 3–6 hours after injection has been reported. Vomiting and transient slight myelosuppression may be seen.

Drug interactions: Do not use concurrently with **vaccines**.

Iodine-containing contrast media (Conray[1]*; Gastrografin[2]*; Gastromiro[5]*; Hexabrix[1]*; Iomeron[5]*; Isovist[2]*; Niopam[5]*; Omnipaque[4]*; Optiray[1]*; Oxilan[3]*; Scanlux[6]*; Ultravist[2]*; Urografin[2]*; Visipaque[4]*) *POM*

Indications: Iodine-containing contrast media (ICM) are positive contrast agents that appear radiopaque on radiographs. They are water-soluble monomers or dimers of tri-iodinated benzoic acid, provided as ionic and non-ionic forms. Both forms may be used for i.v. urography, contrast studies of the lower urinary tract, angiography, arthrography, sino- or fistulography, sialography or dacryocystography.

Specific formulations are also available for contrast studies of the GI tract, and these should only be used for this purpose. Only non-ionic forms should be used for myelography, but note that not all non-ionic forms are licensed for this purpose in man.

Forms: *Injectable:* Produced in a variety of concentrations (see Table). Manufacturers: [1] Mallinkrodt Medical; [2] Schering Health Care; [3] Guerbet Laboratories; [4] Amersham Health; [5] Bracco; [6] Sanochemia U.K.

Constituent	Properties	Trade name	Spinal	Vascular, urinary	GI	Formulations (mg iodine/ml)
Iothalamic acid	Ionic	Conray[1]	–	+	–	141, 202, 282, 400
Sodium meglumine diatrizoate	Ionic	Urografin[2]	–	+	–	146, 292, 370
Sodium meglumine diatrizoate	Ionic	Gastrografin[2]	–	–	+	370
Sodium meglumine ioxaglate	Ionic, Low osmolar	Hexabrix[1]	–	+	–	320
Iohexol	Non-ionic, Low osmolar	Omnipaque[4]	+	+	–	140, 180, 200, 240, 300, 350
Iomeprol	Non-ionic, Low osmolar	Iomeron[5]	+	+	–	150, 200, 250 300, 350, 400
Iopamidol	Non-ionic, Low osmolar	Niopam[5] Scanlux[6]	+	+	–	150, 200, 300, 340, 370 300, 340, 370
Iopamidol	Non-ionic, Low osmolar	Gastromiro[5]	–	–	+	300
Iopromide	Non-ionic, Low osmolar	Ultravist[2]	–	+	–	150, 240, 300, 370
Iodixanol	Non-ionic, Isosmolar	Visipaque[4]	–	+	–	270, 320
Iotrolan	Non-ionic, Isosmolar	Isovist[2]	+	–	(–)[a]	190, 240, 300
Ioxilan	Non-ionic Low osmolar	Oxilan[3]	–	+	–	300, 350
Ioversol	Non-ionic Low osmolar	Optiray[1]	–	+	–	160, 240, 300, 320, 350

a Isovist is intended for myelography. However, it may also, according to the manufacturer's data sheet, be used in body cavities, for arthrography, or for GI use.

Dose: Depends on the contrast examination being performed. Readers are referred to standard radiography texts for details of procedures.

Adverse effects and contraindications: Adverse effects may be seen with any ICM, although the risk is greater with ionic than with non-ionic media. Within the group of ionic ICM, the risk of side-effects is less with Hexabrix, which is low osmolar. Adverse effects reported in man to be associated with i.v. injection of ICM include nausea and vomiting, hypotension, dyspnoea, erythema or urticaria, sensation of heat, cardiac rate or rhythm disturbances, and anaphylactic shock. Seizures or transient motor or sensory dysfunction have been reported in man following myelography. Use of ICM for GI studies in man have resulted in osmotic diarrhoea, dehydration and hypotension. Aspiration of ICM may result in pulmonary oedema. Similar adverse effects have been reported in animals; treatment should be symptomatic. ICM are contraindicated in patients with known or suspected hypersensitivity to iodine-containing preparations of this type. They should be used with care in patients with moderate to severe impairment of renal function, since the main route of excretion is via the kidneys. Abnormalities of fluid or electrolyte balance should be corrected before use. When used intravascularly, catheters should be flushed regularly to minimize the risk of clotting; non-ionic media have less anti-coagulant activity *in vitro* than the ionic preparations.

Drug interactions: In man, the capacity of thyroid tissue to take up iodine has been shown to be decreased for 2 weeks, and sometimes up to 6 weeks, after administration of ICM. Consequently this may affect the use of **iodine** isotopes for the treatment of thyroid disease. In man it has been established that hypersensitivity reactions can be aggravated in patients on **beta-blockers**.

Ipecacuanha (Paediatric ipecacuanha*) *P*

Indications: Ipecacuanha is used to induce emesis.

Forms: *Oral:* 0.7 ml per 10 ml syrup.

Dose: *Cats, Dogs:* 1–2 ml/kg p.o. This equates to 0.07–0.14 ml of ipecacuanha extract per kg. Maximum dose 15 ml of syrup. Allow patient to drink water. Can repeat after 20 minutes if necessary.

Adverse effects and contraindications: Induction of vomiting is contraindicated if the dog is unconscious, fitting, or has a reduced cough reflex, or if the poison has been ingested for more than 2 hours, or if the ingesta contain paraffin, petroleum products or other oily or volatile organic products, due to the risk of inhalation. Induction of emesis is contraindicated if strong acid or alkali has been ingested, due to the risk of further damage to the oesophagus. Ipecacuanha may have a variety of cardiac effects if absorbed.

Drug interactions: Ipecacuanha reduces the effectiveness of **activated charcoal**; do not use together.

Iron (CosmoFer*; Ferrous sulphate*) *PML*

Indications: Iron is used to treat iron-deficiency anaemia associated with iron-deficient diets (rare) or chronic haemorrhage (e.g. GI haemorrhage).

Forms:
Injectable: 50 mg/ml iron dextran (CosmoFer).
Oral: 200 mg $FeSO_4$ tablet (Ferrous sulphate).

Dose:
Cats: 25 mg/kg i.m. weekly prn or 50–100 mg/cat p.o. q24h.
Dogs: 25 mg/kg i.m. weekly prn or 100–300 mg/dog p.o. q24h.
Birds: 10 mg/kg i.m. of iron dextran.

Adverse effects and contraindications: The oral route should be used. The only valid reason for administering iron parenterally is failure of oral therapy due to severe GI adverse effects, continuing severe blood loss or iron malabsorption. Modified release preparations should be avoided as they are ineffective. Iron is absorbed in the duodenum and the release of iron from modified release preparations occurs lower down the GI tract. Parenteral iron may cause arrhythmias, anaphylaxis, shunting of iron to reticuloendothelial stores and iron overload. Its use is contraindicated in patients with hepatic, renal (particularly pyelonephritis) or cardiac disease, and untreated urinary tract infections. Oral iron may cause nausea, vomiting, constipation and diarrhoea.

Isoflurane (Isocare; Isofane; Isoflo; Isoflurane Vet; Vetflurane) *POM*

Indications: Isoflurane, a volatile halogenated ether, is suitable for the induction and maintenance of anaesthesia for all types of surgery and in all species, irrespective of age. Isoflurane is potent and highly volatile, and so should only be delivered from a suitable, calibrated vaporizer.

Forms: 100 ml bottle.

Dose: *Cats, Dogs, Small mammals, Birds, Reptiles:* The *expired* concentration of isoflurane required to maintain surgical anaesthesia in 50% of recipients is about 1.4% in animals, but depends to a large part on other drugs used (*see Drug interactions*). Isoflurane is less soluble in blood than halothane and so changes in vaporizer setting cause more rapid changes in the 'level of anaesthesia', provided other physiological variables remain constant. The cessation of administration results in rapid recovery. Isoflurane crosses the placental barrier and will affect neonates delivered by caesarean operation. The duration of action of non-depolarizing neuromuscular blocking agents is longer in isoflurane, compared with halothane-anaesthetized animals.

Adverse effects and contraindications: Isoflurane has a pungent smell and induction to anaesthesia using chambers or masks may be less well tolerated in small dogs and cats compared to halothane. Isoflurane causes dose-dependent hypotension by causing vasodilation, particularly in skeletal muscle. This adverse effect does not wane with time. Isoflurane is a more potent respiratory depressant than halothane; respiratory depression is also dose-dependent. Isoflurane does not 'sensitize' the myocardium to catecholamines to the extent that halothane does, but can generate cardiac arrythmias in certain conditions. Assertions that isoflurane is safer than halothane in certain 'high–risk' cases should be discounted.

Drug interactions: Opioid agonists, **benzodiazepines** and **N₂O** reduce the concentration of halothane required to achieve surgical anaesthesia.

Isosorbide dinitrate (Cedocard*; Isoket*; Isosorbide*) *POM*

Indications: Isosorbide dinitrate, a nitrate that acts as a venous dilator, is used in the treatment of pulmonary oedema associated with congestive heart failure and mitral regurgitation. It may be beneficial in cases of right-sided congestive heart failure to help reduce ascites and pleural effusion (in combination with standard heart failure medication).

Forms:
Injectable: 1 mg/ml solution for i.v. use (Isoket).
Oral: 5 mg, 10 mg, 20 mg, 40 mg tablets.

Dose:
Cats: 2.5 mg/cat p.o. q12h.
Dogs: 0.1–1 mg/kg p.o. q8–12h.

Adverse effects and contraindications: Adverse effects include hypotension and tachycardia. *See also Glyceryl trinitrate.*

Isotretinoin – see Vitamin A

Itraconazole (Sporanox*) POM

Indications: Itraconazole is a triazole antifungal agent. It inhibits the cytochrome systems involved in the synthesis of ergosterol in fungal cell membranes, causing increased cell wall permeability and allowing leakage of cellular contents. It has a greater selectivity for fungal cytochrome-dependent enzymes than does ketoconazole. Itraconazole is effective in treating aspergillosis, candidiasis, blastomycosis, coccidioidomycosis, cryptococcosis, histoplasmosis and dermatophytosis. It has been used successfully to treat ringworm in Persian cats without the need for clipping. It is widely distributed in the body, although low concentrations are found in tissues with low protein contents, e.g. CSF, ocular fluid and saliva.

Forms: *Oral:* 100 mg capsule; 10 mg/ml solution.

Dose:
Cats, Dogs: 5 mg/kg p.o. q24h. 4–20 weeks of treatment may be needed, dependent upon culture results.
Birds: 10 mg/kg p.o. q12h. Note: It is not well tolerated by African Grey parrots.

Adverse effects and contraindications: Itraconazole is better tolerated than ketoconazole in dogs and cats due to its greater selectivity for fungal cytochrome P450-dependent systems. Blockade of mammalian steroid synthesis does not occur at recommended therapeutic doses. Adverse effects include anorexia, nausea, abdominal pain and hepatic toxicosis; avoid its use if liver disease is present. Drug eruption, ulcerative dermatitis and limb oedema have been reported. Itraconazole is contraindicated in pregnancy. It has a narrow safety margin in birds and should be discontinued if emesis or anorexia occurs.

Drug interactions: Antacids, omeprazole, H_2 antagonists and adsorbents may reduce the absorption of itraconazole. Plasma concentration of **digoxin** may be increased by itraconazole. In man, antifungal imidazoles and triazoles inhibit the metabolism of **antihistamines** (particularly **terfenadine**), **oral hypoglycaemics, anti-epileptics, cisapride** and **cyclosporin.** The significance of these interactions in veterinary species have not been studied.

Ivermectin (Animec*; Bimectin*; Eraquell*; Ivomec*; Oramec*; Panomec*; Rycomec*; Virbamec*) PML

Indications: Ivermectin is a parasiticide used in the management of ectoparasitic and endoparasitic infestations in cats, reptiles and small mammals.

Forms: *Injection:* 1% w/v solution.

Dose:
Cats: 0.2–0.4 mg/kg s.c., p.o. q7–14d on 2–4 occasions.
Small mammals: 0.2–0.4 mg/kg s.c., p.o.
Birds: 0.2 mg/kg i.m., s.c. Dilute 1% solution 1:4.5 ivermectin:water and administer 0.1 ml/kg p.o.
Reptiles (except chelonians)*:* 0.2 mg/kg s.c., p.o.

Adverse effects and contraindications: Use in dogs cannot be recommended, as they are susceptible to the toxic CNS effects and death may occur; collies are particularly susceptible. This susceptibility has been linked to a mutation of the multiple drug resistance (*MDR*) gene, which normally prevents the entry of ivermectin across the blood–brain barrier. **Do not administer to chelonians as an irreversible paralysis may develop.**

Kaolin (BCK; Gastric tablets*; **Kaobiotic**; **Kaogel**; Kaolin and morphine*; Kaolin oral suspension*) *GSL*

Indications: Kaolin is an adsorbent antidiarrhoeal agent with a possible antisecretory effect. It is often combined with antibacterials to treat non-specific diarrhoeas in dogs and cats. BCK may be useful in the management of flatulence and acute poisoning.

Forms: *Oral:* BCK: granules containing 40 mg/g bismuth, 50 mg/g calcium phosphate, 400 mg/g charcoal, 430 mg/g kaolin; Gastric tablets: 160 mg; Kaolin, 10 mg liquorice powder, 40 mg sodium bicarbonate, 0.001 ml peppermint oil per tablet; Kaogel: 0.2 g kaolin and 4.3 mg pectin/ml suspension; Kaopectate: 0.2 g kaolin/ml suspension; Kaolin and morphine: 0.2 g kaolin/ml and 55–80 mg morphine/ml suspension; Kaobiotic: 729 mg kaolin and 8.125 mg neomycin tablet.

Dose: *Cats, Dogs:* BCK: 5–15 ml p.o. q8–12h; Gastric tablets 1–4 tablets q8h; Kaolin suspensions 0.2 g kaolin/kg p.o. q2–6h; Kaobiotic: $^1/_4$ tablet/4 kg p.o. q6h.

Drug interactions: Kaolin may decrease the absorption of **lincomycin**, **trimethoprim** and **sulphonamides**.

Ketamine (**Ketaset**; **Vetalar**) *POM*

Indications: Ketamine is a cyclohexanone derivative used to provide chemical restraint or dissociative anaesthesia. It is useful in reptiles, particularly those who 'breath hold'. 'Dissociative' anaesthesia is associated with mild stimulation of cardiac output and blood pressure, modest respiratory depression, and the preservation of cranial nerve reflexes. For example, the eyes remain open during anaesthesia and should be protected using bland ophthalmic ointment. Used alone, ketamine causes skeletal muscle hypertonicity, and movement may occur that is unrelated to surgical stimulation. These effects are normally controlled by the co-injection of acepromazine, and/or alpha$_2$ agonists, and/or benzodiazepines. Ketamine produces profound visceral and somatic analgesia and inhibits central sensitization to pain through NMDA blockade. Therefore, low doses may be useful throughout the management of severe trauma, before limb amputation or during and after major surgery, when it exerts a marked anaesthetic-sparing effect. It is particularly effective when infused with OP3 agonist drugs.

Forms: *Injectable:* 100 mg/ml solution.

Dose:
Cats:
- Analgesia: 1–2 mg/kg i.m. repeated to effect. For perioperative analgesia add 100 mg ketamine to 500 ml Hartmann's solution and infuse at 0.25 ml/5 kg/min.
- Minor restraint: 11 mg/kg i.m. Lower doses (and fewer side-effects) are possible when other drugs are co-injected.
- Anaesthesia: 22–33 mg/kg i.m. or 2.2–4.4 mg/kg i.v.; may need to supplement with other injectable or inhalational anaesthetics. Anaesthesia occurs in 3–5 minutes with a duration of 20–45 minutes and full recovery in approximately 10 hours (cats can usually attain sitting position within 2 hours).
  Ketamine 5 mg/kg + medetomidine 0.08 mg/kg i.m. – sedation in 5 minutes.
  Ketamine 5–10 mg/kg + midazolam 0.25 mg/kg i.m. – sedation in 2 minutes.

Dogs: For perioperative analgesia add 30 mg ketamine and 3 mg alfentanil to 43.7 ml crystalloid solution and infuse at the animal's weight in ml/h.

Small mammals: Rabbits: 15–35 mg/kg i.m., s.c.; Guinea pigs: 60 mg/kg i.p.; Mice, Rats: 87 mg/kg i.p; Hamsters: 200 mg/kg i.p.; Others: 40–50 mg/kg i.m. May be administered with xylazine 2–5 mg/kg i.m. or 10 mg/kg i.p.or diazepam 2.5 mg/kg i.m., i.p. or medetomidine 0.25–0.5 mg/kg i.m., i.p., s.c. or fentanyl 0.05 mg/kg i.p., s.c.

Birds: Ketamine 15–40 mg/kg (plus diazepam 1.5 mg/kg i.m. or acepromazine 0.5–1 mg/kg) gives 20–30 minutes deep sedation/light anaesthesia.
Ketamine 20 mg/kg plus xylazine 4 mg/kg i.m. provides longer anaesthesia and recovery in 2–3 hours.

Reptiles: 10–50 mg/kg i.m., s.c. Larger reptiles require a smaller dose per kg. Anaesthesia occurs in 10–30 minutes and recovery takes 24–96h.

See Sedation protocols, pages 297–301.

Caution: Ketamine may be abused and so should be stored in a locked cabinet.

Adverse effects and contraindications: Adverse effects include tachycardia, salivation (control with atropine), and muscle hypertonicity. Cardiovascular depression, rather than stimulation, and arrhythmias, may arise in animals with high 'sympathetic' tone, e.g. in 'shocked' animals. Respiratory depression may occasionally be marked. High doses may cause bizarre, though temporary behavioural effects, and proprioceptive deficiencies. In reptiles, doses >110 mg/kg may cause respiratory depression and cardiac arrest.

Ketoconazole (Nizoral*) *POM*

Indications: Ketoconazole is a broad-spectrum imidazole antifungal agent. It acts by inhibiting the synthesis of ergosterol in fungal cell membranes, thus causing increased cell wall permeability and allowing leakage of cellular contents. Ketoconazole is used to treat aspergillosis, candidiasis, blastomycosis, coccidioidomycosis, cryptococcosis, sporotrichosis and dermatophytosis. Ketoconazole also inhibits cytochrome P450-dependent enzymes, resulting in reduced gonadal and adrenal steroid synthesis with negligible effects on mineralocorticoid production. It is used in the management of hyperadrenocorticism (HAC), particularly in the following circumstances: medical management of adrenal tumours; short-term test therapy to provide evidence for or against a diagnosis of HAC in animals with vague test results; and as a primary therapy in dogs that do not tolerate mitotane or trilostane and in cats. Its efficacy in the management of HAC is variable. Ketoconazole may be used in combination with ciclosporin to reduce the dose, and therefore, cost of ciclosporin therapy.

Forms: *Oral:* 200 mg tablet.

Dose:
Cats, Dogs:
- Antifungal therapy: 5–10 mg/kg p.o. q8–12h after meals. Several months of treatment may be required depending on the organism and site of infection. Doses up to 40 mg/kg/day are recommended to treat CNS or nasal infections (often in conjunction with amphotericin B); ketoconazole does not attain therapeutic levels in the CNS at 'normal' doses.
- Hyperadrenocorticism: 5 mg/kg p.o. q12h for 7 days, increasing to 10 mg/kg p.o. q12h for 14 days if no adverse effects seen. Perform an ACTH stimulation test after 14 days and if there is inadequate suppression increase the dose to 15–30 mg/kg p.o. q12h.
Birds: 25–30 mg/kg p.o. q8h for 2 weeks.
Reptiles: 50 mg/kg p.o. q24h for 7 days.

Adverse effects and contraindications: Adverse effects include hepatotoxicity (not recognized in the dog unless high doses are used but routine monitoring of liver function tests is recommended), anorexia, vomiting and alterations in hair coat colour. Ketoconazole possibly has teratogenic effects. Cataract development has been associated with ketaconazole use in dogs.

Drug interactions: The absorption of ketoconazole may be impaired by drugs that increase the pH of gastric contents, e.g. **antacids**, **antimuscarinics** and **H₂ blockers**; stagger dosing of these drugs around ketoconazole dose. Ketoconazole extends the activity of **methylprednisolone**. In man, antifungal imidazoles and triazoles inhibit the metabolism of **antihistamines**, **oral hypoglycaemics** and **antiepileptics**. Concomitant use of ketoconazole is likely to increase blood levels of **ciclosporin**.

Ketoprofen (Ketofen) *POM*

Indications: Ketoprofen is a propionic acid NSAID that acts as a dual inhibitor of COX-1 and lipoxygenase enzymes, thus having potent effects on the vascular and cellular phases of inflammation. It has antipyretic, analgesic and anti-inflammatory effects. It is used to control mild to moderate pain.

Forms:
Injectable: 1% solution.
Oral: 5 mg, 20 mg tablets.

Dose:
Cats, Dogs: 2 mg/kg i.v., i.m., s.c. q24h for up to 3 days;
or 2 mg/kg i.v., i.m., s.c. once, followed by 1 mg/kg p.o. q24h for 4 further days; or 1 mg/kg p.o. q24h for up to 5 days.
Small mammals: Rabbits: 3 mg/kg i.m., s.c. q24h.

Adverse effects and contraindications: Adverse effects are dose-related and reflect the reduction in prostaglandin synthesis. The commonest is GI irritation and ulceration. Renal papillary necrosis is the second most common, particularly if hypotension, dehydration or other nephrotoxic drugs are present. Blood dyscrasias, hepatotoxicity and exacerbation of heart failure may be seen rarely. Do not use if gastric or duodenal ulceration is suspected, in haemorrhagic syndromes, in cases of renal failure or where previous reaction to ketoprofen has occurred. Severe toxicity (usually with an acute overdose) may present with vomiting, pyrexia, metabolic acidosis, depression, coma, seizures and GI bleeding. Treatment of acute toxic ingestion includes emptying the gut, treating the acidosis, alkalinizing urine with sodium bicarbonate and supportive therapy.

Drug interactions: Do not use with **corticosteroids** or other **NSAIDs** (increased risk of GI ulceration). In man there is an increased risk of convulsions if NSAIDs are administered with **fluoroquinolones**. NSAIDs may antagonize the hypotensive effects of **anti-hypertensives** (e.g. **beta-blockers**). The concomitant use of **diuretics** may increase the risk of nephrotoxicity. Do not mix with other substances in the same syringe.

Ketorolac trometamol (Acular*)*POM*

Indications: Ketorolac is a topical NSAID for ophthalmic use. It is useful for anterior uveitis and ulcerative keratitis when topical corticosteroids are contraindicated.

Forms: *Topical:* 0.5% drops in 5 ml bottle.

Dose: *Cats, Dogs:* 1 drop/eye q6–12h depending on severity of inflammation.

Adverse effects and contraindications: As with other topical NSAIDs, ketorolac trometamol may cause local irritation (stinging). Topical NSAIDs can be used in ulcerative keratitis but with caution. They can delay epithelial healing and have been associated with an increased risk of corneal melting. Regular monitoring is advised.

Lactated Ringer's solution (Hartmann's; Compound sodium lactate) (Aqupharm No. 11) *POM*

Indications: Lactated Ringer's solution is an isotonic solution used as a water/electrolyte replacement fluid, particularly if metabolic acidosis is present.

Forms: *Injectable:* Sodium chloride 6 mg/ml, potassium chloride 0.4 mg/ml, calcium chloride 0.27 mg/ml and molar sodium lactate 0.0289 ml solution.

Dose: *Cats, Dogs:* Fluid requirements depend upon the degree of dehydration and ongoing losses. In uncomplicated cases administer at a dose of 50–60 ml/kg/day i.v. Higher doses are required if the animal is dehydrated.
See Parenteral fluids table on page 294 for further details.

Lactulose (Duphalac*; Lactugel*; Lactulose*; Regulose*) *P*

Indications: Lactulose is a galactose/fructose disaccharide not hydrolysable by mammals but metabolized by colonic bacteria, resulting in the formation of low-molecular-weight organic acids (lactic, formic, acetic acids). These acids increase osmotic pressure, causing a laxative effect, acidify colonic contents, and trap ammonia as ammonium ions, which are then expelled with the faeces. It is used to reduce blood ammonia levels in patients with hepatic encephalopathy (HE) and as a safe, gentle osmotic laxative.

Forms: *Oral:* 3.1–3.7 g/5 ml lactulose in a syrup base.

Dose:
Cats: 0.5–5 ml p.o. q8–12h.
Dogs: 5–25 ml p.o. q8h or in acute cases of HE 18–20 ml/kg of a solution comprising 3 parts lactulose to 7 parts water per rectum as a retention enema for 4–8 hours.
Monitor and adjust therapy to produce two or three soft stools per day.
Birds: Appetite stimulant, hepatic encephalopathy: 0.2–1 ml/kg p.o. q8–12h.

Adverse effects and contraindications: Cats do not like the taste of lactulose. Excessive doses cause flatulence, diarrhoea, cramping and dehydration. Reduce the dose if diarrhoea develops. Synergy may occur when lactulose is used with oral antibiotics (e.g. neomycin). Do not use lactulose with other laxatives.

Latanoprost (Xalatan*) *POM*

Indications: Latanoprost is a topical prostaglandin analogue. It reduces intraocular pressure (IOP) by increasing uveoscleral outflow. It can have a profound effect on IOP in the dog, although its effect in the cat is less predictable and should be avoided in this species. It is indicated for primary glaucoma and is useful in emergency treatment of an acute episode. It causes miosis in dogs and cats.

Forms: *Topical:* 50 μg/ml (0.005%) solution.

Dose: *Dogs:* 1 drop/eye once daily (evening), or q12h.

Adverse effects and contraindications: Miosis, conjunctival hyperaemia and mild irritation develop. Increased iridal pigmentation has been noted in man, but not in dogs. Due to the marked miosis, latanoprost is contraindicated in uveitis and anterior lens luxation.

Drug interactions: Do not use in conjunction with **thiomersal**-containing preparations. Often used in conjunction with **dorzolamide**.

Lenograstim (rhG-CSF) (Granocyte*) *POM*

Indications: Lenograstim is recombinant human granulocyte-colony stimulating factor (rhG-CSF). G-CSF is a cytokine produced by bone marrow stromal cells, monocytes/macrophages, fibroblasts and endothelial cells. In man it stimulates granulocyte production and is indicated in the management of neutropenia. Neutrophil counts rise within 24 hours. Following discontinuation, neutrophil counts drop to normal after 5 days. There are few reports on the use of G-CSF in dogs and cats. It is most likely to be used in the management of febrile patients with neutrophil counts < 1×10^9/l.

Forms: *Injectable:* 33.6 million IU (263 µg) vial for reconstitution.

Dose: *Cats, Dogs:* 19.2 million IU/m² i.v. infusion, s.c.

Adverse effects and contraindications: Normal dogs produce neutralizing antibodies to rhG-CSF. This limits repeated use and may result in neutropenia. This does not appear to be the case in canine chemotherapy patients. A variety of adverse effects have been reported in man, including musculoskeletal pain, transient hypotension, dysuria, allergic reactions, proteinuria, haematuria and increased liver enzymes.

Levamisole (Levasure*; Nilverm gold*) *PML* (**Spartakon**) *GSL*

Indications: Levamisole is an anthelmintic that stimulates nicotinic cholinoceptors to cause muscular paralysis and interferes with carbohydrate metabolism in susceptible nematodes. Its paralysing effect allows the worm to be expelled. It is used in the treatment of *Aelurostrongylus abstrusus*, *Oslerus osleri* and *Capillaria aerophilia* in cats and dogs, and *Ascaridia columbiae* and *C. obsignata* in racing and show pigeons. In pigeons the use of levamisole should be combined with good environmental hygiene.

Forms:
Injectable: 30 mg/ml, 75 mg/ml solution.
Oral: 20 mg tablet (Spartakon – licensed for use in pigeons only), 15 mg/ml suspension.

Dose:
Cats: Aelurostrongylus abstrusus: 15 mg/kg p.o. q48h for 3 treatments, then 30 mg/kg p.o. 3 days later, then 60 mg/kg p.o. 2 days later. *Capillaria aerophilia*: 4.4 mg/kg s.c. for 2 days, then 8.8 mg/kg s.c. once 2 weeks later; or 5 mg/kg p.o. q24h for 5 days followed by 9 days of no therapy. Repeated twice.
Dogs: Capillaria aerophilia: 7–12 mg/kg p.o. q24h for 3–7 days. *Oslerus osleri*: 7–12 mg/kg p.o. q24h for 20–45 days.

Birds: 10 mg/kg i.m., s.c., 10–20 mg/kg p.o.; repeat in 14 days. Prophylaxis in Pigeons: 20 mg/bird p.o. twice a year. Do not provide any food for 24 hours prior to treatment. Treat all birds in a loft simultaneously. *Reptiles:* Snakes: 10 mg/kg s.c. once; chelonians: 5 mg/kg s.c. once. Repeat every 2 weeks if necessary until test negative for parasites.

Adverse effects and contraindications: Adverse effects in dogs include vomiting, diarrhoea, panting, shaking, agitation, agranulocytosis, dyspnoea, pulmonary oedema and immune-mediated skin lesions. Adverse effects in cats include hypersalivation, excitement, mydriasis and vomiting. Overdosage may lead to respiratory depression requiring artificial ventilation with oxygen. Vomiting commonly occurs in adult and young racing pigeons 1–2 hours after dosing.

Drug interactions: Levamisole's toxic effects may be enhanced by **neostigmine** or **organophosphates**. In reptiles do not use with chloramphenicol.

Levothyroxine (T4, L–Thyroxine) (Soloxine) *POM*

Indications: Levothyroxine is used to treat hypothyroidism. It is a synthetic form of thyroxine. In birds it is used to induce moult.

Forms: 0.1 mg, 0.2 mg, 0.3 mg, 0.5 mg, 0.8 mg tablets.

Dose: *Cats, Dogs:* 0.02–0.04 mg/kg/day. Alternatively dose at 0.5 mg/m^2 body surface area daily. Dose once or divided twice a day according to response. Monitor serum T4 levels pre-dosing and 4–8 hours after dosing.
Birds: 0.02 mg/kg p.o. q24h. Dissolve 1 mg tablet in 28.4 ml water and give 0.4–0.5 ml/kg q24h.
See page 293 for conversion of body weight to surface area (m^2).

Adverse effects and contraindications: The use of levothyroxine is contraindicated in cases of adrenal insufficiency. Cases of pre-existing cardiac disorders require lower doses initially. Symptoms of overdosage include tachycardia, excitability, nervousness and excessive panting.

Drug interactions: In man many drugs may affect thyroid function tests including **anabolic steroids**, **antithyroid drugs**, **barbiturates**, **corticosteroids**, **diazepam**, **heparin**, **insulin**, **mitotane** (op'–DDD), **oestrogens**, **phenylbutazone**, **propranolol** and **thiazides**. The actions of **catecholamines** and **sympathomimetics** are enhanced by thyroxine. Thyroid hormones increase the catabolism of vitamin K-dependent clotting factors, thereby potentiating the anticoagulant effects of **warfarin**. Diabetic patients receiving thyroid hormones may have altered **insulin** requirements; monitor carefully during the initiation of therapy. **Oestrogens** may increase thyroid requirements by increasing thyroxine-binding globulin. The therapeutic effect of **digoxin** and **digitoxin** may be reduced by thyroid hormones. Tachycardia and hypertension may develop when **ketamine** is given to patients receiving thyroid hormones.

Lidocaine (Lignocaine) (EMLA*; Intubeaze; Lignadrin; Lignavet; Lignocaine; Lignol; Locaine; Locovetic) *POM*

Indications: Lidocaine is an amide-linked local anaesthetic with a rapid onset and an intermediate duration of action. Lidocaine can be used for topical, infiltration, i.v. regional, conduction and regional anaesthesia, including extradural and spinal injection. Topical application to the skin is used prior to venipuncture or catheter placement. The inclusion of adrenaline prolongs duration of action. Lidocaine is also a class 1B anti-arrhythmic agent. It decreases the rate of ventricular firing, action potential duration, absolute refractory period and increases relative refractory period. It is the drug of choice for treating certain ventricular arrhythmias. Infusions of lidocaine reduce the inhaled concentrations of anaesthetic required to achieve surgical anaesthesia and prevents central sensitization to noxious surgical stimuli.

Forms:
Injectable: 2% (20 mg/ml) solution for injection. Note: Some products contain adrenaline, do not use them i.v.
Topical: 2% solution (Intubeaze); 2.5% cream (EMLA).

Dose:
Cats:
- Local anaesthesia: Apply to affected area (small gauge needle) with an appropriate volume (usually 1–5 ml) prn.
- Topical laryngeal anaesthesia (prior to tracheal intubation): 0.1–0.3 ml of the 2% solution sprayed on to the back of the throat. Allow 30–90 seconds before attempting intubation.
- Oesophagitis: 2 mg/kg p.o. q4–6h.
- Ventricular arrhythmias: 0.25–1 mg/kg i.v. slowly followed by a constant i.v. infusion of 0.01–0.04 mg/kg/min.
- Topical skin: Apply thick layer of cream to skin and cover with a bandage for 30 mins–1 h prior to venipuncture.

Dogs:
- Local anaesthesia: Apply to affected area (small gauge needle) with an appropriate volume (usually 1–5 ml) prn.
- Oesophagitis: 2 mg/kg p.o. q4–6h.
- Ventricular arrhythmias: 2–8 mg/kg i.v. in 2 mg/kg boluses followed by a constant i.v. infusion of 0.025–0.1 mg/kg/min.
- Intra-operative analgesia and anaesthetic-sparing: constant infusion of 0.05–0.2 mg/kg/m.
- Topical skin: Apply thick layer of cream to skin and cover with a bandage for 30 mins–1 h prior to venipuncture.

To prepare a 1 mg/ml solution add 1 g (50 ml of 2% solution) to 1 litre of 5% dextrose). In small dogs and cats a less concentrated solution may be used for greater accuracy. **Do not use solutions containing adrenaline for i.v. use.**

Adverse effects and contraindications: Adverse effects include depression, seizures, muscle fasciculations, vomiting, bradycardia and hypotension. If the reactions are severe, decrease or discontinue administration. Seizures may be controlled with i.v. diazepam or pentobarbital. Monitor the ECG carefully during therapy. Rapid i.v. injection may cause hypotension. Cats tend to be more sensitive to CNS effects. The CFC propellant used in aerosol preparations (Xylocaine) is alleged to have caused laryngeal oedema in cats. The effect of lidocaine may be antagonized by hypokalaemia.

Drug interactions: Lidocaine is physically compatible with all standard i.v. solutions and many other drugs. **Cimetidine** and **propranolol** may prolong serum lidocaine clearance if administered concurrently. **Procainamide** administered with lidocaine may cause additive CNS effects. Other **anti-arrhythmics** may cause increased myocardial depression. Large doses of lidocaine may prolong **suxamethonium**-induced apnoea.

Lignocaine – see Lidocaine

Lincomycin (Lincocin) *POM*

Indications: Lincomycin is a lincosamide antibiotic active against Gram-positive cocci (including penicillin-resistant staphylococci) and many obligate anaerobes. It is bacteriostatic or bactericidal, depending on the organism and drug concentration. The lincosamides are particularly indicated for staphylococcal bone and joint infections. Being weak bases, they are ion-trapped in fluid that is more acidic than plasma and are therefore concentrated in prostatic fluid, milk and intracellular fluid. Clindamycin is more active than lincomycin, particularly against obligate anaerobes, and is better absorbed from the gut.

Forms:
Injectable: 100 mg/ml solution for i.v. or i.m. use.
Oral: 100 mg, 500 mg tablets.

Dose: *Cats, Dogs:* 22 mg/kg i.m. q24h or 11 mg/kg i.m. q12h or 11–22 mg/kg i.v. q8–12h or 22 mg/kg p.o. q12h or 15 mg/kg p.o. q8h.
Birds: 100 mg/kg i.m. q12h, 75 mg/kg p.o. q12h.

Adverse effects and contraindications: Human patients on lincomycin may develop colitis (diarrhoea). Although not a major veterinary problem, patients developing diarrhoea (particularly if it is haemorrhagic) while taking the medication should be monitored carefully. Administer lincomycin on an empty stomach. Toxicity is a possibility in patients with liver disease; weigh the risk *versus* the potential benefits before use of this drug in such patients. Rapid i.v. administration should be avoided since this can result in collapse due to cardiac depression and peripheral neuromuscular blockade. **Lincosamides are highly toxic to rabbits, guinea pigs and hamsters,** death occurring due to overgrowth of toxin-producing strains of *Clostridium* spp.

Drug interactions: The action of **neuromuscular blocking agents** may be enhanced if given with lincomycin. The absorption of lincomycin may be reduced by **kaolin**.

Liothyronine (T3, L–Tri–iodothyronine) (Tertroxin*) POM

Indications: Liothyronine is a synthetic form of thyroid hormone. It is used to treat hypothyroidism where levothyroxine has been unsuccessful, and in the diagnosis of feline hyperthyroidism (T3 suppression test).

Forms: *Oral:* 20 μg tablets.

Dose:
Cats: T3 suppression test:
Take a sample for thyroxine (T4) estimation at 0 hours. Administer 20 μg T3 p.o. every 8 hours for 7 doses, giving the last dose on the morning of the third day. 4 hours after the last dose take a sample for T4 estimation. In the normal cat, serum T4 levels will be suppressed by 50% or greater with an absolute decrease in serum T4 of 19 nmol/l. Hyperthyroid cats show little or no decrease in serum T4 concentration.
Dogs: 2–6 μg/kg p.o. q8–12h.

Adverse effects and contraindications: Symptoms of overdosage include tachycardia, excitability, nervousness and excessive panting.

Drug interactions: These are as for levothyroxine.

Lithium carbonate (Camcolit*; Liskonum*; Priadel*) POM

Indications: Lithium carbonate stimulates bone marrow stem cells, causing an increase in the production of haematopoietic cell lines, particularly granulocytes. It may be useful in the treatment of idiopathic aplastic anaemia, cytotoxic drug-induced neutropenia or thrombocytopenia, oestrogen-induced bone marrow suppression or cyclic haematopoiesis. Experimental studies show that lithium may prevent neutropenia associated with cytotoxic drugs when administered concomitantly. Clinical trials showing this are lacking.

Forms: *Oral:* 250 mg, 400 mg tablets.

Dose: *Dogs:* 11 mg/kg p.o. q12h. There is a lag phase of up to 4 weeks before its effects may be seen.

Adverse effects and contraindications: Adverse effects include nausea, diarrhoea, muscle weakness, fatigue, polyuria and polydipsia. The release of T3 and T4 may be blocked by lithium; assess thyroid status every 6 m. Avoid the use of lithium in patients with renal impairment (nephrotoxic at high doses), cardiac disease and conditions with sodium imbalance (e.g. hypoadrenocorticism). The recommended serum lithium concentration is 0.5–1.8 mmol/l; assess every 3 months if possible (may be available through NHS hospitals). **Lithium is toxic to cats.**

Drug interactions: The excretion of lithium may be reduced by **ACE inhibitors**, **loop diuretics**, **NSAIDs** and **thiazides**, thus increasing the risk of toxicity. Lithium toxicity is made worse by sodium depletion; avoid concurrent use with **diuretics**. The excretion of lithium may be increased by **theophylline**. Lithium antagonizes the effects of **neostigmine** and **pyridostigmine**. Neurotoxicity may occur if lithium is administered with **diltiazem** or **verapamil**.

Lomustine (CCNU) (Lomustine*) POM

Indications: Lomustine is an alkylating agent in the nitrosourea family. It is highly lipid-soluble, allowing rapid transport across the blood–brain barrier. In man lomustine has been used in the treatment of primary and metastatic brain tumours. Its use in this context in animals is less well defined but the drug has been reported to have some efficacy in the treatment of metastatic mast cell tumours and refractory lymphoma.

Forms: *Oral:* 40 mg capsule.

Dose:
Cats: A dose of 60 mg/m^2 p.o. q21d has been suggested but it is not well established. If using this drug in the cat, specialist advise should be sought prior to its use.
Dogs: 50–90mg/m^2 p.o. q21 days.
See page 293 for body weight to m^2 conversion table.

Adverse effects and contraindications: Myelosuppression is the dose-limiting toxicity, with neutropenia developing 7 days after administration. Neutropenia may be severe and life-threatening at the higher end of the dose range in some dogs. GI and hepatic toxicity have been reported infrequently.

Drug interactions: Lomustine requires hepatic microsomal enzyme hydroxylation for the production of anti-neoplastic metabolites. It should be used with caution in dogs being treated with agents that induce liver enzyme activity, e.g. **phenobarbital**.

Loperamide (Imodium*; Loperamide*; Norimode*) *POM*

Indications: Loperamide is an opioid derivative that reduces GI motility. It is used in the management of non-specific acute and chronic diarrhoea, and irritable bowel syndrome. Its action is as for diphenoxylate.

Forms: *Oral:* 2 mg capsule, 0.2 mg/ml syrup.

Dose: *Cats, Dogs:* 0.04–0.2 mg/kg p.o. q8–12h.

Adverse effects and contraindications: Use with care in cats as excitability may be seen. Constipation will occur in some cases.

Lufenuron (**Program**) *POM*

Indications: Lufenuron is a benzylphenyl urea derivative. It is a larvicidal drug (blocks the formation of larval chitin), indicated for the management of flea infestations in dogs and cats.

Forms:
Oral: 23.1 mg, 67.8 mg, 204.9 mg, 409.8 mg tablets; 7% suspension in ampoules.
Injectable: 40 mg/0.4 ml, 80 mg/0.8 ml.

Dose:
Cats: 30 mg/kg in food once monthly; 40 mg (in cats weighing up to 4.5 kg) or 80 mg (in cats >4.5 kg) s.c. every 6 months.
Dogs: 10 mg/kg tablet in food once monthly.
Note: Insecticides that kill adult fleas will be required if there is a heavy initial infestation. Adult fleas may be seen for a short time following initial administration.

Adverse effects and contraindications: Administer the drug on a full stomach as food is necessary to facilitate the drug's absorption from the GI tract.

Drug interactions: Lufenuron is compatible with other flea control products.

Lysine (L-Lysine) *GSL*

Indications: Lysine is an amino acid that antagonizes arginine, an amino acid required in viral replication. It has a beneficial effect in the management of human herpes simplex infection and has been used in the management of feline herpesvirus infection. However, there is limited clinical evidence as to its efficacy in treating FHV-1.

Forms: *Oral:* 250 mg, 500 mg tablets.

Dose: *Cats:* 250–500 mg q12–24h.

Adverse effects: Do not use preparations containing propylene glycol as they may be toxic to cats. Diarrhoea may be seen. Cats are very sensitive to arginine deficiency and dietary arginine must not be reduced.

Magnesium sulphate (Magnesium sulphate*) *POM*

Indications: Magnesium sulphate is used in man for the emergency treatment of serious arrhythmias, especially in the presence of hypokalaemia (when hypomagnesaemia may be present). In animals magnesium salts have been used to treat unresponsive ventricular dysrhythmias, as a chemical defibrillator and in the management of severe hypotension.

Forms: *Injectable:* 50% solution containing 2 mmol magnesium per ml. Dilute to a 20% or lower solution prior to use.

Dose: *Cats, Dogs:* 0.4–0.5 mmol/kg/day by continuous rate infusion has been advocated. The dose in man is 8 mmol/person over 10–15 minutes followed by an i.v. infusion of 1 mmol/kg over 24 hours. There are few reports on the use of this drug in companion animals.

Mannitol (Mannitol*) *POM*

Indications: Mannitol is an osmotic diuretic that elevates the osmolality of glomerular filtrate, causing water to be retained within the nephron and increasing the excretion of sodium and chloride. It is indicated to: promote diuresis in the early stages of oliguric renal failure; promote excretion of toxic substances; decrease intraocular pressure; and help decrease cerebral oedema. Its effect on intraocular pressure lasts for approximately 5 hours and additional therapy is then needed. It is not suitable for the mobilization of local or general oedema as it may cause cardiac overload. Mannitol acts as a free radical scavenger and may be useful in managing reperfusion injury.

Forms: *Injectable:* 10%, 15%, 20%, 25% solutions for i.v. infusion.

Dose: *Cats, Dogs:*
- Acute glaucoma or acute cerebral oedema: 1–2 g/kg i.v. infusion over 30 min. Withhold water for the first few hours after administering. May repeat 2–4 times over next 48 hours; monitor for dehydration.
- Early oliguric renal failure (as an alternative to using furosemide and dopamine): 0.25–0.5 g/kg i.v. over 5–10 min. Rehydrate the patient prior to the use of mannitol.

If crystals have formed in the vial, they may be resolubilized by warming the vial in a hot water bath; cool to body temperature before administration.

Adverse effects and contraindications: Mannitol should not be used in patients with cerebral haemorrhage, severe congestive heart failure, pulmonary oedema or anuric renal failure (before rehydration). Monitor electrolyte and fluid balance. It is recommended that an in-line i.v. filter be used when infusing concentrated mannitol. The osmolality of the 25% solution is 1375 mOsm/l. Do not add KCl or NaCl to concentrated (20 or 25%) mannitol solutions as a precipitate may form.

Marbofloxacin (Marbocyl) *POM*

Indications: Marbofloxacin is a fluoroquinolone antimicrobial agent with a broad spectrum of activity. It is a bactericidal antibiotic inhibiting bacterial DNA gyrase. It is active against mycoplasmas and many Gram-positive and Gram-negative organisms including *Pasteurella* spp., *Staphylococcus* spp., *Pseudomonas aeruginosa*, *Klebsiella* spp., *Escherichia coli*, *Proteus* spp. and *Salmonella* spp. The bactericidal effect is concentration-dependent, particularly against Gram-negative bacteria, meaning that pulse dosing regimens may be effective. The fluoroquinolones are effective against beta–lactamase-producing bacteria. Marbofloxacin is relatively ineffective in treating obligate anaerobic infections. The fluoroquinolones are highly lipophilic drugs that attain high concentrations within cells in many tissues and are particularly effective in the management of soft tissue, urogenital (including prostatitis) and skin infections. Resistance development is low.

Forms:
Injectable: 100 mg, 200 mg powder for reconstitution.
Oral: 5 mg, 20 mg, 80 mg tablets.

Dose:
Cats, Dogs: 2 mg/kg i.v., s.c., p.o. q24h.
Birds: 10 mg/kg p.o. q24h.

Adverse effects and contraindications: Cartilage abnormalities have been reported following the use of other fluoroquinolones in growing animals. Such abnormalities have not been specifically reported following the use of marbofloxacin. Some animals show GI signs (nausea, vomiting). Use with caution in epileptics until further information is available, as fluoroquinolones potentiate CNS adverse effects when administered concurrently with NSAIDs in man. High doses of enrofloxacin have resulted in reports of retinal blindness in cats. Although not reported with marbofloxacin, caution should be exercised before using dose rates above those recommended by the manufacturer for cats.

Drug interactions: Adsorbents and **antacids** containing cations (**Mg²⁺, Al³⁺**) may bind to fluoroquinolones, preventing their absorption from the GI tract. The absorption of fluoroquinolones may be inhibited by **sucralfate** and **zinc salts**; doses should be at least 2 hours apart. **Enrofloxacin** increases plasma **theophylline** concentrations. Preliminary data suggests this does not occur with marbofloxacin unless used in patients with renal insufficiency. **Cimetidine** may reduce the clearance of fluoroquinolones and should be used with caution in combination.

Mebendazole (Telmin*; Vermox*) *PML*

Indications: Mebendazole is a broad-spectrum benzimidazole anthelmintic indicated for the treatment of *Toxocara canis*, *T. cati*, *Toxascaris leonina*, *Trichuris vulpis*, *Uncinaria stenocephala*, *Ancylostoma caninum*, *Taenia pisiformis*, *T. hydatigena*, *Echinococcus granulosus* and *Taeniaformis hydatigena*.

Forms: *Oral:* 100 mg/g granules (Telmin); 20 mg/ml suspension (Vermox).

Dose:
Cats, Dogs:
Ascarids: BW <2 kg: 50 mg p.o. q12h for 2 consecutive days; ≥2 kg: 100 mg p.o. q12h for 2 consecutive days.
Other helminths: BW <2 kg: 50 mg p.o. q12h for 5 days; 2–30 kg: 100 mg p.o. q12h for 5 consecutive days; >30 kg: 200 mg p.o. q12h for 5 consecutive days.
Small mammals: 50 mg/kg p.o. q12h for 2 consecutive days.

Adverse effects and contraindications: Mebendazole may cause diarrhoea. Reports of hepatotoxicity may be due to idiosyncratic reactions.

Medetomidine (Domitor) *POM*

Indications: Medetomidine is an alpha$_2$-adrenergic agonist producing dose-dependent sedation, muscle relaxation and visceral analgesia. It is used alone for chemical restraint, sedation and pre-anaesthetic medication. In combination with other drugs, conditions of surgical anaesthesia may be produced. Pre-anaesthetic medication with medetomidine has a marked sparing effect on the dose of induction and maintenance agents used. It counteracts muscle rigidity associated with 'dissociative anaesthesia'. It can be used in conjunction with acepromazine and opioids to improve the 'stopping power' of chemical restraint mixtures for dangerous animals. It has marked pre-emptive analgesic effects.

Forms: *Injectable:* 1 mg/ml solution for i.v., i.m. or s.c. use.

Dose:
Cats: Moderate sedation: 0.05–0.1 mg/kg i.v., i.m., s.c.
Deep sedation: 0.1–0.15 mg/kg i.v., i.m., s.c.
Dogs: Premedication: 0.01–0.02 mg/kg i.v., i.m., s.c.
Slight sedation: 0.01–0.03 mg/kg i.v., i.m., s.c.
Moderate/deep sedation and analgesia: 0.03–0.08 mg/kg i.v., i.m., s.c.
Small mammals: 0.5 mg/kg i.m., i.p., s.c.; Rabbits: 0.25–0.5 mg/kg s.c., i.m. Lower dose when in combination with ketamine and/or butorphanol to 0.1–0.25 mg/kg.

Effects can be reversed by atipamezole.
Note: The higher doses required to achieve the desired effect in excited and/or aggressive animals may cause considerable physiological perturbation. When high doses are likely to be necessary, it is safer to use medetomidine/opioid combinations.
See Sedation protocols, pages 297–301.

Adverse effects and contraindications: Medetomidine appears to depress cardiopulmonary function in a dose-dependent manner and should not be used in animals with cardiopulmonary disease. Prolonged effects caused by high doses in normal animals, and low doses in animals with liver dysfunction should be terminated with atipamezole; severe hypothermia will develop in cold conditions. Diuresis and muscle tremors may be seen after injection. Medetomidine may cause vomiting, and should not be used when gagging or vomiting may cause undesirable increases in intracranial or intra-ocular pressure. Spontaneous arousal from deep sedation with medetomidine can occur in dogs. It should not be used in pregnant animals, nor in animals likely to require or receiving sympathomimetic amines, e.g. **isoprenaline**, **dobutamine**. Intramuscular injection is painful.

Medroxyprogesterone acetate (Promone-E) *POM*

Indications: Medroxyprogesterone is a long-acting progestogen used to treat feline psychogenic alopecia, dermatitis and eosinophilic keratitis, to decrease libido in male dogs, to manage prostatic hypertrophy, and to control oestrus in the bitch and queen. When used in the management of feline skin disease, ensure effective topical and environmental parasite controls are instituted before considering progestagen therapy. It is used in birds to manage feather plucking.

Forms:
Injectable: 50 mg/ml suspension.
Oral: 5 mg tablet.

Dose:
Cats:
- Psychogenic dermatitis: 10 mg/kg s.c. q3 months prn.
- Prevention of oestrus: 5 mg/cat/wk commencing in dioestrus or anoestrus.

Dogs:
- Prevention of oestrus in bitches: <5 kg 12.5 mg/dog, 5–8 kg 25 mg/dog, 8–12 kg 36 mg/dog, >12 kg 3 mg/kg s.c. Inject 6–8 weeks before oestrus is due.
- Interruption of oestrus: Once pro-oestral bleeding has started, 10 mg/dog p.o. q24h for 4 days then 5 mg/dog p.o. q24h for 12 days. Use a doubled dose for bitches >15 kg.
- Prostatic hypertrophy: 50–100 mg/dog s.c. every 3–6 months.

Birds:
- Persistent ovulation: 5–10 mg/kg i.m., s.c.
- Feather plucking, sexual behavioural problems: 25–50 mg/kg i.m. Repeat in 4–6 weeks if necessary.

Adverse effects and contraindications: The use of medroxyprogesterone acetate in the treatment of behavioural disorders in cats and dogs, and specifically of feline spraying, is not recommended; alternative treatments are available. Subcutaneous injections may cause a permanent local alopecia, skin atrophy and depigmentation. Adverse effects include temperament changes (listlessness and depression), increased thirst or appetite, cystic endometrial hyperplasia/pyometra, diabetes mellitus, adrenocortical suppression, reduced libido (males), mammary enlargement/neoplasia and lactation. As progestins may cause elevated levels of growth hormone in the dog, acromegaly may develop. Because of adrenocortical suppression, glucocorticoids may need to be given to patients if a stress factor (e.g. surgery, trauma) is introduced. Do not use in pregnancy. As the adverse effects are of a serious nature and in some cases permanent, carefully weigh the risks *versus* benefits of using this drug.

Megestrol acetate (Megoestrol acetate) (Ovarid) *POM*

Indications: Megestrol acetate is an oral progestogen, indicated for the prevention and postponement of oestrus in the bitch and queen, the management of pseudopregnancy and oestrogen-dependent mammary tumours in the bitch, miliary dermatitis, eosinophilic granuloma and eosinophilic keratitis in the cat. When used in the management of feline skin disease, ensure effective topical and environmental parasite controls are instituted before considering progestagen therapy.

Forms: *Oral:* 5 mg, 20 mg tablets.

Dose:
Cats:
- Progestogen-responsive skin disorders (eosinophilic alopecia, granuloma, miliary dermatitis): 2.5–5 mg p.o. q48–72h until response and then reduce dose to 2.5–5 mg once a week.
- Prevention of oestrus: 2.5 mg/cat p.o. weekly for up to 30 weeks or 5 mg/cat for 3 days at signs of calling.

Dogs:
- Prevention of oestrus: Begin during first 3 days of pro-oestrus at 2 mg/kg p.o. q24h for 8 days or 2 mg/kg p.o. q24h for 4 days followed by 0.5 mg/kg p.o. q24h for 16 days.
- Postponement of oestrus: 0.5 mg/kg p.o. q24h for a maximum of 40 days. Commence treatment preferably 14 days (minimum 7 days) before the effect is required.
- False pregnancy: 2 mg/kg p.o. q24h for 5–8 days commencing when signs of false pregnancy are first seen.
- Treatment of oestrogen-dependent mammary tumours: 2 mg/kg p.o. q24h for 10 days, or 2 mg/kg p.o. q24h for 5 days, then 0.5–1 mg/kg p.o. q24h for 10 days.

Adverse effects and contraindications: Do not administer on more than two consecutive occasions or in bitches with reproductive tract disease, pregnancy or mammary tumours (unless oestrus-dependent). The major adverse effects include temperament changes (listlessness), increased thirst or appetite, cystic endometrial hyperplasia/pyometra, diabetes mellitus, adrenocortical suppression, mammary enlargement/neoplasia and lactation. As progestins may cause elevated levels of growth hormone in the dog, acromegaly may develop. Because of adrenocortical suppression, glucocorticoids may need to be given if a stress factor is introduced. The use of progestogens in the management of behavioural disorders in cats and dogs is not recommended; alternative treatments are available. As the adverse effects are of a serious nature and in some cases permanent, carefully weigh the risks *versus* benefits of using this drug.

Meglumine antimonate (Glucantime*) *POM*

Indications: Meglumine antimonate, a pentavalent antimonate, is the first-choice treatment for canine leishmaniasis. Animals may be clinically normal after treatment but remain carriers and follow-on treatment with allopurinol may be beneficial.

Forms: *Injectable:* 300 mg/ml solution. See www.leishmania.co.uk for supplies.

Dose: *Dogs:* 100 mg/kg s.c., i.m., slow i.v. q24h until clinical remission achieved. Treat for 20 days; rest for 10–15 days; then treat for a further 10 days. **Seek expert advice when treating leishmaniasis**.

Adverse effects and contraindications: Do not use where severe liver or renal dysfunction exists. Intolerance is rare but it is recommended to start with half dosage and gradually increase to an effective dose.

Melatonin (Melatonin*; Regulin*) *POM*

Indications: Melatonin is synthesized in the pineal gland and is involved in the neuroendocrine control of photoperiod dependant moulting. The mechanism of action is unknown, but it may act either directly on hair follicles, or by altering levels of MSH or prolactin. It has been used with success in the management of recurrent flank alopecia, pattern alopecia and alopecia X.

Forms:
Injectable: 18 mg subcutaneous implants (Regulin).
Oral: 3 mg tablets (Melatonin). Melatonin tablets are obtainable from health food stores in the USA. However, as unlicensed medicines their use in the UK must be supported by a Special Treatment Authorization.

Dose: *Dogs:* Implants: 18–36 mg subcutaneously once: 3–6 mg q8h p.o. until hair coat is normal. Treatment may have to be repeated.

Adverse effects and contraindications: Dogs receiving implants may rarely experience sterile abscess or granuloma formation. Other effects are uncommon.

Meloxicam (Metacam) *POM*

Indications: Meloxicam is an NSAID that preferentially inhibits COX-2 enzyme thereby limiting the production of prostaglandins involved in inflammation. It is a poor inhibitor of COX-1 enzyme and as such is safer than some other NSAIDs. Meloxicam has antipyretic, analgesic, anti-inflammatory and anti-platelet effects. It is used to control mild to moderate pain and inflammation associated with the musculoskeletal system. Its analgesic activity is enhanced if administered pre-emptively.

Forms:
Injectable: 5 mg/ml solution.
Oral: 1.5 mg/ml suspension.

Dose:
Cats: 0.3 mg/kg s.c., p.o. then 0.1 mg/kg p.o. q24h for 4 days, then 1 drop/cat p.o. q24h thereafter.
Dogs: 0.2 mg/kg s.c., p.o. once only for 1 day then 0.1 mg/kg p.o. q24h thereafter.
Small mammals: Rabbits: 0.3–0.6 mg/kg s.c., p.o.; Rats: 1–2 mg/kg s.c., p.o.; Mice: 2 mg/kg s.c. p.o.
Birds: 0.1–0.2 mg/kg s.c., p.o. q24h.

Adverse effects and contraindications: As meloxicam preferentially inhibits the COX-2 enzyme, adverse effects are less severe than those seen with some other **NSAIDs**. General adverse effects associated with **NSAID** use include GI irritation and ulceration, renal papillary necrosis, particularly if hypotension, dehydration or other nephrotoxic drugs are present, nausea, diarrhoea and fluid retention, which may precipitate cardiac failure. Although these are less likely to develop following the use of meloxicam it is prudent not to use this drug if gastric or duodenal ulceration is suspected, in haemorrhagic syndromes, in cases of cardiac or renal failure or in dehydrated, hypovolaemic or hypotensive patients (increased risk of nephrotoxicity). Do not administer meloxicam to pregnant animals.

Drug interactions: Do not use with **corticosteroids** or other **NSAIDs** (increased risk of GI ulceration). In man there is an increased risk of convulsions if NSAIDs are administered with **fluoroquinolones**. NSAIDs may antagonize the hypotensive effects of **anti-hypertensives** (e.g. **beta-blockers**). The concomitant use of **diuretics** may increase the risk of nephrotoxicity. Do not mix with other substances in the same syringe. The concurrent use of meloxicam with **diuretics** or **aminoglycosides** may increase the risk of nephrotoxicity. Meloxicam may cause false low **T3** and **T4** values.

Melphalan (Alkeran*) *POM*

Indications: Melphalan is an alkylating agent used to treat multiple myeloma and may also be used as a substitute for cyclophosphamide in the treatment of canine lymphoma.

Forms: *Oral:* 2 mg tablet.

Dose: *Cats, Dogs:*
- Myeloma: 1–2 mg/m^2 p.o. q24h for 3–6 weeks then reduce gradually. Often used with prednisolone 40 mg/m^2 p.o. q24h for 7–14d then 20 mg/m^2 p.o. q48h.
- Lymphoma: 5 mg/m^2 p.o. q48h.

See page 293 for conversion of body weight to surface area (m^2).

Adverse effects and contraindications: Adverse effects include leucopenia, thrombocytopenia, anorexia, nausea and vomiting.

Mepivacaine (Intra-epicaine*) *POM*

Indications: Mepivacaine is an amide-linked local anaesthetic with pharmacological properties similar to those of lidocaine; it is of equivalent anaesthetic potency but has a slightly longer duration of action. It has less intrinsic vasodilator activity than lidocaine and is thought to be less irritant to tissues It may be used for infiltration and extradural anaesthesia, to produce conduction blockade and intra-articular analgesia.

Forms: *Injectable:* 2.0% solution without vasodilator or antimicrobial preservative.

Dose: *Cats, Dogs:* Inject the minimal volume required to achieve effect. Toxic doses for mepivacaine have not been established in companion animals.

Adverse effects and contraindications: It is slightly less toxic than lidocaine but should probably not be used in near-term animals or neonates, as its activity is prolonged in the fetus. Inadvertent i.v. injection may cause convulsions and/or cardiac arrest. The former may be controlled with i.v. diazepam.

Methadone (Methadone*) *POM* Schedule 2 Controlled Drug

Indications: Methadone is a synthetic mu(OP3) opioid agonist used as a pre-anaesthetic agent and for short-term pain control. It has similar effects and duration of action to morphine. It may be mixed with acepromazine to produce neuroleptanalgesia for minor procedures, or pre-anaesthetic medication. As with other analgesics, methadone is most effective when given before noxious stimulation begins and in conjunction with other analgesic drugs. In equi-analgesic doses the pattern and incidence of side-effects produced by methadone and morphine are similar, although the incidence of vomiting seems to be lower. Its sedative and euphoric effects are less marked than those produced by morphine. It is often used with a tranquillizer (e.g. diazepam) to produce deep sedation.

Forms: *Injectable:* 10 mg/ml solution.

Dose:
Cats: 0.1 mg/kg i.v., i.m.
Dogs: 0.1–0.5 mg/kg i.m., 0.1 mg/kg i.v. prn.

Adverse effects and contraindications: Attempts to treat severe pain may be unsuccessful. In common with other opioids, methadone may constrict branches of the pancreatic duct and should not be used in dogs with pancreatitis. CNS toxicity (hyperaesthesia in cats) or respiratory depression may occur at very high doses or with an overdose. Hyperaesthesia may be controlled with low (0.01 mg/kg i.v.) doses of acepromazine. Intravenous methadone may cause histamine release. Other toxic effects may be reversed using naloxone, providing that the antagonism of analgesia is desirable and/or justified.

Drug interactions: Other **CNS depressants** (e.g. **anaesthetics**, **antihistamines**, **barbiturates**, **phenothiazines**, **tranquillizers**) may cause increased CNS or respiratory depression when used concurrently with the narcotic analgesics. Because narcotic analgesics can increase biliary tract pressure, plasma amylase or lipase levels may be increased up to 24 hours after narcotic administration.

Methenamine hippurate (Hexamine hippurate)
(Hiprex*; **Methenamine and sodium acid phosphate**) *POM*

Indications: Methenamine is a urinary antiseptic used in the long-term control of recurrent urinary tract infections. It should not be used alone as it is only bacteriostatic. It requires an acidic urine to be effective.

Forms: *Oral:* 150 mg methenamine and 116 mg monosodium phosphate tablet; 1 g methenamine hippurate (Hiprex) tablet.

Dose:
Cats: 1 tablet methenamine/sodium acid phosphate p.o. q24h or 250 mg methenamine p.o. q12h.
Dogs: 1–3 tablets methenamine/sodium acid phosphate p.o. q24h or 500 mg methenamine p.o. q12h.

Adverse effects and contraindications: Methenamine may cause GI disturbances, bladder irritation or a rash. Its use is contraindicated with severe renal impairment, dehydration and metabolic acidosis.

Drug interactions: Efficacy is reduced when drugs that alkalinize urine (**potassium citrate**) are used concurrently.

Methimazole (Felimazole) *POM*

Indications: Methimazole is a thioglyxaline that interferes with the synthesis of thyroid hormones by inhibiting peroxidase-catalysed reactions (blocks oxidation of iodide), the iodination of tyrosyl residues in thyroglobulin, and the coupling of mono- or di-iodotyrosines to form T3 and T4. There is no effect on iodine uptake and it does not inhibit peripheral de-iodination of T4 to T3. It is used to control thyroid hormone levels in cats with hyperthyroidism. As a veterinary licensed product, methimazole has replaced carbimazole as the drug of choice for treatment of feline hyperthyroidism.

Forms: *Oral:* 2.5 mg, 5 mg tablet.

Dose: *Cats:* 2.5 mg/cat p.o. q12h. Two to three weeks of treatment are generally needed to establish euthyroidism. Monitor therapy on the basis of serum thyroxine concentrations (4–6 hours after dosing) and adjust dose accordingly for long-term medical management. Assess haematology, biochemistry and serum total T4 after 3, 6, 10 and 20 weeks and thereafter every 3 months, adjusting dosage as necessary.

Adverse effects and contraindications: Do not use in pregnant or lactating queens. Vomiting and inappetence/anorexia may be seen and are often transient. Pruritus and haematological abnormalities (e.g. neutropenia) are seen. Occasional hepatopathies and immunological adverse effects (cytopaenias, serum anti-nuclear antibodies) can be seen. Treatment of hyperthyroidism can decrease glomerular filtration rate, thereby raising serum urea and creatinine values, and occasionally unmask occult renal failure.

Drug interactions: Phenobarbital may reduce clinical efficacy. **Benzimidazole** drugs reduce hepatic oxidation and may lead to increased circulating drug concentrations.

Methionine (Methionine*) *P*

Indications: Methionine is a urinary acidifier used in the management of struvite urolithiasis. It is also an antidote to paracetamol poisoning if given within 12 hrs of ingestion.

Forms: *Oral:* 250 mg tablets.

Dose:
- Urine acidification:
  Cats: 200 mg/cat p.o. q8h.
  Dogs: 200 mg–1 g/dog p.o. q8h.
  Adjust the dose until urine pH is 6.5 or lower.
- Paracetamol poisoning: *Cats, Dogs:* 2.5 g/animal p.o. followed by 3 further doses of 2.5 g/animal q4h.

Adverse effects and contraindications: Overdosage may lead to metabolic acidosis. There is an increased risk of acidosis if used with other urinary acidifying treatments. Methionine should not be used in animals with renal failure or severe hepatic disease or in the young.

Methocarbamol (Robaxin*) *POM*

Indications: Methocarbamol is a centrally acting skeletal muscle relaxant with a generalized CNS depressant activity; it does not relax skeletal muscles directly. It is used in the treatment of tetanus and some toxicities (e.g. strychnine) and as a general muscle relaxant for muscular spasms.

Forms: *Oral:* 750 mg tablets.

Dose: *Cats, Dogs:* 20–45 mg/kg p.o. q8h. Very high doses may be required for tetanus. It is recommended that the dose should not exceed 330 mg/kg, although serious toxicity or death has not been reported after overdoses.

Adverse effects and contraindications: Adverse effects include salivation, emesis, lethargy, weakness and ataxia.

Drug interactions: As methocarbamol is a CNS depressant, additive depression may occur when given with other **CNS depressant agents**.

(s)-Methoprene (Frontline Combo) *POM*

Indications: (s)-Methoprene is an insect growth regulator that is directly and indirectly ovicidal. It prevents contamination of the environment of treated animals with the immature stages of fleas. It does not kill adult fleas.

Forms: *Topical:* Spot-on 12% w/v in combination with Fipronil.

Methotrexate (Methotrexate*) *POM*

Indications: Methotrexate is an antimetabolite antineoplastic agent that competitively inhibits folic acid reductase. Folic acid is reduced by this enzyme to tetrahydrofolic acid, required for DNA synthesis and cellular replication. Methotrexate may be used to treat lymphomas and some solid tumours, although its use is often limited by toxicity. In human medicine it is used to treat refractory rheumatoid arthritis, although data is lacking with regards its use in canine/feline immune-mediated polyarthritides.

Forms: *Oral:* 2.5 mg, 10 mg tablets.

Dose: *Cats, Dogs:* 2.5 mg/m^2 p.o. q24h. Adjust the frequency of dosing according to toxic effects.
See page 293 for conversion of body weight to surface area (m^2).

Caution: Wear gloves when administering and handling tablets.

Adverse effects and contraindications: Adverse effects (particularly with high doses) include GI ulceration, hepatotoxicity, nephrotoxicity and haemopoietic toxicity. Monitor haematological parameters.

Drug interactions: Methotrexate is highly bound to serum albumin and thus may be displaced by **phenylbutazone**, **phenytoin**, **salicylates**, **sulphonamides** and **tetracycline**, resulting in increased blood levels and toxicity. **Folic acid supplements** may inhibit the response to methotrexate. Methotrexate increases the cytotoxicity of **cytarabine**. Cellular uptake is decreased by **hydrocortisone**, **methylprednisolone** and **penicillins**, and is increased by **vincristine**. Concurrent use of **NSAIDs** increases the risk of haematological, renal and hepatic toxicity.

Methylene blue – see Methylthioninium chloride

Methylphenidate hydrochloride (Ritalin*) *POM*

Indications: Methylphenidate is a stimulant used in the treatment of canine hyperkinesis and narcolepsy.

Forms: *Oral:* 10 mg tablet.

Dose: *Dogs:*
Hyperkinesis: 2–4 mg/kg p.o. q8–12h.
Narcolepsy: 0.25 mg/kg as required.

Adverse effects and contraindications: Contraindicated in patients with epilepsy, cardiovascular disease and glaucoma. Adverse effects include convulsions and elevated blood pressure. In animals unaffected by canine hyperkinesis there is an increase in heart rate and respiratory rate and the risk of anorexia, tremors, aggression, insomnia and hyperthermia.

Methylprednisolone (**Depo-Medrone**; **Medrone**; **Solu-Medrone**) *POM*

Indications: Methylprednisolone is a corticosteroid with 5 times the anti-inflammatory potency of hydrocortisone and 20% more potency than prednisolone. On a dose basis, 0.8 mg methylprednisolone is equivalent to 1 mg prednisolone. Methylprednisolone has minimal mineralocorticoid activity. It is used as an anti-inflammatory agent and in the management of shock. Methylprednisolone is suitable for alternate-day use.

Forms:
Injectable: Methylprednisolone acetate 40 mg/ml suspension (Depo-Medrone); 125 mg, 500 mg powder for reconstitution (Solu-Medrone).
Oral: 2 mg, 4 mg tablets.

Dose:
Cats:
- Asthma: 1–2 mg/kg (depot injection) i.m. q1–3wks.
- Inflammation/flea allergy: 5 mg/kg i.m. (depot injection) every 2 months or 1 mg/kg p.o. q24h reducing to 2–5 mg/cat p.o. q48h.

Dogs:
- Inflammation: Initially 1.1 mg/kg i.m. (depot injection) q1–3wks or 0.2–0.5 mg/kg p.o. q12h.
- Immunosuppression: 1–3 mg/kg p.o. q12h reducing to 1–2 mg/kg p.o. q48h.
- CNS trauma: 30 mg/kg i.v. within 8 hours of trauma, followed by 15 mg/kg i.v. 2 and 6 hours later, followed by 2.5 mg/kg as an i.v. infusion for 48 hours.

Doses should be tapered to the lowest effective dose.

Adverse effects and contraindications: Prolonged use of methylprednisolone suppresses the hypothalamic–pituitary axis (HPA) and causes adrenal atrophy. Animals on chronic therapy should be tapered off steroids when discontinuing the drug. Catabolic effects of glucocorticoids lead to weight loss and cutaneous atrophy. Iatrogenic hyperadrenocorticism may develop with long-term use. Vomiting and diarrhoea may be seen and GI ulceration may develop. Glucocorticoids may increase urine glucose levels and decrease serum T3 and T4. **Do not use in pregnant animals.** Systemic corticosteroids are generally contraindicated in patients with renal disease and diabetes mellitus. Impaired wound healing and delayed recovery from infections may be seen.

Drug interactions: There is an increased risk of GI ulceration if used concurrently with **NSAIDs**. Hypokalaemia may develop if **amphotericin B** or potassium-depleting diuretics (**furosemide, thiazides**) are administered concomitantly with corticosteroids. **Insulin** requirements are likely to increase in patients taking glucocorticoids. The metabolism of corticosteroids may be enhanced by **phenobarbital** or **phenytoin**.

Methyltestosterone (Orandrone; Sesoral) *POM*

Indications: Methyltestosterone is an androgenic steroid used in the management of deficient sex drive in male animals, reversal of feminization in male dogs caused by the oestrogenic effects of testicular tumours (once the tumour has been removed), oestrogen-dependent mammary tumours, oestrus suppression in the bitch, false pregnancy in the bitch, testosterone-responsive incontinence in neutered male dogs and anaemia of chronic renal failure. Its use has also been suggested for the management of feline endocrine alopecia, alopecia due to hypogonadism, and senile alopecia in male dogs. Its value as a supportive anabolic agent in cases of debility or senile decline or in the management of anaemia is controversial. Note that Sesoral is only authorized for use in the management of false pregnancy.

Forms: *Oral:* 5 mg methyltestosterone tablet (Orandrone); 4 mg methyltestosterone and 0.005 mg ethinylestradiol tablet (Sesoral).

Dose: *Cats, Dogs:* Orandrone 0.5 mg/kg (to nearest 2.5 mg) p.o. q24h; Sesoral: 0.34 mg/kg p.o. then 0.17 mg/kg p.o. q12h for 5 days.

Adverse effects and contraindications: Do not use if liver damage, renal damage or congestive heart failure present. Avoid use in pregnant or breeding animals. Alopecia may develop in some cats. Methyltestosterone may cause increased serum creatinine levels and creatinine excretion.

Drug interactions: The **insulin** requirements in diabetic patients may be altered. Androgens suppress the activity of clotting factors II, V, VII, and X and thus increase the bleeding tendency in patients on **anticoagulant** therapy.

Methylthioninium chloride (Methylene blue)
(Methylthioninium chloride*) *GSL*

Indications: Methylthioninium chloride acts as an electron donor to methaemoglobin reductase. It is used in the management of methaemoglobinaemia.

Forms: *Injectable:* 10 mg/ml (1% solution).

Dose: *Dogs:* 1–10 mg/kg i.v. of a 1% solution slowly once. Use an in-line filter if possible.

Adverse effects and contraindications: Methylthioninium chloride may cause a Heinz body haemolytic anaemia and renal failure; do not use unless adequate renal function is demonstrated.

Metoclopramide (Gastrobid Continus*; Maxolon*; Metoclopramide*) *POM*

Indications: Metoclopramide acts as an anti-emetic and an upper GI prokinetic stimulant. Distal intestinal motility is not significantly affected. It inhibits vomiting by blocking dopamine at the chemoreceptor trigger zone whilst increasing oesophageal sphincter pressure, the tone and amplitude of gastric contractions and peristaltic activity in the duodenum and jejunum, and relaxing the pyloric sphincter by sensitizing tissues to acetylcholine. There is no effect on gastric, pancreatic or biliary secretions and nor does metoclopramide depend on an intact vagal innervation to affect motility.

Forms:
Injectable: 5 mg/ml solution.
Oral: 10 mg, 15 mg tablet; 1 mg/ml syrup.

Dose:
Cats, Dogs: 0.5–1 mg/kg i.m., s.c., p.o. q6–8h or 1–2 mg/kg i.v. over 24 hours as a slow infusion.
Small mammals: Ferrets, Rabbits, Guinea pigs: 0.5–1 mg/kg s.c., p.o. q6–8h.
Birds: 0.2–0.4 mg/kg i.v., i.m., s.c. q6–8h.
Reptiles: 0.06 mg/kg p.o. q24h. Chelonians: 1–10 mg/kg p.o. q24h.

Adverse effects and contraindications: Do not use metoclopramide where GI obstruction or perforation is present or for longer than 72 hours without a definitive diagnosis. It is relatively contraindicated in epileptic patients. Adverse effects are unusual, although more common in cats than dogs, and include changes in mentation (depression, nervousness, restlessness) and behaviour. As metoclopramide blocks dopamine it may cause sedation and extrapyramidal effects (movement disorders characterized as slow to rapid twisting movements involving the face, neck, trunk or limbs). Cats may exhibit signs of frenzied behaviour or signs of disorientation. Metoclopramide reduces renal blood flow, which may exacerbate pre-existing renal disease.

Drug interactions: The activity of metoclopramide may be inhibited by antimuscarinic drugs (e.g. **atropine**) and **narcotic analgesics**. The effects of metoclopramide may decrease (e.g. **cimetidine**, **digoxin**) or increase (e.g. **oxytetracycline**) drug absorption. The absorption of nutrients may be accelerated, thereby altering **insulin** requirements and/or timing of its effects. **Phenothiazines** may potentiate the extrapyramidal effects of metoclopramide. The CNS effects of metoclopramide may be enhanced by **narcotic analgesics** or **sedatives**. Metoclopramide antagonizes **cabergoline**.

Metronidazole (Flagyl*; Metrolyl*; Metronidazole*; **Stomorgyl**)
POM

Indications: Metronidazole is a synthetic nitroimidazole with antibacterial and antiprotozoal activity. It is used to treat anaerobic infections, giardiasis and other protozoal infections, and in the management of hepatic encephalopathy. Metronidazole may have effects on the immune system by modulating cell-mediated immune responses. It is absorbed well from the GI tract and diffuses into many tissues including bone, CSF and abscesses. Its mechanism of action on protozoans is unknown but in bacteria it appears to be reduced spontaneously under anaerobic conditions to compounds that bind to DNA and cause cell death. Spiramycin (a constituent of Stomorgyl) is active against Gram-positive aerobes including *Staphylococcus* spp., *Streptococcus* spp., *Bacillus* spp. and *Actinomyces* spp. Metronidazole has been used as an appetite stimulant in reptiles.

Forms:
Injectable: 5 mg/ml i.v. infusion.
Oral: 200 mg, 400 mg, 500 mg tablets; 40 mg/ml oral solution
25 mg metronidazole and 46.9 mg spiramycin tablets, 125 mg metronidazole and 234.4 mg spiramycin tablets, 250 mg metronidazole and 469 mg spiramycin tablets (Stomorgyl).

Dose:
Cats: Flagyl: 8–10 mg/kg p.o. q12h. Injectable solution may be given intrapleurally to treat empyema.
Stomorgyl: 12.5 mg metronidazole and 23.4 mg spiramycin/kg q24h for 5–10 days.
Dogs: Flagyl: 15–25 mg/kg p.o. q12h or 10 mg/kg s.c., slow i.v. infusion q12h. Use higher doses, 25 mg/kg p.o. q12h, for protozoal infections. Injectable solution may be given intrapleurally to treat empyema.
Stomorgyl: 12.5 mg metronidazole and 23.4 mg spiramycin/kg q24h for 5–10 days.
Small mammals: Ferrets: 20 mg/kg p.o. q24h. Rabbits, Guinea pigs, Chinchillas: 40 mg/kg p.o. q24h. Other rodents: 20–60 mg/kg p.o. q24h.
Birds: 10 mg/kg i.m. q12h or 20–50 mg/kg p.o. q12h.
Reptiles: Various dose rates are suggested by different authors ranging from 20 mg/kg to 100–275 mg/kg p.o. q24h. Most dose recommendations are in the range 20–50 mg/kg p.o. q24–48h.

Adverse effects and contraindications: Some texts recommend doses in excess of 25 mg/kg. There is a greater risk of adverse effects with rapid i.v. infusion or high total doses. Adverse effects in animals are uncommon and are generally limited to vomiting, CNS toxicity (nystagmus, ataxia, knuckling, head tilt and seizures), hepatotoxicity and haematuria. Prolonged therapy or the presence of pre-existing hepatic disease may predispose to CNS toxicity. Use with caution in the first trimester of pregnancy as it may be teratogenic. **Do not**

administer to Indigo or King Snakes due to toxicity. Use with caution in chinchillas as anecdotally it has been associated with liver failure.

Drug interactions: The one-stage prothrombin (OSPT) time in patients on **warfarin** may be prolonged by metronidazole. **Phenobarbital** or **phenytoin** may enhance the metabolism of metronidazole. **Cimetidine** may decrease the metabolism of metronidazole and increase the likelihood of dose-related adverse effects. Spiramycin should not be used concurrently with other antibiotics of the **macrolide** group.

Mexiletine (Mexitil*) POM

Indications: Mexiletene is a class 1b anti-dysrhythmic. It has similar characteristics to lidocaine and tocainide. It can be combined with beta-blockers.

Forms: *Oral:* 50 mg, 200 mg capsules; 25 mg/ml solution.

Dose: *Dogs:* 4–8 mg/kg p.o. q8–12h.

Adverse effects and contraindications: Adverse effects include nausea, vomiting (following oral dosage – administer with food to alleviate this), depression, convulsions, tremor, nystagmus, bradycardia, hypotension, jaundice and hepatitis.

Drug interactions: The absorption of mexiletine may be delayed by **atropine** and **opioid analgesics**. Mexiletine excretion may be reduced by **acetazolamide** and alkaline urine and increased by urinary acidifying drugs (e.g. **methionine**). The action of mexiletine may be antagonized by **hypokalaemia**. **Cimetidine** decreases the rate of mexilitene elimination.

Miconazole (Malaseb; Surolan) POM

Indications: Miconazole is an imidazole antifungal agent that has activity against *Cryptococcus*, *Candida* and *Coccidioides*. It is used topically in the management of fungal skin and ear infections, including dermatophytosis.

Forms: *Topical:* 2% cream/powder (Daktarin); 2% shampoo (Malaseb); 23 mg/ml suspension with prednisolone, polymyxin (Surolan).

Dose: *Cats, Dogs:*
- Fungal otitis: 2–12 drops in affected ear q12–24h.
- Dermatophytosis: Apply topically to affected area. Continue for 2 weeks after a clinical cure and negative fungal cultures.

Midazolam (Midazolam*) POM

Indications: Midazolam is a short-acting water-soluble benzodiazepine agent. Compared with diazepam it is more potent, has a shorter onset and duration of action, and is less irritant to tissues. It is used with ketamine to offset muscle hypertonicity and with opioids and/or acepromazine for pre-anaesthetic medication in the critically ill. It provides unreliable sedation on its own, although it will sedate depressed animals.

Forms: 1 mg/ml, 5 mg/ml solutions for injection.

Dose:
Cats, Dogs: 0.066–0.3 mg/kg i.v., i.m., s.c. or 0.25 mg/kg midazolam + ketamine 5–10 mg/kg ± acepromazine (0.025–0.05 mg/kg) i.m., or 0.2 mg/kg midazolam + 2 mg/kg ketamine i.v.
Small mammals: Rabbits, Ferrets, Chinchillas: 1 mg/kg i.v., 2 mg/kg i.m.; Rodents: 5 mg/kg i.v., i.m., i.p. If used with ketamine or fentanyl, lower doses may be sufficient.
Birds: 0.8–3 mg/kg i.m., i.v.
See Sedation protocols, pages 297–301.

Adverse effects and contraindications: In man i.v. administration of midazolam has been associated with respiratory depression and severe hypotension. Excitement may occasionally develop.

Drug interactions: Concurrent use of midazolam with **antihistamines**, **barbiturates**, **opioid analgesics**, or **CNS depressants** may enhance the sedative effect. **Opioid analgesics** may increase the hypnotic and hypotensive effects of midazolam. Midazolam decreases the dose of **inhalational anaesthetics**. **Erythromycin** inhibits the metabolism of midazolam.

Mifepristone (Mifegyne*) POM

Indications: Mifepristone is a progesterone antagonist, acting on progesterone receptors. It is used to terminate pregnancy in bitches.

Forms: *Oral:* 200 mg tablet.

Dose: *Dogs:* 2.5–3.5 mg/kg p.o. q12h for 5 days after day 32 of pregnancy.

Adverse effects and contraindications: Nausea and vomiting may be seen.

Drug interactions: Avoid concurrent use of **NSAIDs** until 12 days after mifepristone treatment.

Milbemycin (**Milbemax**; **Program plus**) *POM*

Indications: The milbemycins are fermentation products of *Streptomyces hygroscopicus*. Milbemycin oxime is a mixture of the A4 and A3 oximes of milbemycin D. It is a parasiticide active against *Dirofilaria immitis* (3rd and 4th larval stages) and adult forms of *Ancylostoma caninum*, *A. tubaeforme*, *Toxacara canis*, *T. cati*, *Toxascaris leonina* and *Trichuris vulpis*. It is also active against *Angiostrongylus vasorum*, *Crenosoma vulpis*, *Sarcoptes scabei*, *Pneumonyssoides caninum*, *Cheyletiella* and *Demodex* (unlicensed uses). However, milbemycin in the form of Program Plus is not suitable for the treatment of demodicosis.

Forms: *Oral:* 2.3 mg, 5.75 mg, 11.5 mg, 23 mg tablets co-formulated with lufenuron (Program plus). 2.5 mg, 4 mg, 12.5 mg tablets co-formulated with praziquantel (Milbemax).

Dose:
Cats: 2 mg/kg p.o. once (Milbemax).
Dogs: 0.5 mg/kg p.o. once.
Administer with food or immediately after feeding.
In heartworm areas medicate within one month of the appearance of mosquitos and administer the last dose one month after the mosquito season finishes. Where a dog is to travel to a heartworm area begin dosing within one month of arrival and give last dose after the dog has left the region.

Adverse effects and contraindications: Pale mucous membranes and increased intestinal transit times have been observed in some dogs. At large overdoses (25 times the normal monthly dose) toxic reactions including ataxia, pyrexia and periodic recumbency have been recorded in Rough Collies.

Milrinone (Primacor*) *POM*

Indications: Milrinone is a bipyridine phosphodiesterase F-III inhibitor, increasing cAMP concentrations in myocardium. It acts as a positive inotrope and has mild arteriodilating properties. By bypassing the beta receptors increased contractility may be maintained chronically. Milrinone is not in common usage.

Forms: *Injectable:* 1 mg/ml solution.

Dose: *Dogs:* Constant rate infusion: 1–10 µg/kg/min

Adverse effects and contraindications: Milrinone may be arrhythmogenic. Monitor blood pressure, heart rate, ECG, CVP, urine output and fluid/electrolyte status. Long-term beneficial effects are not proven. It may cause rupture of chordae tendinae in chronic mitral valve disease.

Mineral products (Additrace*) *POM*

Indications: Trace element solutions containing essential minerals are used when prolonged parenteral nutritional support is anticipated.

Forms: *Injectable:* Contains iron, zinc, manganese, copper, chromium, selenium, molybdenum, fluorine and iodine ions.

Dose: *Cats, Dogs:* 5–10 ml/l of parenteral nutrition solution. Seek expert advice before giving parenteral nutrition.

Minocycline (Minocycline*) *POM*

Indications: Minocycline is a lipid-soluble tetracycline with antibacterial (bacteriostatic), antirickettsial, antimycoplasmal and antichlamydophila activity. It has the broadest spectrum of all the tetracyclines. Its rate of excretion is not affected by renal function as it is cleared by hepatic metabolism and is therefore recommended when tetracyclines are indicated in animals with renal impairment. Being extremely lipid-soluble, it penetrates well into prostatic fluid and bronchial secretions.

Forms: *Oral:* 50 mg, 100 mg capsules or tablets.

Dose: *Cats, Dogs:* 5–15 mg/kg p.o. q12h.

Adverse effects and contraindications: Adverse effects of minocycline include nausea, vomiting and diarrhoea.

Drug interactions: Absorption of minocycline is reduced by **antacids**, **calcium**, **magnesium** and **iron salts**, and **sucralfate**. **Phenobarbital**, **phenytoin** and **primidone** may increase its metabolism, decreasing plasma levels.

Misoprostol (Cytotec*) *POM*

Indications: Misoprostol, a synthetic prostaglandin E_1 analogue, inhibits gastric acid secretion and increases bicarbonate and mucus secretion, epithelial cell turnover and mucosal blood flow. It prevents and promotes healing of gastric and duodenal ulcers, particularly those associated with the use of NSAIDs. Some reports suggest it may not prevent gastric ulceration caused by methylprednisolone. It may also be useful in the management of canine atopy.

Forms: *Oral:* 200 μg tablet.

Dose:
Cats: 5 μg/kg p.o. q8h.
Dogs: 2–7.5 μg/kg p.o. q6–8h.
Note: In man doses of up to 20 μg/kg p.o. q6–12h are used to manage pre-existing NSAID-induced gastric ulceration, whilst doses of 2–5 μg/kg p.o. q6–8h are used prophylactically to prevent ulceration.

Adverse effects and contraindications: Adverse effects include diarrhoea, abdominal pain, nausea, vomiting and abortion. **Do not use in pregnant animals**. Combinations with an NSAID (e.g. diclofenac, Naproxen) are available for man, but are not suitable for small animals because of different NSAID pharmacokinetics.

Drug interactions: Use of misoprostol with **gentamicin** may exacerbate renal dysfunction.

Mitotane (op'–DDD) (Lysodren*) *POM*

Indications: Mitotane is effective in the management of pituitary-dependent hyperadrenocorticism (HAC; Cushing's syndrome) in cats and dogs and adrenal gland hyperplasia/adenoma in ferrets. It has been used in the management of adrenal-dependent HAC, but with poor success. However, its use has been superceded by the licensed product **trilostane**. Mitotane causes severe progressive necrosis of the zona fasciculata and zona reticularis, thereby reducing the production of adrenal cortical hormones. The zona glomerulosa, and thus production of aldosterone, is relatively spared. Its efficacy in cats is very variable, with many showing no response at non-toxic levels.

Forms: *Oral:* 500 mg tablet or capsule.
Mitotane is unavailable in the UK. It may be imported. An STA is required from the VMD; justification for its preference to the authorized product, trilostane, required, including an adverse drug reaction report for trilostane.

Dose:
Cats, Dogs:
- Pituitary-dependent HAC: 30–50 mg/kg p.o. q24h for 7–10 days (to effect) then weekly to fortnightly. In diabetic animals the initial dose should be reduced to 25–35 mg/kg p.o. q24h. The addition of prednisolone at a dose of 0.1–0.2 mg/kg p.o. q24h may help decrease the adverse effects associated with acute endogenous steroid withdrawal.
- Inoperable adrenal carcinomas: As above but may require 50–150 mg/kg p.o. q24h.

Small mammals: Ferrets: 50 mg/ferret p.o. q24h for 7 days, then 50 mg p.o. q72h until clinical signs resolve.

Mitotane should be given with food to improve its absorption from the intestinal tract.
Caution: Wear gloves when handling this drug.

Adverse effects and contraindications: Monitor diabetic animals closely as they may have rapidly changing insulin requirements during the early stages of therapy. Adverse effects include anorexia, vomiting, diarrhoea and weakness; generally associated with too rapid a drop in plasma cortisol levels. They usually resolve with steroid supplementation. Acute-onset neurological signs may be seen 2–3 weeks after initiation of therapy, possibly due to rapid growth of a pituitary tumour. Provide supplemental glucocorticoids during periods of stress. Following the initial 7–10 days therapy an ACTH stimulation test should be performed to monitor the efficacy of therapy. Approximately 5% of dogs require permanent glucocorticoid and mineralocorticoid replacement therapy if given mitotane overdose.

Drug interactions: Barbiturates and **corticosteroids** increase the hepatic metabolism of mitotane. There may be enhanced CNS depression with concurrent use of **CNS depressants**. **Spironolactone** blocks mitotane's action.

Montmorillonite (Diarsanyl) *GSL*

Indications: Montmorillonite is used as an intestinal protectant and adsorbent in animals with diarrhoea. It acts in a similar way to kaolin but is a trilamellar smectite clay with superior adsorbent properties. It is combined in Diarsanyl with simple sugars and electrolytes to help compensate for GI electrolyte loss and energy deficiency.

Forms: *Oral:* Paste in 10, 24 and 60 ml multi-dose syringes; 4.5 g montmorillonite, 2.5 g lactose, 2.5 g dextrose, 2.5 g glycerine, 0.4 g citric acid, 35.8 mg/kg sodium, 3.9 mg/kg potassium, 9.2 mg/kg magnesium, 3.9 calcium, 66.4 mg/kg phosphorus per 10 ml of paste.

Dose:
Cats: 1 ml p.o. q12h.
Dogs: BW <7 kg: 1 ml p.o. q12h; 7–17 kg: 2 ml p.o. q12h; 18–30 kg: 4 ml p.o. q12h; 31–60 kg: 10 ml p.o. q12h

Adverse effects: Unknown, but likely to be constipation.

Morphine (Morphine*; Oramorph*) *POM* Schedule 2 Controlled Drug

Indications: Morphine is a mu (OP3) agonist primarily used to improve sedation of pre-anaesthetic medication and for the management of perioperative and severe traumatic pain. Its euphoric and sedative effects make it the most suitable drug for severe pain management. It is most effective when given before noxious stimulation begins. Prolonged pain can be controlled by repeated injections or by infusion. It has an onset of action of 10–15 minutes with a duration of analgesia of approximately 1–4 hours. It has a greater duration of effect in cats. Morphine may be used to provide extradural analgesia.

Forms:
Injectable: 10 mg/ml, 15 mg/ml, 20 mg/ml, 30 mg/ml solutions.
Oral: 10 mg, 30 mg, 60 mg, 100 mg tablets.

Dose:
Cats: 0.1–0.5 mg/kg i.m., s.c. prn or q6–8h.
Dogs: 0.25–2 mg/kg i.v., i.m., s.c. prn or q4–6h. For extradural use 0.1 mg/kg is dissolved in 0.26 ml/kg sterile saline and injected extradurally over 30–60 seconds. There is a latent period of 30–60 minutes following extradural administration. Its duration is 10–23 hours.
Cats, Dogs: Post-operative analgesia: add morphine to fluids such that provision of maintenance fluid requirements (3–4 ml/kg/h) simultaneously delivers 0.1–0.3 mg/kg/h morphine (depending upon the discomfort level).
Small mammals: Ferrets: 0.5–5 mg/kg i.m., s.c. q6h; Rabbits, Guinea pigs: 2–5 mg/kg i.m., s.c. q2–4h; Rats, Gerbils, Hamsters, Mice: 2.5 mg/kg i.m., s.c. q2–4h.

Note: The dose of morphine is determined by the degree of pain present; the greater this is, the higher the dose that may be used safely without risk of adverse effects.
See Sedation protocols, pages 297–301.

Adverse effects and contraindications: Morphine is a more potent emetic than other opioid analgesics, and although the act of vomiting does not appear to cause distress in either cats or dogs, morphine should not be used when gagging or vomiting may cause undesirable increases in intracranial or intraocular pressure. Morphine may constrict branches of the pancreatic duct and so should not be used in dogs with pancreatitis. Adverse effects in cats (hyperaesthesia) are only seen in gross overdosage, and may be controlled with acepromazine. Rapid i.v. injection in dogs may cause histamine release (transient tachycardia and hypotension), nervous agitation and respiratory stimulation. High doses given by other routes will potentiate the respiratory depressant effects of other CNS depressant drugs. Adverse, or prolonged effects may be treated with naloxone only if the antagonism of analgesia is justified.

Drug interactions: Enhanced CNS or respiratory depression may occur with other **CNS depressants** (**anaesthetics**, **antihistamines**, **barbiturates**, **phenothiazines**, **tranquillizers**). As narcotic analgesics can increase biliary tract pressure, plasma amylase or lipase levels may be increased for up to 24 hours after drug administration.

Mupirocin (Bactroban*) POM

Indications: Mupirocin (pseudomonic acid A) is an antibacterial used in the management of bacterial skin infections; especially those associated with *Staphylococcus* spp. Mupirocin has a novel chemical structure unrelated to any other known class of antibiotic. It blocks protein synthesis in bacteria by inhibiting bacterial isoleucyl-tRNA synthetase. As a consequence of this unique mode of action, mupirocin lacks cross-resistance with other antibacterial agents and exhibits activity against multiresistant strains of bacteria. Uses for mupirocin include canine acute moist dermatitis, intertrigo (fold pyoderma), callus pyoderma and canine and feline acne. Low-level resistance to mupirocin is emerging. It is generally indicated for the management of resistant infections. Do not use for longer than 10 days to avoid the development of resistance. Mupirocin inhibits growth of several pathogenic fungi, including a range of dermatophytes and *Pityrosporum* spp. and topical application may be useful in controlling such infections, although data are currently lacking as to its efficacy *in vivo*.

Forms: *Topical:* 2% cream, ointment.

Dose: *Cats, Dogs:* Apply to infected areas 3 times daily.

Adverse effects and contraindications: Application in man has been associated with stinging. Avoid if renal impairment present.

Nalbuphine (Nubain*) POM

Indications: Nalbuphine is an opioid agonist/antagonist. It may be used as an analgesic *per se*, or to antagonize some of the adverse effects of pre-administered opioid agonists, without complete reversal of analgesia (sequential analgesia). Its sedative and euphoric effects are less marked than those produced by morphine.

Forms: *Injectable:* 10 mg/ml solution.

Dose:
Dogs: 0.1–0.2 mg/kg i.v., i.m., s.c.
Small mammals: 1–4 mg/kg i.m., s.c. q4–8h.

Adverse effects and contraindications: Attempts to treat severe pain with nalbuphine may be unsuccessful and alternative analgesic modalities, e.g. local anaesthetics, NSAIDs, should be considered. In common with other opioids, nalbuphine may constrict branches of the pancreatic duct and so should not be used in dogs with pancreatitis. Adverse effects include respiratory depression. Severe effects should be treated with naloxone.

Drug interactions: Barbiturate anaesthetics, **phenothiazines** and **tranquillizers** may enhance nalbuphine's central nervous and respiratory depression.

Naloxone (Naloxone*; Narcan*) *POM*

Indications: Naloxone is a pure narcotic antagonist, devoid of respiratory depressant or any other adverse effect. In animals, it can be used to identify persistent activity of opioid agonist drugs. The i.v. injection of a low naloxone dose will cause a transient elevation of consciousness when persistent opioid activity contributes to an unexpectedly prolonged recovery from anaesthesia. When no response occurs it may be assumed that the problem results from other drugs or physiological problems like hypothermia. It is used to treat gross overdosage with opioid agonist/antagonist drugs, e.g. butorphanol, nalbuphine.

Forms: *Injectable:* 0.02 mg/ml, 0.4 mg/ml solution.

Dose:
Dogs: 0.015–0.04 mg/kg i.v., i.m., i.t., s.c.
Small mammals: 0.01–0.1 mg/kg i.v., i.p.

Adverse effects and contraindications: Naloxone not only antagonizes exogenous opioids, but incapacitates endogenous pain modulating systems. Its indiscriminate use in animals which have undergone major surgery or trauma will expose the recipient to acute, severe discomfort. In such cases, the effects of opioid overdose, i.e. respiratory depression, should be managed by endotracheal intubation and artificial ventilation. The duration of action of naloxone is shorter than that of opioid agonists, and so repeated injections are normally required to prevent renarcotization.

Nandrolone (**Laurabolin**; **Nandrolin**; **Retarbolin**) *POM*

Indications: Nandrolone is a testosterone derivative with anabolic and anti-catabolic actions. It is indicated wherever excessive tissue breakdown or extensive repairs processes are proceeding. Its use has also been advocated in the management of aplastic anaemia and anaemia associated with renal failure.

Forms: *Injectable:* 10 mg/ml, 25 mg/ml, 50 mg/ml (in oil).

Dose: *Cats, Dogs:* 1–5 mg/kg i.m., s.c. q21 days. Maximum dose of 20–25 mg for the **cat** and a maximum dose of 40–50 mg in the **dog**.

Adverse effects and contraindications: Monitor haematology to determine the efficacy of treatment and liver enzymes to monitor for hepatotoxicity. Do not use in breeding bitches or queens, in pregnant animals or those with liver disease or diabetes mellitus. Androgenic effects may develop. Use in immature animals may result in early closure of epiphyseal growth plates.

Drug interactions: The concurrent use of anabolic steroids with **adrenal steroids** may potentiate the development of oedema.

Natamycin (Mycophyt*) *POM*

Indications: Natamycin is an antifungal antibiotic active against *Trichophyton, Microsporum, Aspergillus, Pityrosporum canis* and *Candida* spp. It is used topically to control fungal infections of the skin and external ear canal.

Forms: *Topical:* Powder for preparation of a suspension containing 0.01% w/v natamycin.

Dose: *Cats, Dogs:* Mycophyt should be made up according the manufacturer's recommendations and applied to the whole body by sponging or the affected area.

Adverse effects and contraindication: None reported.

Drug interactions: Do not use Mycophyt with **other topical preparations**.

Neomycin (**Auroto**; **Dermobion**; **Hydrocortisone and neomycin**; **Kaobiotic**; Maxitrol*; **Neopen**; Nivemycin*; **Oterna**; **Panolog**; **Vetodale**) *POM*

Indications: Neomycin, an aminoglycoside antibiotic, is bactericidal and active against Gram-negative bacteria, although some *Staphylococcus* and *Enterococcus* species are sensitive. All obligate anaerobic bacteria and many haemolytic streptococci are resistant. Aminoglycosides operate a concentration-dependent cell killing mechanism, leading to a marked post-antibiotic effect; they are more active in an alkaline environment. As neomycin is extremely nephrotoxic and ototoxic it is used topically for infections of the skin, ear or mucous membranes, or orally to reduce intestinal bacterial population in the management of hepatic encephalopathy. As with other aminoglycosides it is not absorbed after oral administration unless GI ulceration is present. This drug has been used (often combined with antimuscarinic agents) in the treatment of non-specific bacterial enteritides. However, other antibacterial drugs, if required at all, are better indicated than neomycin for such use.

Forms:
Oral: 8.125 mg (Kaobiotic), 175 mg, 500 mg tablets (Nivemycin). Kaobiotic also contains sulfadiazine, sulphaguanidine, sulphamerazine, sulphathiazole, kaolin and pectin.
Topical: Many dermatological, ophthalmic and otic preparations contain 0.25–0.5% neomycin.

Dose:
Cats: Oral: 5.5–10 mg/kg p.o. q12h.
Ophthalmic: 1 drop/eye q6–8h.
Otic: 2–12 drops/ear or apply liberally to skin q4–12h.
Dogs:
Hepatic encephalopathy with dietary protein restriction and lactulose:
Oral: 20 mg/kg p.o. q6h or per rectum as a retention enema.
Ophthalmic: 1 drop/eye q6–8h.
Otic: 2–12 drops/ear or apply liberally to skin q4–12h.
Small mammals: 5–50 mg/kg p.o. q12h or topically 2 drops/eye, 2–12 drops/ear or apply liberally to skin q4–12h.

Adverse effects and contraindications: Systemic toxicity, ototoxicity and nephrotoxicity may very occasionally occur following prolonged high-dose oral therapy or where there is severe GI ulceration/ inflammatory bowel disease, as sufficient neomycin may be absorbed. Some patients may develop a severe diarrhoea/malabsorption syndrome and bacterial or fungal superinfections.

Drug interactions: Absorption of **digoxin**, **methotrexate**, **potassium** and **vitamin K** may be decreased by neomycin. Other ototoxic and nephrotoxic drugs, e.g. **furosemide** and **gentamicin** should be used with caution in patients on oral neomycin therapy.

Neostigmine (Neostigmine*) *POM*

Indications: Neostigmine is an anticholinesterase drug; inhibition of acetylcholinesterase prolongs the action of acetylcholine. In comparison with edrophonium, it has a slower onset but a longer duration of action. It is used to treat acute myaesthenic crises when difficulty in breathing and swallowing (megaoesophagus) are seen. It is also used to antagonize non-depolarizing neuromuscular blocking agents. For this purpose, it is most useful when long-acting neuromuscular blocking agents such as pancuronium have been used.

Forms:
Injectable: 2.5 mg/ml solution.
Oral: 15 mg tablet.

Dose: *Cats, Dogs:*
- Myasthenic crisis: 0.01–0.1 mg/kg i.v., i.m., s.c., interval dependent upon duration of response. For longer term use 0.1–0.25 mg/kg p.o. q4h (total daily dose not to exceed 2 mg/kg).
- Antagonism of non-depolarizing neuromuscular blocking agents: Neostigmine (0.05 mg/kg) is mixed with glycopyrronium (0.01 mg/kg) and injected i.v. over 2 minutes once signs of spontaneous recovery from 'block', e.g. diaphragmatic 'twitching', are present. Continued ventilatory support should be provided until full respiratory muscles activity is restored. If glycopyrronium is unavailable, atropine (0.04 mg/kg) is given i.v., followed by neostigmine (0.05 mg/kg) as soon as heart rate rises.

Adverse effects and contraindications: Adverse effects of anticholinesterases are due to their parasympathomimetic action. Muscarinic effects include increased GI motility, salivation, gastric secretion and bradycardia. Severe bradyarrhythmias, even asystole, occur if neostigmine is used to antagonize neuromuscular block without the co-administration of antimuscarinic drugs. If an overdose occurs or if cholinergic signs become severe, treatment with atropine (0.05 mg/kg) may be indicated. Neostigmine produces a therapeutic effect for 4 hours. As it produces marked adverse effects, use pyridostigmine for long-term management of acute myaesthenic crises.

Drug interactions: Aminoglycosides, clindamycin, lincomycin and **propranolol** may antagonize the effect of neostigmine. Neostigmine enhances the effect of **suxamethonium** but antagonizes the effect of **non-depolarizing muscle relaxants**.

Netilmicin (Netillin*) *POM*

Indications: Netilmicin is an aminoglycoside antibiotic active against many Gram-negative microorganisms, even some resistant to gentamicin. It should be reserved for infections caused by gentamicin-resistant organisms or where gentamicin resistance is a high probability, where it is an alternative to amikacin. It is ineffective in sites of low oxygen tension (abscesses, exudates), making all obligate anaerobic bacteria resistant. Aminoglycosides are bactericidal and their mechanism of killing is concentration-dependent, leading to a marked post-antibiotic effect, allowing pulse-dosing regimens to be used to limit toxicity. Experience with netilmicin is limited in veterinary medicine.

Forms: *Injectable:* 10, 50, 100 mg/ml solutions.

Dose: *Cats, Dogs:* 1–2 mg/kg i.v. (infuse over 30 min), i.m., s.c. q8h.

Adverse effects and contraindications: Netilmicin is nephrotoxic and ototoxic, and can potentiate neuromuscular blockade. Monitoring serum netilmicin levels should be considered to ensure therapeutic levels and minimize toxicity, particularly in neonates, geriatric patients and those with reduced renal function.

Drug interactions: Avoid the concurrent use of other nephrotoxic, ototoxic or neurotoxic agents (e.g. **amphotericin B**, **cisplatin**, **furosemide**). Increase monitoring and adjust dosages when these drugs must be used together. Aminoglycosides may be chemically inactivated by **beta-lactam antibiotics** (e.g. **penicillins**, **cephalosporins**) or **heparin** when mixed *in vitro*. The effect of non-depolarizing muscle relaxants (e.g. **atracurium**, **pancuronium**, **tubocurarine**, **vecuronium**) may be enhanced by aminoglycosides. Synergism may occur when aminoglycosides are used with **penicillins** or **cephalosporins.**

Nicergoline (Fitergol) *POM*

Indications: Nicergoline blocks serotonin and dopamine receptors and is an alpha-adrenergic antagonist, primarily acting through alpha$_1$ adrenoceptors. Its reported effects are to promote cerebral vasodilatation, thereby improving cerebral oxygenation and to have a neuroprotective action. Nicergoline is indicated for the treatment of age-related behavioural disorders such as diminished vigour and vigilance, fatigue and sleep disorders.

Forms: *Oral:* 5 mg tablet.

Dose: *Dogs:* 0.25–0.5 mg/kg q24h administered in the morning. It may be administered as a solution.

Drug interactions: Do not administer nicergoline within 24 hours of alpha$_2$ agonists (**xylazine**, **medetomidine**, **romifidine**). Concurrent use of other **vasodilators** may cause hypotension.

Nicotinamide (Nicotinamide*) *GSL*

Indications: Administration of nicotinamide (Vitamin B3) with oxytetracycline or doxycycline has been used in the management of immune-mediated dermatoses in the dog. Its mechanism is unknown, although nicotinamide blocks antigen IgE-induced histamine release, and inhibits phosphodiesterase activity and protease release. In combination with tetracyclines it has also been used in the management of discoid lupus, lupoid onychodystrophy, panniculitis and GSD metatarsal fistulae.

Forms: *Oral:* 50 mg, 500 mg tablets.

Dose: *Dogs:* 500 mg q8h for dogs >10kg, reducing to q12h then q24h.

Adverse effects and contraindications: Adverse effects are uncommon, although vomiting, anorexia, lethargy and diarrhoea have been reported.

Nitenpyram (Capstar) *GSL*

Indications: Nitenpyram is a neonicotinoid insecticide used in the treatment of fleas on dogs and cats. It kills adult fleas within 30 minutes of oral dosing.

Forms: *Oral:* 11.4 mg, 57 mg tablets.

Dose: *Cats, Dogs:* Minimum recommended dose 1 mg/kg p.o. once; repeat as required.

Nitrofurantoin (Nitrofurantoin*) *POM*

Indications: Nitrofurantoin is a nitrofuran antibacterial. It is reduced in the bacterial cell by nitroreductase enzymes to form products that interact with bacterial DNA and cause strand breakage. It is bacteriostatic at low and bactericidal at high concentrations. It is well absorbed following oral administration but rapidly excreted in urine. As a consequence therapeutic levels are not attained in serum or most tissues but are attained in the urinary tract. The concentration of nitrofurantoin is highest in alkaline urine. However, urine should not be alkalinized as the activity of nitrofurantoin is significantly decreased. Nitrofurantoin has activity against many Gram-positive and Gram-negative bacteria.

Forms: *Oral:* 50, 100 mg tablet; 25 mg/5ml oral suspension.

Dose: *Cats, Dogs:* 4 mg/kg p.o. q8h.
Prophylaxis: management of recurrent urinary tract infection: 3–4 mg/kg every day after micturition and last thing at night.

Adverse effects and contraindications: The use of nitrofurantoin is contraindicated in patients with significant renal impairment, as serum levels rise with an increased risk of serious toxicity. In man nitrofurantoin may rarely cause a peripheral neuritis, pulmonary complications, hepatotoxicity, emesis, diarrhoea and GI bleeding. High oral doses may cause thrombocytopenia, anaemia and leucopenia with prolonged bleeding times. Since nitrofurans are mutagenic, they should not be given to pregnant animals.

Drug interactions: The bioavailability of nitrofurantoin may be increased by **antimuscarinic drugs** and **food** as they delay gastric emptying time and increase absorption of this weak acid from the stomach.

Nitroglycerine – see Glyceryl trinitrate

Nitroprusside (Nitroprusside sodium*) *POM*

Indications: Nitroprusside is a very potent direct arteriolar and venous dilator that acts independently of the autonomic innervation. It is rapidly metabolized to cyanide and nitric oxide. It markedly lowers systemic and pulmonary vascular resistance and systemic arterial blood pressure, thereby increasing cardiac output and reducing ventricular filling pressure. It is indicated for the short-term management of severe systemic hypertensive crises, acute life-threatening heart failure secondary to mitral or aortic regurgitation and severe refractory CHF, often in combination with dopamine or dobutamine.

Forms: *Injectable:* 50 mg ampoule for reconstitution giving a 10 mg/ml solution.

Dose: *Cats, Dogs:* To prepare solution for injection: Add 2–3 ml 5% dextrose to vial. Add dissolved solution to 1 litre of 5% dextrose and promptly protect solution from light (aluminium foil or other opaque covering). The administration set need not be protected from light. The resultant solution containing 50 μg/ml of nitroprusside, is stable for 24 hours after reconstitution and will have a brownish tint. Discard if it turns blue, dark red or green. Do not add other drugs to nitroprusside solutions. Give 1–15 μg/kg/min i.v. constant infusion using flow control device to provide accurate dose. Start at lower rates and titrate up according to effect. A dose of 3 μg/kg/min controls most patients. Monitor blood pressure continuously and avoid extravasation at the i.v. site. Do not administer for longer than 24 hours to reduce the problem of thiocyanate toxicity.

Adverse effects and contraindications: Once the infusion ceases, blood pressure will return to pretreatment levels within 1–10 minutes. Excessive doses, prolonged therapy, depletion of hepatic thiosulphate supply, or severe hepatic or renal insufficiency may lead to profound hypotension, cyanide or thiocyanate toxicity. Withdraw the drug gradually following prolonged use as sudden withdrawal may cause a rebound increase in systemic vascular resistance and ventricular filling pressures. Initiate oral vasodilator therapy prior to discontinuation. Monitor acid/base status to evaluate therapy and to detect metabolic acidosis (early sign of cyanide toxicity). Administer vitamin B12 parenterally as this may prevent cyanide toxicity. Thiocyanate toxicity may cause delirium; monitor serum thiocyanate levels in patients on prolonged therapy if possible, especially those with concurrent renal dysfunction; plasma thiocyanate concentrations above 10 mg/dl are toxic.

Drug interactions: The hypotensive effects of nitroprusside may be enhanced by **anaesthetics**, **beta-blockers** (e.g. **propranolol**), **calcium-channel blockers** (e.g. **diltiazem**), **corticosteroids**, **diuretics** and **NSAIDs**. **Sympathomimetics** may cause an additive tachycardia.

Nitroscanate (**Lopatol**; **Nitroscanate**; **Troscan**) *GSL*

Indications: Nitroscanate is a broad-spectrum anthelmintic. It is highly effective in a single dose against common canine nematodes and cestodes including *Toxocara canis, Toxascaris leonina, Ancylostoma caninum, Uncinaria stenocephala, Taenia ovis, T. hydatigena, T. pisiformis* and *Dipylidium caninum*. At the recommended dose nitroscanate gives limited control of *Echinococcus granulosus*. It is not effective against *Trichuris vulpis*.

Forms: *Oral:* 100 mg, 500 mg tablets.

Dose: *Dogs:* 50 mg/kg p.o. with one-fifth of the daily food ration in the morning. Nitroscanate tablets should be given whole. Give remaining food ration after 8 hours.

Adverse effects and contraindications: Adverse effects include vomiting in dogs and CNS disturbances (ataxia and disorientation) in cats; **do not use in cats**. Nitroscanate is irritant and tablets should not be crushed, broken or divided.

Nitrous oxide (Nitrous oxide*) *POM*

Indications: Nitrous oxide is an odourless gas used with oxygen to 'carry' volatile anaesthetics, e.g. halothane, for the induction and maintenance of anaesthesia. At the onset of anaesthesia it accelerates the uptake of volatile anaesthetic and speeds induction. During the maintenance period it reduces the inspired concentration of volatile anaesthetic required to achieve surgical anaesthesia, and thus lowers the adverse effects of the latter. Because less volatile drug is required over a given period of time, recovery from anaesthesia is more rapid.

Forms: *Inhalation:* 100% gas.

Dose: *Cats, Dogs, Small mammals, Birds:* Inspired concentrations of 50–70%.

Caution: Prolonged exposure of theatre staff to nitrous oxide may cause a megaloblastic anaemia due to interference with vitamin B12.

Adverse effects and contraindications: Nitrous oxide displaces oxygen in inspired breath; when concentrations >70% are used, atmospheric hypoxia may occur. Nitrous oxide should not be used in conditions in which lung pathology, and/or hypoventilation is likely to impair blood oxygenation. Nitrous oxide is relatively impotent and concentrations <50 % have little, if any, effect in animals. The delivery of safe concentrations of nitrous oxide in oxygen depend on accurate, calibrated flow meters. The inspired concentration of oxygen may fall to critically low levels when nitrous oxide is used in rebreathing anaesthetic breathing systems, i.e. 'circle' and 'to-and-fro' systems, especially when low-flow, or 'closed' systems are employed. Do not use in such systems unless the inspired oxygen level can be measured on a 'breath-for-breath' basis. Nitrous oxide rapidly enters air-filled spaces within the body, increasing their volume and/or pressure. This may critically aggravate conditions such as closed pneumothorax, or GDV complex, when space distension may prevent ventilation. Nitrous oxide is rapidly evolved from blood when its administration ends, and may dilute alveolar oxygen levels to an extent that precludes adequate blood oxygenation. So-called 'diffusion hypoxia' is prevented by enriching inspired gas with 100% oxygen for 5–10 minutes after nitrous oxide administration is discontinued.

Nizatidine (Axid*) POM

Indications: Nizatidine is a potent H_2 receptor antagonist that reduces gastric acid secretion; it may have a gastric prokinetic effect. It is used to treat gastroduodenal ulceration and severe reflux oesophagitis.

Forms:
Injectable: 25 mg/ml solution.
Oral: 150, 300 mg capsules.

Dose: *Cats, Dogs:* 1 mg/kg i.v. q12h; 2.5 mg/kg p.o. q12–24h.

Adverse effects and contraindications: There is little information on the use of this drug in veterinary medicine. No adverse effects reported yet, but slow i.v. injection is recommended.

Normal saline – see Parenteral fluids table, page 294

NPH Insulin – see Insulin

Nystatin (**Canaural**; Nystatin*; Nystan*; **Panolog**) POM

Indications: Nystatin is an antifungal agent with a broad spectrum of activity but noted for its activity against *Candida*, particularly *C. albicans*.

Forms:
Oral: 100,000 IU/ml suspension.
Topical: Various topical products.

Dose:
Cats, Dogs: Apply to affected areas q8–12h.
Birds: Juvenile birds: 1–2 drops p.o. after each feed. Older birds: 100,000 IU/300 g p.o. q12–24h.
Reptiles: 100,000 IU/kg p.o. q24h for 10 days.

Octreotide (Sandostatin*; Sandostatin LAR*) *POM*

Indications: Octreotide is a long-acting analogue of the hypothalamic hormone somatostatin. It may be useful in the management of gastric, enteric and pancreatic endocrine tumours (e.g. insulinoma, gastrinoma) and acromegaly as it potentially inhibits hormonal release, although variable responses have been reported in veterinary medicine. Tumours not expressing somatostatin receptors will not respond.

Forms: *Injectable:* 50, 100, 200, 500 μg/ml solution; depot preparation: 10 mg, 20 mg, 30 mg vial.

Dose: *Cats, Dogs:* 10–20 μg/animal s.c. q8–12h. There is limited information on the use of this drug in dogs and cats. In man doses up to 200 μg/person q8h are used. Similar doses of the aqueous preparation may be required in animals, but dosages for the depot preparation are not known.

Adverse effects and contraindications: Adverse effects recorded in man include GI disturbances (anorexia, vomiting, abdominal pain, bloating, diarrhoea and steatorrhoea), hepatopathy and pain at injection sites.

Oestradiol – see Estradiol

Oestriol – see Estriol

Ofloxacin (Exocin*) *POM*

Indications: Ofloxacin is a topical fluoroquinolone for ophthalmic use when other antibacterial agents are ineffective. It is active against many ocular pathogens, including *Staphylococcus* spp. and *Pseudomonas aeroginosa*, although there is increasing resistance amongst some staphylococcal and streptococcal organisms.

Forms: *Topical:* 0.3% solution.

Dose: *Cats, Dogs:* Apply 1 drop to affected eye q6h.

Adverse effects and contraindications: May cause local irritation after application.

Olsalazine (Dipentum*) *POM*

Indications: Olsalazine is a dimer of 5-aminosalicylic acid (5-ASA), used in the management of colitis. It may be used in patients sensitive to sulfasalazine. Olsalazine is cleaved by colonic bacteria into 5-ASA which has a local anti-inflammatory effect.

Forms: *Oral:* 250 mg capsule.

Dose: *Dogs:* 10–20 mg/kg p.o. q12h.

Adverse effects and contraindications: Do not use in patients sensitive to salicylates.

Omeprazole (Losec*) *POM*

Indications: Omeprazole is a proton pump inhibitor. It is 10 times more potent than cimetidine in inhibiting gastric acid secretion and has a longer duration of activity (>24 hours). It is used in the management of gastric hyperacidity, GI ulcers and the Zollinger–Ellison syndrome (gastrinoma). Lansoprazole, rabeprazole and pantoprazole are similar drugs but have no known clinical advantage over omeprazole. Esomeprazole (Nexium) is a newer preparation containing only the active isomer.

Forms:
Oral: 10 mg, 20 mg, 40 mg capsules, tablets.
Injectable: 40 mg vial for reconstitution for i.v. injection. Discard remainder after use.

Dose:
Cats: 0.75–1 mg/kg p.o. q24h.
Dogs: 0.5–1.5 mg/kg i.v., p.o., q24h for a maximum of 8 weeks.

Adverse effects and contraindications: Adverse effects include nausea, diarrhoea, constipation and skin rashes. Chronic suppression of acid secretion has caused hypergastrinaemia in laboratory animals leading to mucosal cell hyperplasia, rugal hypertrophy and the development of carcinoids, and so treatment for a maximum of 8 weeks has been recommended. An i.v. preparation of rabeprazole is available, but has caused pulmonary oedema in dogs at high doses.

Drug interactions: Omeprazole may enhance the effects of **phenytoin**.

Ondansetron (Zofran*) *POM*

Indications: Ondansetron is a serotonin (5-hydroxytryptamine) antagonist and has potent anti-emetic effects. It is indicated for the management of nausea and vomiting in patients who are unable to tolerate, or whose signs are not controlled by, other drugs. Granisetron, dolasetron and tropisetron are similar drugs but have yet to be extensively used in animals.

Forms:
Injectable: 2 mg/ml solution.
Oral: 4 mg, 8 mg tablets; 4 mg/5 ml syrup.

Dose: *Cats, Dogs:* 0.5 mg/kg i.v. loading dose followed by 0.5 mg/kg/h infusion for 6h or 0.5–1 mg/kg p.o. q12–24h.

Adverse effects and contraindications: In man, constipation, headaches, occasional alterations in liver enzymes and, rarely, hypersensitivity reactions have been reported.

Ophthalmic irrigant (Balanced salt solution*) *P*

Indications: Balanced salt solution is an isotonic non-irritant sterile solution for general ophthalmic irrigation. It can be used as an extraocular and intraocular irrigant.

Forms: Balanced salt solution contains: 0.64% sodium chloride, 0.39% sodium acetate, 0.17% sodium citrate, 0.048% calcium chloride, 0.03% magnesium chloride, 0.075% potassium chloride.

Dose: Irrigate as required.

Orbifloxacin (Orbax) *POM*

Indications: Orbifloxacin is a fluoroquinolone antimicrobial agent with a broad spectrum of activity. It is a bactericidal drug, inhibiting DNA gyrase, and its action is concentration-dependent meaning that pulse dosing regimens may be effective. It is particularly active against mycoplasmas, many Gram-negative organisms and some Gram-positive organisms including *Pasteurella* spp., *Staphylococcus* spp., *Pseudomonas aeruginosa*, *Klebsiella* spp., *Escherichia coli*, *Proteus* spp. and *Salmonella* spp. The fluoroquinolones are effective against beta-lactamase-producing bacteria. Orbifloxacin is ineffective in treating obligate anaerobic infections. It is a highly lipophilic drug attaining high concentrations within cells in many tissues and is particularly effective in the management of soft tissue, urogenital (including prostatic) and skin infections. Resistance development is rare.

Forms: *Oral:* 6.25 mg, 25 mg, 75 mg tablets.

Dose: *Dogs:* 2.5 mg/kg p.o. q24h.

Adverse effects and contraindications: Cartilage abnormalities have been reported following the use of other fluoroquinolones in growing animals. Such abnormalities have not been specifically reported following the use of orbifloxacin. These drugs should be used with caution in epileptics until further information is available from dogs, as they potentiate CNS adverse effects when administered concurrently with **NSAIDs** in man. Caution should be exercised before using dose rates above those recommended by the manufacturer. The potential adverse effects of orbifloxacin on the canine retina have not been studied (*see Enrofloxacin*).

Drug interactions: Absorbents and **antacids** containing cations (Mg^{2+}, Al^{3+}) may bind fluoroquinolones preventing their absorption from the GI tract. Their absorption may also be inhibited by **sucralfate** and **zinc salts**; separate dosing by at least 2 hours. Fluroquinolones increase plasma **theophylline** concentrations. **Cimetidine** may reduce the clearance of fluoroquinolones and so should be used with caution with these drugs.

Oxazepam (Oxazepam*) POM Schedule 2 Controlled Drug

Indications: Oxazepam is a benzodiazepine that has been used as an appetite stimulant, particularly where cyproheptadine is unsuccessful.

Forms: *Oral:* 10 mg, 15 mg, 30 mg tablets.

Dose: *Cats, Dogs:* 0.2–0.4 mg/kg p.o. q24h.

Drug interactions: The metabolism of oxazepam may be decreased and excessive sedation may occur if given with **cimetidine**.

Oxymetazoline (Afrazine*) P

Indications: Oxymetazoline is a sympathomimetic drug that acts as a nasal decongestant by causing vasoconstriction of mucosal blood vessels.

Forms: Paediatric nasal drops: 0.025% solution.

Dose: *Cats, Dogs:* 1 drop/nostril q12h for maximum 48 hours.

Adverse effects and contraindications: As the effects of this drug wear off a rebound phenomenon develops due to secondary vasodilation. This results in a subsequent temporary increase in nasal congestion.

Oxytetracycline (**Duphacycline**; **Engemycin**; **Oxycare**) POM

Indications: Oxytetracycline, a bacteriostatic antibiotic, inhibits the growth of many Gram-positive and Gram-negative bacteria, rickettsiae, mycoplasms, spirochaetes and other microbes. It inhibits protein synthesis and is selectively concentrated by bacterial cells. Oxytetracycline in combination with nicotinamide has been used in the management of immune-mediated conditions, including discoid lupus erythematosus and lupoid onychodystrophy. The tetracyclines vary in their lipid solubility. Doxycycline and minocycline are the most lipid-soluble and penetrate into most tissues and body fluids. Oxytetracycline is less lipid-soluble, is excreted unchanged in urine and bile and undergoes enterohepatic recirculation.

Forms:
Injectable: 50 mg/ml solution.
Oral: 50 mg, 100 mg, 250 mg tablets.
Feed supplement and soluble powders also available.

Dose:
Cats, Dogs: 7–11 mg/kg i.v. (cat only), i.m., s.c. q24h; 10–20 mg/kg
p.o. q8h. Give orally on an empty stomach.
Small mammals: Ferrets, Hamsters, Gerbils: 20 mg/kg i.m. q12h;
Rabbits, Chinchillas: 15 mg/kg i.m. q12h; Guinea pigs: 5 mg/kg i.m.
q12h; Rats: 20 mg/kg i.m. q8–12h; Mice 100 mg/kg s.c. q12h.
Birds: Parrots: 50 mg/kg i.m. q24h; Other birds: 50 mg/kg i.m. q48–72h.
Oral dosing for prophylaxis 500 mg/kg soft food, 2.5 g/l drinking water.

Adverse effects and contraindications: Adverse effects include
vomiting, diarrhoea, depression, hepatotoxicity (rare), fever, hypotension
(following i.v. administration) and anorexia (cats). Only use in cats when
no other agent is suitable. Prolonged use may lead to development of
superinfections. Although not well documented in veterinary medicine,
tetracyclines induce dose-related functional changes in renal tubules in
several species, which may be exacerbated by dehydration,
haemoglobinuria, myoglobinuria or concomitant administration of other
nephrotoxic drugs. Severe tubular damage has occurred following the
use of outdated or improperly stored products and occurs due to the
formation of a degradation product. Tetracyclines stain teeth of children
when used in the last 2–3 weeks of pregnancy or the first month of life.
Although this phenomenon has not been well documented in animals, it
does occur in dogs and it is prudent to restrict the use of tetracyclines in
all young animals. Avoid oral dosing in birds, other than for prophylaxis,
as tetracyclines are poorly absorbed from the GI tract, rapidly lose
potency in drinking water and put birds off drinking water due to their
taste. Injectable preparations in birds may cause toxicity or muscle
necrosis and the concentrated injectable depot formulations used for
cattle and sheep should never be given to small animals. **Oral
tetracyclines may cause GI disturbances and death in guinea pigs.**

Drug interactions: The bactericidal action of the **penicillins** may be
inhibited by oxytetracycline. **Antacids** containing divalent or trivalent
cations (Mg^{2+}, Ca^{2+}, Al^{3+}), **food** or **milk products** bind tetracycline,
reducing its absorption. Tetracyclines may increase the nephrotoxic
effects of methoxyflurane. The GI effects of tetracyclines may be
increased if administered concurrently with **theophylline** products.

Oxytocin (Oxytocin Leo; Oxytocin S; Pituitary extract [synthetic]) *POM*

Indications: Oxytocin is a synthetic oxytocin. It stimulates smooth
muscle contraction in the oestrogen-sensitized uterus and is used to

induce parturition when uterine inertia is present (as long as no obstruction is present), to evacuate uterine contents, to decrease haemorrhage following parturition and to promote the 'let-down' of milk.

Forms: *Injectable:* 10 IU/ml solution.

Dose:
Cats:
- Obstetric indications: 2–5 IU i.m., s.c.
- Milk let-down: 1–10 IU i.m., s.c.

Dogs:
- Obstetric indications: 2–10 IU i.m., s.c.
- Milk let-down 2–20 IU i.m., s.c.

Small mammals: 0.2–3 IU/kg s.c., i.m.
Birds: Egg retention: 3–6 IU/kg i.m.
Reptiles: Egg retention: 2–10 IU/kg after 1–2 ml 10% calcium gluconate/kg p.o. q24h for 4 doses.

Keep vial in refrigerator and warm syringe contents before injecting.

Adverse effects and contraindications: Initially use low dosages as overstimulation of the uterus can be hazardous to both mother and fetuses.

Drug interactions: Severe hypertension may develop if used with **sympathomimetic pressor amines**.

Pamidronate (Pamidronate*) *POM*

Indications: Pamidronate is a bisphosphonate that is adsorbed onto hydroxyapatite crystals, so slowing their rate of growth and dissolution. It is used to treat acute moderate to severe hypercalcaemia when other therapeutic regimens are ineffective, or in long-term therapy of chronic hypercalcaemia.

Forms: *Injectable:* 3, 6, 9 mg/ml concentrate for i.v. infusion.

Dose: *Dogs:* 0.9–1.3 mg/kg i.v. infusion over 24h once.

Adverse effects and contraindications: Adverse effects include nausea, diarrhoea, hypocalcaemia, hypophosphataemia, hypomagnasaemia and hypersensitivity reactions.

Drug interactions: Concurrent use of **aminoglycosides** may result in severe hypocalcaemia.

Pancreatic enzyme (Lypex*; **Pancrex-Vet**; **Tryplase**) *GSL*

Indications: Pancreatic enzymes (lipase, protease, amylase) are used to control signs of exocrine pancreatic insufficiency.

Forms: *Oral:* Powder containing not less than 1400 IU free protease, 20,000 IU lipase and 24,000 IU amylase per gram; capsules containing not less than 9000 IU amylase, 13,000 IU lipase and 450 IU protease.

Dose:
Cats: 1 teaspoonful of powdered non-enteric coated pancreatic extract mixed thoroughly with each meal. Adjust dose as necessary.
Dogs: At least 1–1.5 teaspoonfuls of powdered non-enteric coated pancreatic extract per 100 g of food or per 10 kg body weight per meal. Mix thoroughly with food. Best results are usually obtained by feeding only 2 or 3 meals/day. Use the manufacturer's recommendations as the minimum required initially; the dose may be reduced empirically once a satisfactory response is achieved. Efficacy may be augmented by antibiotic control of secondary bacterial overgrowth. Concomitant administration of acid blockers is not cost-effective.
Birds: One capsule/kg q24h mixed in food.

Note: Enteric coated preparations are less effective than powdered non-enteric coated pancreatic extracts. A new enteric coated preparation (Lypex) has not been fully evaluated. Uncrushed tablets are also generally ineffective. If used, crush tablets and break open capsules.

Caution: Powder spilled on hands should be washed off or skin irritation may develop. Avoid inhaling powder as it causes mucous membrane irritation and may trigger asthma attacks in susceptible individuals.

Adverse effects and contraindications: High doses may cause diarrhoea and GI cramping. Contact dermatitis of the lips is occasionally seen with powdered enzyme.

Drug interactions: The effectiveness may be diminished by **antacids** (**magnesium hydroxide, calcium carbonate**).

Pancuronium (Pancuronium*) *POM*

Indications: Pancuronium is a non-depolarizing neuromuscular blocking agent with a medium to long duration of activity. It produces mild vagolysis (increases heart rate) and may cause slight increases in blood pressure. It is suitable for cases requiring medium to long periods of profound skeletal muscle relaxation, i.e. >45 minutes, especially when modest cardiovascular stimulation is desired. Duration of effect is dose-dependent, but varies markedly between individuals. Pancuronium is used in patients undergoing mechanical ventilation and is favoured when it is important to maintain cardiac output.

Forms: *Injectable:* 2 mg/ml.

Dose: *Cats, Dogs:* 0.05–0.1 mg/kg i.v.; initially use higher dose, repeat doses at increments of 0.01 mg/kg. Repeated doses may be cumulative and lead to difficulty in antagonism.

Adverse effects and contraindications: Neuromuscular blocking agents **must not be used** if the provision of adequate anaesthesia and analgesia cannot be guaranteed and the means for adequate lung ventilation are unavailable. Neuromuscular blockade with pancuronium should always be antagonized with an antimuscarinic/anticholinesterase combination. Because of its potency and duration of action, neostigmine is preferred to edrophonium. If an overdose is given or if prolonged blockade occurs, use neostigmine to antagonize the effect of pancuronium.

Drug interactions: The following agents may antagonize the effects of pancuronium: **anticholinesterases** (**pyridostigmine**, **neostigmine**), **azathioprine**, **clindamycin**, **lincomycin**, **potassium** and **theophylline**. As **suxamethonium** may enhance muscular relaxation, delay the administration of pancuronium until the effects of suxamethonium begin to diminish. The action of pancuronium may be increased or intensified by some **antibiotics** (e.g. **aminoglycosides**, **clindamycin**, **lincomycin**), **inhalational anaesthetics** (e.g. **halothane**), **magnesium salts** and **quinidine**. Duration of action is longer when **isoflurane** (rather than **halothane**) is used to maintain anaesthesia.

Papaveretum (Papaveretum*) *POM* Schedule 2 Controlled Drug

Indications: Papaveretum (Omnopon) is a narcotic analgesic. It comprises a mixture of the alkaloids of opium, containing the equivalent of anhydrous morphine 85.5%, anhydrous codeine 6.8% and papaverine 7.8%. It is used as an analgesic, a sedative or as pre-anaesthetic medication, either alone or in combination with acepromazine and/or hyoscine (scopolamine). It has a similar effect to morphine with an onset of action of 15–60 minutes and a duration of 4 hours. Its sedative and euphoric effects are similar to those produced by morphine.

Forms: *Injectable:* 7.7 mg/ml, 15.4 mg/ml papaveretum solutions; 15.4 mg/ml papaveretum and 0.4 mg/ml hyoscine (scopolamine) solution. 7.7 mg/ml solution provides the equivalent of 5 mg anhydrous morphine/ml. 15.4 mg/ml solution provides the equivalent of 10 mg anhydrous morphine/ml.

Dose:
Cats: 0.2–1.0 mg/kg i.m., s.c.
Dogs: 0.2–3 mg/kg i.m., s.c.
See Sedation protocols, pages 297–301.

Adverse effects and contraindications: Severe adverse effects should be treated with **naloxone**. High doses may lead to respiratory depression. Papaveretum has similar adverse effects to morphine but is less likely to cause vomiting.

Drug interactions: Enhanced CNS or respiratory depression may occur with other **CNS depressants** (**anaesthetics**, **antihistamines**, **barbiturates**, **phenothiazines**, **tranquillizers**). As narcotic analgesics can increase biliary tract pressure, plasma amylase or lipase levels may be increased for up to 24 hours after drug administration.

Paracetamol (Acetaminophen) (Paracetamol*) *POM*

Indications: Paracetamol is an NSAID, although not a cyclo-oxygenase inhibitor. It modulates the concentration of prostaglandin intermediates. Its main use is as an antipyretic and to control mild to moderate somatic pain; it has poor anti-inflammatory effects. Paracetamol produces few GI side effects and can be administered to patients with gastric ulceration. Do not use in cats as they lack glucuronyl transferase enzymes required to metabolize the drug.

Forms: *Oral:* 500 mg tablet; 120 mg/5 ml, 250 mg/5 ml oral suspension.

Dose:
Dogs: 10 mg/kg p.o. q12h.
Small mammals: 1–2 mg/ml of drinking water (use flavoured products).

Adverse effects and contraindications: Do not use in cats. The main concern with paracetamol is hepatotoxicity.

Drug interactions: Metoclopramide enhances paracetamol's absorption thereby enhancing its effects.

Paraffin (**Katalax**; Lacri–Lube*; Liquid paraffin*) *GSL*

Indications: Paraffin (mineral oil) is a laxative used to manage constipation. It is also a lipid-based tear substitute that mimics the lipid portion of the tear film and helps to prevent evaporation of tears. Paraffin is a long-acting ocular lubricant and is used when frequency of treatment is not easy. It is beneficial in the management of keratoconjunctivitis sicca, during general anaesthesia and for eyelid paresis.

Forms:
Oral: White soft paraffin paste (Katalax); liquid paraffin.
Topical: 3.5 g, 5 g ophthalmic ointment (Lacri–Lube).

Dose:
Cats:
- Constipation: Adults 1 inch Katalax paste p.o. q12–24h; kittens $^1/_2$ inch Katalax paste p.o. q12–24h.
- Ocular: Apply to eye at night, or q6–8h prn.

Dogs:
- Constipation: 1–2 tablespoons per meal as required.
- Ocular: Apply to eye at night or q6–8h prn.

Birds: 4 ml/kg orally, per cloaca.

Adverse effects and contraindications: As paraffin is tasteless, normal swallowing may not be elicited if syringing orally. Thus inhalation and subsequent lipoid pneumonia is a significant risk. Paraffin ointment may blur vision, although not often a problem in dogs/cats.

Penicillamine (Penicillamine*) *POM*

Indications: D-Penicillamine is an orally administered chelating agent that binds copper, mercury and lead. In dogs it has been used mainly for treating copper-associated hepatopathy in Bedlington Terriers and the oral treatment of lead poisoning. It has also been used in the treatment of primary biliary cirrhosis, idiopathic chronic active hepatitis and cystinuria (decreases cystine excretion by combining with cystine to form the soluble complex cystine–D-penicillamine disulphide). D-Penicillamine may be used in the management of lead toxicity in birds when injecting EDTA is too difficult or long-term chelation is required.

Forms: *Oral:* 125 mg, 250 mg tablets.

Dose:
Dogs:
- Lead poisoning: Patients commonly receive CaEDTA before receiving penicillamine at 100–110 mg/kg p.o. q24h on an empty stomach for 1–2 weeks. Stop treatment for 1 week and resume until blood lead levels are normal (at end of 'rest' week). If adverse effects occur, the daily dose may be divided and given q6–8h or reduced to 33–55 mg/kg p.o. q24h.
  Dogs who fail to tolerate the lower dose regimens may be pre-treated with anti-emetic drugs (phenothiazines or antihistamines) 30–60 minutes before treating with penicillamine.
- Copper-associated hepatitis in Bedlington Terriers: 125–250 mg p.o. q24h given on an empty stomach 30 minutes before feeding. Must be given for months to be effective.
- Chronic hepatitis: 10–15 mg/kg p.o. q12h.
- Cystinuria: 10–15 mg/kg p.o. q12h.

Birds: Lead poisoning: 55 mg/kg p.o. q12h.

Adverse effects and contraindications: Adverse effects in the dog include anorexia, vomiting, pyrexia and nephrotic syndrome. Serious adverse effects that have been described in people given penicillamine include leucopenia, thrombocytopenia, skin rashes and lupus-like reactions.

Drug interactions: The absorption of penicillamine is decreased if administered with **antacids**, **food**, or **iron** or **zinc salts**. An increase in the renal and haematological effects of penicillamine have been recorded in people receiving it with **cytotoxic drugs** or **gold**.

Penicillin G (Benzyl Penicillin) (Crystapen*; Depocillin; Depomycin forte; Neopen) POM

Indications: Penicillin G is a beta-lactamase-susceptible, beta-lactam antibiotic. It binds to penicillin-binding proteins involved in cell wall synthesis, decreasing bacterial cell wall strength and rigidity, and affecting cell division, growth and septum formation. It is bactericidal. As animal cells lack a cell wall the beta-lactam antibiotics are safe. Penicillin G has a narrow spectrum of activity and is susceptible to acid degradation in the stomach. It is used parenterally to treat infections caused by sensitive organisms (e.g. *Streptococcus* spp., *Clostridium* spp., *Borrelia borgderferi* and fusospirochaetes). The sodium salt is absorbed well from s.c. or i.m. sites. Procaine penicillin is sparingly soluble, providing a 'depot' from which it is slowly released. When used for 'blind' therapy of undiagnosed infections penicillins may be given in conjunction with gentamicin with or without metronidazole.

Forms: *Injectable:* Penicillin G sodium: 300 mg powder; Procaine penicillin: 300 mg/ml suspension; Several compound preparations are available containing Penicillin G procaine penicillin and dihydrostreptomycin.

Dose:
Cats, Dogs: Penicillin G sodium 15–25 mg/kg i.v., i.m. q4–6h; Penicillin G procaine 10–15 mg/kg i.m., s.c. q12h.
Small mammals: Rabbits: 40,000 IU/kg (= 40 mg/kg) s.c. once every 7 days (x 3 doses) for *Treponema cuniculi* infection. For other infections 40,000 IU/kg (40 mg/kg) s.c. q24h.

As penicillin kills in a time-dependent fashion, it is important to maintain tissue concentrations above the MIC for the organism throughout the interdosing interval.

Adverse effects and contraindications: 600 mg of penicillin G sodium contains 1.7 mEq of Na^+. This may be clinically important for patients on restricted sodium intakes. After reconstitution penicillin G sodium is stable for 7 days if refrigerated, 24 hours if not. The i.m. administration of concentrations >600 mg/ml may cause discomfort. Patients with significant renal or hepatic dysfunction may need dosage adjustment. **Do not administer penicillins to hamsters, gerbils, guinea pigs or chinchillas**. Use with caution in rabbits but it has been used long-term for treatment of abscesses and osteomyelitis. Procaine is toxic to rats and mice.

Drug interactions: Avoid the concomitant use of bacteriostatic antibiotics. The **aminoglycosides** may inactivate penicillins when mixed in parenteral solutions. Penicillin and **aminoglycosides** act synergistically. **Procaine** can antagonize the action of **sulphonamides** and so procaine penicillin G should not be used with them.

Penicillin V (Phenoxymethylpenicillin)
(Phenoxymethylpenicillin*) *POM*

Indications: Penicillin V is a beta-lactamase-susceptible, beta-lactam antibiotic. Its mode of action is as for Penicillin G. Penicillin V is administered orally as it is more resistant to acid degradation than penicillin G and is better absorbed. As it has a narrow spectrum of activity, its use is limited to the treatment of infections caused by *Streptococcus* spp., *Clostridium* spp., *Borrelia borgderferi* and fusospirochaetes. Serious infections should be treated with parenteral penicillin G as the absorption of penicillin V is unpredictable. Penicillin V may be used later in the course of therapy. When used for 'blind' therapy of undiagnosed infections penicillins may be administered with gentamicin with or without metronidazole.

Forms: *Oral:* 250 mg (= 400,000 IU) tablets; 25 mg/ml solution.

Dose: *Cats, Dogs:* 10–30 mg/kg p.o. q8–12h.

As phenoxymethyl penicillin kills in a time-dependent fashion, dosing regimens should be designed to maintain tissue concentrations above the MIC for the bacterium throughout the interdosing interval.

Adverse effects and contraindications: Each gram of penicillin V contains 2.6 mEq of K^+. This may be clinically significant in patients on a reduced potassium intake. Patients with significant renal or hepatic dysfunction may need dosage adjustment. **Do not administer penicillins to hamsters, gerbils, guinea pigs, chinchillas or rabbits.**

Drug interactions: Avoid the concomitant use of bacteriostatic antibiotics (**erythromycin, oxytetracycline**).

Pentamidine isethionate (Pentacarinat*) *POM*

Indications: Pentamidine isethionate is an antiprotozoal drug, indicated for the treatment of leishmaniasis when resistance to the pentavalent antimony drugs (meglumine antimonate and sodium stibogluconate) has occurred. It is an aromatic diamidine that kills protozoans by interacting with DNA. It is rapidly taken up by the parasites by a high-affinity energy-dependent carrier.

Forms: *Injectable:* 300 mg vials of powder for reconstitution.

Dose: *Dogs:* 3–4 mg/kg i.m. on alternate days for a maximum of 10 treatments. Never give by rapid i.v. injection. **Seek expert advice before treating leishmaniasis**.

Caution: Care should be taken by staff handling this drug as it is a highly toxic agent. Similar precautions to those recommended when handling cytotoxic agents used in cancer chemotherapy should be taken.

Adverse effects and contraindications: Adverse reactions include pain and necrosis at the injection site, hypotension, nausea, salivation, vomiting and diarrhoea. Hypoglycaemia and blood dyscrasias are also reported in man. Never give by rapid i.v. injection due to cardiovascular effects. Pentamidine is a toxic drug and the potential to cause toxic damage to kidney and liver in particular should be carefully considered prior to use. Contraindicated in animals with impaired liver or kidney function.

Pentazocine (Fortral*; Pentazocine*) *POM* Schedule 3
Controlled Drug

Indications: Pentazocine is a mixed agonist/antagonist (weak) opioid used for short-term management of mild to medium pain in dogs. It has little sedative effect, only a slight effect on the GI tract and causes less respiratory depression than morphine. It can be given with acepromazine to produce neuroleptanalgesia, for minor sedation or pre-anaesthetic medication. After i.v. injection it has a rapid onset (2–5 minutes) and a short (45–60 minutes) duration of action. Unlike most other opioid agonists it increases heart rate.

Forms:
Injectable: 30 mg/ml for i.v., i.m. or s.c. use.
Oral: 25 mg tablet; 50 mg capsule.

Dose:
Dogs: 1–3 mg/kg i.m., 2–6 mg/kg p.o. repeated q3–4h prn.
Small mammals: 5–10 mg/kg s.c. q4h prn.

Adverse effects and contraindications: Rapid i.v. injection, alone or with acepromazine, may cause marked excitement. Pentazocine should not be used in cats as it tends to cause stimulation. It is ineffective in the management of severe pain.

Drug interactions: Barbiturate anaesthetics may cause additive respiratory or CNS depression if used with pentazocine.

Pentobarbital (Pentobarbitone) (Dolethal; Euthatal; Lethobarb; Pentobarbital; Pentoject) *POM* Schedule 3 Controlled Drug

Indications: Pentobarbital is a short-acting barbiturate that may be used as an i.v. anaesthetic, to control acute seizures or for euthanasia.

Forms: Injectable solutions for euthanasia: 200 mg/ml.

Dose:
Cats, Dogs:
- Status epilepticus: A dose of 20 mg/kg is prepared. Give aliquots of 3 mg/kg i.v. every 90 seconds until the seizure is controlled. The 'end-point' of administration is the cessation of seizure activity, i.e. not surgical planes of anaesthesia. Repeat q4–8h prn.
- Anaesthesia: 25–30 mg/kg i.v. slowly.

All species: Euthanasia: 150 mg/kg i.v. (or i.p. in small mammals and exotic birds) as rapidly as possible or to effect.

Drug interactions: The following increase the effect of pentobarbital, **antihistamines** and **opioids**.

Pentosan polysulphate (Cartrophen) *POM*

Indications: Pentosan polysulphate is a semi-synthetic polymer with a molecular weight of 2000. It binds to damaged cartilage matrix comprising aggregated proteoglycans and stimulates the synthesis of new aggregated glycosaminoglycan molecules. Its ability to inhibit a range of proteolytic enzymes may be of particular importance.

Forms: *Injectable:* 100 mg/ml solution.

Dose: *Dogs:* 3 mg/kg s.c. q5–7 days on four occasions; 10–20 mg/joint intra-articularly.

Adverse effects and contraindications: Do not use if septic arthritis is present or if renal or hepatic impairment exists. As pentosan polysulphate may induce spontaneous bleeding, its use in animals which have bleeding disorders is contraindicated.

Pentoxifylline (Oxpentifylline) (Trental*) *POM*

Indications: Pentoxifylline, a methylxanthine derivative, exerts peripheral vasodilatory actions and has immunological effects. It has been used in veterinary medicine to treat canine familial dermatomyositis, allergic contact dermatitis and vasculitis. There is evidence of its value in the treatment of interface dermatoses including lupoid onychodystropy and metatarsal fistula in German Shepherd Dogs.

Forms: *Oral:* 400 mg tablets.

Dose: *Dogs:* 10 mg/kg p.o. q8–24h.

Adverse effects and contraindications: Mild vomiting and diarrhoea have been reported.

Pethidine (Pethidine) *POM* Schedule 2 Controlled Drug

Indications: Pethidine is a pure mu (OP3) agonist with a fast onset (10–15 minutes) and a short duration of action (30–45 minutes). It is effective in suppressing mild to moderate pain, particularly that arising from GI, biliary or urogenital smooth muscle spasm. Although its sedative and euphoric effects are less marked than those produced by morphine, pethidine/acepromazine mixtures produce useful neuroleptanalgesia for minor procedures, or pre-anaesthetic medication. Unlike other opioid agonists it increases heart rate. In man, pethidine causes less biliary tree spasm than morphine, which suggests that it may be the most useful opioid analgesic for dogs with pancreatitis. Pethidine rarely causes vomiting so is preferred in cases with increased intracranial or intraocular pressure.

Forms: *Injectable:* 50 mg/ml solution.

Dose:
Cats: 5–10 mg/kg i.m., s.c. prn or q4–6h.
Dogs: 2–10 mg/kg i.m., s.c. prn or q3–4h.
Small mammals: 10–20 mg/kg i.m. q2h.
See Sedation protocols, pages 297–301.

Adverse effects and contraindications: Adverse effects in cats (hyperaesthesia) are only seen in gross overdosage and may be controlled with acepromazine. Rapid i.v. injection in dogs causes marked histamine release (tachycardia and hypotension). Intramuscular injections may occasionally cause urticarial reactions. Pethidine should not be used in animals at risk from histamine release, e.g. certain skin allergies, 'asthma' and possibly those with mast cell tumours. Histamine-based reactions should be treated with chlorphenamine, or adrenaline in critical cases. Adverse, or prolonged non-histaminoid effects, e.g. respiratory depression, may be treated with naloxone only if the antagonism of analgesia is justified. Respiratory depression is seen at very high doses.

Drug interactions: Increased CNS or respiratory depression if pethidine is used with other **CNS depressants** (**anaesthetics, antihistamines, barbiturates, phenothiazines, tranquillizers**). The metabolism of pethidine is inhibited by **cimetidine,** thereby sustaining high plasma concentrations. As narcotic analgesics may increase biliary tract pressure, plasma amylase and lipase levels may be increased for up to 24 hours after narcotic administration. Pethidine is preferred to morphine for control of pain with pancreatitis.

Phenobarbital (Phenobarbitone) (Epiphen; Phenobarbital*)
POM Schedule 3 Controlled Drug

Indications: Phenobarbital is a long-acting barbiturate used in the management of seizures and occasionally as a tranquillizer. It acts as an anticonvulsant by increasing the threshold of electrical excitability required for seizure discharge and by decreasing the duration of after discharges in the motor cortex. Its mechanism of action is through enhanced responsiveness to the inhibitory postsynaptic effects of GABA, as well as inhibition of the excitatory neurotransmitter glutamate. It is the initial drug of choice for treating idiopathic seizure disorders in both dogs and cats and is used adjunctively for the emergency treatment of acute seizure disorders secondary to other causes (e.g. strychnine toxicity, tetanus, meningitis). In a behavioural context phenobarbital is used in the treatment of the behavioural signs of limbic epilepsy, such as sudden-onset aggressive responses and fear reactions. Some authors suggest the use of phenobarbital in combination with propranolol in the management of fear and phobia-related behaviour problems.

Forms:
Injectable: 200 mg/ml solution.
Oral: 15 mg, 30 mg, 60 mg, 100 mg tablets.

Dose:
Cats, Dogs:
• Initial therapy for idiopathic epilepsy: 1–2.5 mg/kg p.o. q12h (cats); 1–8 mg/kg p.o. q12h (dogs). With chronic therapy, induction of the hepatic microsomal enzyme system results in a decreased half-life. As a result, the dose may need to be increased or doses may need to be given more frequently (q8h). Trough phenobarbital levels should be assessed every 6 or 12 months. Some authors suggest that animals with inadequate seizure control should not be considered refractory to phenobarbital therapy until doses exceeding 10 mg/kg q12h with therapeutic serum levels have been achieved.

- Adjunctive therapy of status epilepticus (or severe recurring seizures): 5–30 mg/kg (start at low end of dose range) i.v. over 5–10 minutes. Maximum anti-seizure activity may take up to 30 minutes. Dose may be increased and repeated at 30-minute intervals until seizures controlled or a total dose of 30 mg/kg given. For each 3 mg/kg given, serum concentration increases by 21.5 μmol/l. Thus, a total dose of 18 mg/kg may be necessary to achieve a concentration approximately in the middle of the therapeutic range (130 μmol/l; see therapeutic range below) in dogs that have not had prior therapy. In dogs already receiving phenobarbital, higher doses may be necessary. If using with diazepam, administer i.m. to avoid cardiovascular and respiratory depression.

Adverse effects and contraindications: Adverse effects include sedation, ataxia, polyphagia and PU/PD. Polyphagia and PU/PD are likely to persist throughout therapy. Ataxia and sedation occur commonly following initiation of therapy but usually resolve within 1 week, although they may continue if high doses are used. Raised ALT and AST levels are common. However, some cases on chronic, high dose therapy may develop a life-threatening hepatopathy; monitor serum bile acids every 6 months and perform pre- and postprandial bile acid tests if in doubt. Neutropenia, thrombocytopenia, anaemia and splenomegaly have been reported in dogs. Monitor serum phenobarbital levels, if toxicity or lack of seizure control is encountered, 2 hours before (trough) and 2 hours after (peak) dosing. Therapeutic serum levels vary with different laboratories, but are in the region of 65–172 μmol/l. When withdrawing phenobarbital, reduce the dose gradually. If switching from phenobarbital to primidone, 1 mg of phenobarbital is equivalent to 3.8 mg primidone. Abrupt withdrawal may precipitate seizures.

Drug interactions: The effect of phenobarbital may be increased by other **CNS depressants** (**antihistamines, narcotics, phenothiazines**). Phenobarbital may enhance the metabolism of, and therefore decrease the effect of, **corticosteroids, beta-blockers, metronidazole** and **theophylline**. Phenobarbital may decrease the absorption of **griseofulvin**; avoid giving them together. Barbiturates may enhance the effects of other **antiepileptics**. **Cimetidine, ketoconazole** and **chloramphenicol** increase serum phenobarbital concentration through inhibition of the hepatic microsomal enzyme system.

Phenoxybenzamine (Dibenyline*) POM

Indications: Phenoxybenzamine, an alpha-adrenergic blocker, irreversibly blocks presynaptic and postsynaptic receptors, producing a so-called chemical sympathectomy. It has no effect on the parasympathetic system. Phenoxybenzamine is used in small animal practice for the treatment of reflex dyssynergia and the treatment of severe hypertension in animals with pheochromocytoma prior to surgery (in conjunction with a beta-blocker).

Forms: *Oral:* 10 mg capsule.

Doses:
Cats: 0.5–1 mg/kg p.o. q12h for 5 days before evaluating efficacy.
Dogs:
- Reflex dyssynergia: 0.25–1 mg/kg p.o. q8–24h for a minimum of 5 days.
- Hypertension associated with phaeochromocytoma: 0.2–1.5 mg/kg p.o. q12h for 10–14 days prior to surgery starting at a low dosage and increasing until the hypertension is controlled. Propranolol 0.15–0.5 mg/kg p.o. q8h is administered concurrently to prevent a hypertensive crisis.

The only oral dosage form available is a 10 mg capsule; round to the nearest 2.5 mg dose.

Adverse effects and contraindications: Always use phenoxybenzamine and a beta-blocker (e.g. propranolol) when treating phaeochromocytomas, as beta blockade without concurrent alpha blockade may lead to a hypertensive crisis. Adverse effects associated with alpha-adrenergic blockade include, hypotension, miosis, tachycardia and nasal congestion. Use with extreme caution in animals with pre-existing cardiovascular disease.

Drug interactions: There is an increased risk of a first dose hypotensive effect if administered with **beta-blockers** or **diuretics**. Phenoxybenzamine will antagonize effects of alpha-adrenergic sympathomimetic agents (e.g. **phenylephrine**).

Phentolamine (Rogitine*) *POM*

Indications: Phentolamine is a competitive alpha-adrenergic blocking agent. It is short acting and has immediate onset of action when given i.v. It is primarily indicated for the emergency treatment of extravasation injuries associated with dopamine, phenylephrine or noradrenaline, and in the management of hypertensive crises associated with phaeochromocytomas.

Forms: *Injectable:* 10 mg/ml solution.

Dose: *Cats, Dogs:*
- Antidote for extravasation injuries secondary to dopamine, phenylephrine or noradrenaline: Dilute 5 mg of phentolamine in 10 ml of normal saline. Using a fine needle, liberally infiltrate the exposed area. Immediate effects should be seen (hyperaemia); must be used within 12 hours of injury.
- Hypertension: 0.02–0.1 mg/kg i.v. bolus followed by an i.v. infusion.

Adverse effects and contraindications: Hypotension.

Drug interactions: The hypertensive and vasoconstricting effects of **adrenaline** and **noradrenaline** are blocked by phentolamine. Enhanced hypotension when administered with many drugs.

Phenylbutazone (**Companazone**; **Phenogel**; **Phenycare**; **Phenylbutazone**) *POM*

Indications: Phenylbutazone is an NSAID that inhibits COX-1 enzyme, limiting prostaglandin production. NSAIDs have antipyretic, analgesic, anti-inflammatory and antiplatelet effects. Phenylbutazone is used to control mild to moderate pain and inflammation in osteoarthritic conditions.

Forms: *Oral:* 100 mg, 200 mg tablets.

Dose:
Cats: 6–8 mg/kg i.v., i.m., p.o. q12h.
Dogs: 2–20 mg/kg i.v., i.m., p.o. q8–12h. Maximum dose 800 mg.

Adverse effects and contraindications: Adverse effects of NSAIDs are dose-related and reflect the reduction in prostaglandin synthesis. The commonest adverse effect is GI irritation and ulceration. Renal papillary necrosis (renal failure) is also a serious adverse effect, particularly if hypotension, dehydration or other nephrotoxic drugs are present. Phenylbutazone may infrequently induce bone marrow suppression (including aplastic anaemia). Nausea, vomiting, diarrhoea, hepatotoxicity (cholestasis and parenchymal damage) and fluid retention, which may precipitate cardiac failure, may develop rarely. Do not use if gastric or duodenal ulceration is suspected, in haemorrhagic syndromes or in cases of cardiac, hepatic or renal disease. Severe toxicity (usually with an acute overdose) may present with vomiting, pyrexia, metabolic acidosis, depression, coma, seizures and GI bleeding. Treatment of acute toxic ingestion includes emptying the gut, treating the acidosis, alkalinising urine with sodium bicarbonate and supportive therapy.

Drug interactions: Do not use with **corticosteroids**, **methoxyflurane** or other **NSAIDs** (increased risk of toxic effects). In man there is an increased risk of convulsions if NSAIDs are administered with **fluoroquinolones**. NSAIDs may antagonize the hypotensive effects of **anti-hypertensives** (e.g. **beta-blockers**). The concomitant use of **diuretics** may increase the risk of nephrotoxicity. Do not mix with other substances in the same syringe. Phenylbutazone may cause false low **T3** and **T4** values. Phenylbutazone displaces a variety of protein-bound drugs including **anaesthetics**, thereby potentiating their effects.

Phenylephrine (Minims phenylephrine*; Phenylephrine*) POM

Indications: Phenylephrine is an alpha$_1$ selective adrenergic agonist that causes peripheral vasoconstriction when given i.v., resulting in increased diastolic and systolic blood pressure, a small decrease in cardiac output and an increased circulation time. It is used in conjunction with fluid therapy, to treat hypotension secondary to drugs or vascular failure. Phenylephrine has minimal effects on cardiac beta receptors. When applied topically to the eye phenylephrine causes vasoconstriction and mydriasis (pupil dilation). Ophthalmic uses include mydriasis prior to intraocular surgery (often in conjunction with atropine), differentiation of involvement of superficial conjunctival vasculature from deep episcleral vasculature (by vasoconstriction), and in the diagnosis of Horner's syndrome (denervation hypersensitivity).

Forms:
Injectable: 1% (10 mg/ml) s.c., i.m. or slow i.v.
Ophthalmic: 2.5%, 10% solutions.

Dose: *Cats, Dogs:*
- Hypotension: Correct blood volume then infuse 0.01 mg/kg very slowly i.v. q15 minutes. Continuously monitor blood pressure if possible.
- Ophthalmic use: 1 drop approximately 2h before intraocular surgery. 1 drop as a single dose for vasoconstriction. 1 drop to both eyes for diagnosis of Horner's syndrome.

Adverse effects and contraindications: Vasoconstrictors should be used with care. Although they raise blood pressure, they do so at the expense of perfusion of vital organs (e.g. kidney). In many patients with shock, peripheral resistance is already high and to raise it further is unhelpful. Adverse effects include hypertension, tachycardia or reflex bradycardia. Extravasation injuries can be serious (necrosis and sloughing) and may be treated with phentolamine.

Drug interactions: There is a risk of arrhythmias if phenylephrine is used in digitalized patients or with volatile anaesthetic agents. When used concurrently with **oxytocic agents** the pressor effects may be enhanced, leading to severe hypertension.

Phenylpropanolamine/Diphenylpyraline (Propalin) POM

Indications: Phenylpropanolamine is a sympathomimetic amine that stimulates alpha-adrenergic receptors. In the lower urinary tract it increases urethral outflow resistance. It is used to treat incontinence secondary to urinary sphincter incompetence. The peripheral vasoconstrictive qualities of this agent may be useful in the management of nasal congestion.

Forms: *Oral:* 50 mg phenylpropanolamine/ml syrup (Propalin).

Dose: *Cats, Dogs:* Propalin: 1 mg/kg p.o. q8h or 1.5 mg/kg p.o. q12h.

Adverse effect and contraindications: Incontinence may recur if doses are delayed or missed. The onset of action may take several days. Adverse effects may include restlessness, aggressiveness, irritability and hypertension.

Phenytoin (Epanutin*; Phenytoin*)*POM*

Indications: Phenytoin is an antiepileptic drug that diminishes the spread and propagation of focal neural discharges. Its action appears to arise from a stabilizing effect on synaptic junctions and it depresses motor areas of the cortex without depressing sensory areas. It is used to control most forms of epilepsy in man. However, in dogs it is metabolized very rapidly such that very high doses need to be given often, whereas cats metabolize the drug very slowly and toxicity easily develops. These undesirable pharmacokinetic properties make it a secondary agent in veterinary medicine.

Forms: *Oral:* 25 mg, 50 mg, 100 mg capsules, 6 mg/ml suspension.

Dose: *Dogs:* 10–35 mg/kg p.o. q6–8h.

Adverse effects and contraindications: This drug is most effective if used in combination with phenobarbital or primidone. It cannot be recommended for use as a sole agent. Monitoring of serum levels is useful in cases when either efficacy or toxicity are in question. Adverse effects include ataxia, vomiting, peripheral neuropathy, liver failure, toxic epidermal necrolysis, pyrexia, lupus erythematosus and delirium. Monitor liver function yearly in patients on chronic therapy. Oral absorption may be enhanced and GI effects decreased if given with food. Abrupt withdrawal may precipitate seizures.

Drug interactions: Many interactions are reported in the human literature. The plasma concentration of phenytoin may be increased by **cimetidine, diazepam, metronidazole, phenylbutazone, sulphonamides** and **trimethoprim**. The absorption, effects or plasma concentration of phenytoin may be decreased by **antacids, barbiturates** and **calcium**. The metabolism of **corticosteroids, doxycycline, theophylline** and **thyroxine** may be increased by phenytoin. The analgesic properties of **pethidine** may be reduced by phenytoin whereas the toxic effects may be enhanced. Concomitant administration of two or more anti-epileptics may enhance toxicity without a corresponding increase in anti-epileptic effect.

Pheromones – Dog Appeasing (DAP) (D.A.P.*)

Indications: DAP is a synthetic formulation reproducing the effects of the 'appeasing pheromone' isolated from the intermammary sulcus of the bitch and naturally secreted by the mother shortly after birth. The applications of DAP are varied. It has been specifically advocated in a prophylactic role for assisting young puppies in settling into their new homes. It is also used in a management role in cases of anxiety-based behavioural disorders, such as separation anxiety, where stress-related behaviour signs, e.g. destructive behaviour, inappropriate vocalization, house soiling and excessive licking, are displayed. In addition it has been found to be extremely effective as part of the approach to fear-related behaviours in dogs, including sound sensitivity and fear of noises, such as fireworks. In such cases DAP is recommended as an adjunct to desensitization and counter-conditioning programme, and the manufacturer recommends the use of the 'Sounds Scary' range of CDs. Other applications include the management of transfer of adult dogs from familiar to unfamiliar surroundings and the management of stress during potentially challenging situations, such as interacting with strangers.

Forms: *Environmental:* Diffuser/Pump spray solution.

Administration: *Dogs:* Diffuser: The diffuser is active over an area of approx 50–70 m². If the total target area exceeds this, a second diffuser should be used. One vial will last for approximately 4 weeks if the device is left switched on 24 hrs/day. Do not repeatedly switch the diffuser on and off – it is designed to be left on at all times. The diffuser should be placed in the room most frequently occupied by the dog and, in the management of behavioural disorders, where the inappropriate behaviour most frequently occurs. For management of sound-related phobias, such as fireworks, the diffuser should be placed in the designated den, which has been provided for the dog to hide in. It should be switched on two weeks before an anticipated phobic event and left on until two weeks after the event. When used to support the process of desensitization during the treatment of sound phobia the diffuser should be left on throughout the period when behavioural therapy is being carried out. For behaviour problems involving hyperattachment to the owner, a treatment period of 3 months is recommended.

Environmental spray: DAP spray can be used inside and outside the home environment. It can be used in cars, hospitalization cages, kennels, indoor pens or refuge areas and applied directly on to bedding. It should not be sprayed directly on to animals or near an animal's face. It can be sprayed with the bottle in an upside down position. In the house DAP spray can compliment the use of the diffuser device where a more local application is needed. Spray 8–10 pumps of DAP on to the required surface 15 minutes before results are expected and before the dog is introduced into the environment to allow the alcohol carrier to evaporate. The effect should last for 1–2 hours, although each animal will respond individually. The application can be renewed after 1–2 hours or when the effects appear to be reducing.

Pheromones – Feline F3 fraction (Feliway*)

Indications: Feline F3 is known as the 'familiarization pheromone' and it is believed to provide a feeling of security for cats in unfamiliar or stressful situations. It is a synthetic analogue of the F3 fraction of the 'feline facial pheromones'. The major applications are for the management of indoor urine marking, inappropriate scratching and stress during transportation. It is also extremely useful in decreasing stress associated with confinement in hospitalization cages and rescue and cattery establishments. It has also been shown to decrease stress during introduction to a new home. Additional indications include management of situational anxiety-related disorders. It can be very effective during handling for anaesthesia induction and during other medical examinations when the spray is applied to the consulting or preparation table.

Forms: *Environmental:* Diffuser: 10% pump spray solution. The diffuser is active over an area of approx 50–70 m². One vial is active for 4 weeks.

Administration: *Cats:* Diffuser: The diffuser is active over an area of approximately 50–70 m². If the total target area exceeds this, a second diffuser should be used. One vial will last for approximately 4 weeks if the device is left switched on 24 hours per day. Do not repeatedly switch the diffuser on and off – it is designed to be left on at all times. The diffuser should be placed in the room most frequently occupied by the cat and, in the case of management of behavioural disorders, where the inappropriate behaviour most frequently occurs.

Pump spray: Feliway is applied to the environment in locations where the inappropriate behaviour is occurring and in locations that are of behavioural significance. When being used as a familiarization signal for cats in potentially stressful situations, or in new environments, the spray should be applied 30 minutes before the cat has access to the area. In the case of management of existing urine marking, one dose (one depression of the nozzle) should be applied daily from about 10 cm from the soiled site at a height of about 20 cm from the floor. The bottle should be kept upright during application. In multicat households the spray should be applied 2–3 times/day on previously marked sites and once a day on other locations which are of behavioural significance. When using to prevent urine marking, spray once per day in locations of behavioural significance. For best results allow the spray to come to room temperature before it is applied and adjust cleaning regimes for indoor marking. Allow 24 hours between cleaning, with biological washing powder followed by surgical spirit, and the application of the feliway spray.

Adverse effects and contraindications: There are no specific contraindications. The pump spray should not mark or stain but it is sensible to patch test furniture, carpets, etc. before using extensively.

Pheromones – Feline F4 fraction (Felifriend*)

Indications: This is a synthetic analogue of the F4 fraction of the feline facial 'pheromones', used to familiarize cats to people towards whom they show apprehensive or fearful behaviour. The primary use is to improve tolerance of handling during veterinary examination and grooming. It may also be used to increase tolerance between cats but is not specifically licensed for use in inter-cat situations.

Forms: *Topical:* 10% pump spray solution; impregnated handwash.

Dose: *Cats:*
- Familiarization to people: Apply 2 sprays of the solution (or handwash) to the palm of each hand and rub the hands and wrists together as required. Place the hands 20 cm in front of the cat's nose and wait for one minute before initiating contact.
- Familiarization to cats: Apply 2 sprays of the pump spray solution on to a compress and apply to the flank and neck regions of each cat. It is best to avoid using the pump spray in front of the cat since this can lead to fear responses, which make application very difficult. Wait for at least one minute after application before introducing the cats to each other and ensure that they are supervised.

Do not spray close to the animal's head, specifically in the region of the eyes.

Adverse effects and contraindications: In some cases a paradoxical increase in agitation and aggression is witnessed. If cats exhibit vocalization and threatening behaviour towards people after the application terminate the contact and reintroduce the hands slowly. Stop if aggression continues. Use in interactions between cats should be carried out with caution, as a paradoxical increase in agitation and aggression may occur.

Phosphate (**Toldimphos**) (**Foston**; Phosphate–Sandoz*) *POM*

Indications: Phosphate is used in the management of hypophosphataemia.

Forms:
Injectable: Foston: 140 mg/ml phosphate (toldimphos, an organically combined phosphorus preparation).
Oral: Phosphate–Sandoz: Effervescent tablets containing 1.936g sodium acid phosphate, 350 mg sodium bicarbonate, 315 mg potassium bicarbonate, equivalent to 500 mg (16.1 mmol) phosphate, 468.8 mg (20.4 mmol) sodium and 123 mg (3.1 mmol) potassium.

Dose: *Cats, Dogs:* 140–280 mg q48h i.m., s.c. for 5–10 doses; 0.5–2 mmol/kg/day p.o.

Phosphate enema solution (Fleet enema*; Fletchers' Phosphate Enema*) *P*

Indications: Phosphate enema solution is a cathartic used to initiate rapid emptying of the colon in dogs.

Forms: 133 ml bottle containing 21.4 g sodium acid phosphate and 9.4 g sodium phosphate (Fleet). 128 ml bottle containing 12.8 g sodium acid phosphate and 10.24 g sodium phosphate (Fletchers').

Dose: *Dogs:* >10 kg: 128 ml per rectum; 4–10 kg: 60–118 ml per rectum.

Adverse effects and contraindications: This enema is contraindicated for use in cats or small dogs as they may develop electrolyte abnormalities (hypocalcaemia and hyperphosphataemia) which can be fatal.

Phytomenadione – see Vitamin K

Pilocarpine (Pilocarpine*; Pilogel*; Sno Pilo*) *POM*

Indications: Pilocarpine is a parasympathomimetic miotic producing miosis in 10–15 minutes for 6–8h. It increases lacrimation and can be used in the management of neurogenic KCS. It increases aqueous outflow and has been used in the management of glaucoma; this role has been superceded by other topical drugs, such as dorzolamide and latanoprost.

Forms: *Ocular:* 0.5%, 1%, 2%, 3%, 4% solutions, 4% gel. Most common concentration used in dogs is 1%.

Dose: *Dogs:* Open-angle glaucoma: 1 drop 1% solution q12h.
Neurogenic KCS: 1 drop 1% solution p.o. q12h.
Higher doses have been recommended in the dog for neurogenic KCS (2 drops 2% solution/10 kg as initial dose) but signs of systemic toxicity may occur.

Adverse effect and contraindications: Conjunctival hyperaemia (vasodilation) and local irritation (due to low pH). It should not be used in cases of uveitis or anterior lens luxation. Pilocarpine is rarely used for ophthalmic purposes in the cat due to potential toxicity. Signs of systemic toxicity include vomiting and diarrhoea.

Pimobendan (Vetmedin) *POM*

Indications: Pimobendan sensitizes the myocardium to calcium, producing a positive inotropic effect whilst improving myocardial oxygen economy. The compound also has phosphodiesterase III and V inhibiting effects that lead to peripheral arterio- and venodilatation. It is indicated for the management of congestive cardiac failure in the dog, particularly when there is evidence of reduced myocardial contractility.

Forms: *Oral:* 1.25 mg, 2.5 mg, 5 mg capsules.

Dose: *Dogs:* 0.2–0.6 mg/kg p.o. q24h one hour before food.

Adverse effects and contraindications: Pimobendan is contraindicated in hypertrophic cardiomyopathy and in cases where augmentation of cardiac output via increased contractility is not possible (e.g. aortic stenosis). A moderate positive chronotropic effect and vomiting may occur in some cases, which may be avoided by dose reduction.

Drug interactions: The positive inotropic effects are attenuated by drugs such as **beta-blockers** and **calcium-channel blockers.** No interaction with **digitalis glycosides** has been noted.

Piperacillin (Tazocin*) POM

Indications: Piperacillin is a ureidopenicillin, classified with ticarcillin as an antipseudomonal penicillin. It acts by binding to penicillin-binding proteins near bacterial cell walls, thereby decreasing bacterial cell wall strength and rigidity, and affecting cell division, growth and septum formation. As mammalian cells lack a cell wall the beta-lactam antibiotics are extremely safe. Piperacillin is reserved for serious life-threatening infections (e.g. endocarditis or septicaemia) caused by *Pseudomonas aeruginosa* and *Bacteroides fragilis* in neutropenic patients, although it has activity against other Gram-negative bacilli including *Proteus* spp. For pseudomonal septicaemias, anti-pseudomonal penicillins should be given with an aminoglycoside (e.g. gentamicin) as there is a synergistic effect. Piperacillin should usually be combined with a beta-lactamase inhibitor and is co-formulated with tazobactam.

Forms: *Injectable:* 2.25 g, 4.5 g powder (2 g or 4 g piperacillin sodium and 0.25 g or 0.5 g tazobactam (Tazocin)).

Dose: *Cats, Dogs:* 50–100 mg/kg by slow i.v. injection/infusion q8h.
Birds: 100–150 mg/kg i.m. q8–12h.
Reptiles: 50–100 mg/kg i.m. q24h.

Adverse effects and contraindications: Nausea, diarrhoea and skin rashes are the commonest adverse effects in man. Painful if given by i.m. injection. The sodium content of each formulation may be clinically important for patients on restricted sodium intakes.

Drug interactions: Piperacillin enhances the effects of **non-depolarizing muscle relaxants.** **Gentamicin** inactivates piperacillin if mixed in the same syringe. Clinical experience with this drug is limited.

Piperazine (**Biozine**; **Endorid**; **Piperazine**) *GSL*

Indications: Piperazine, an anti-ascaridal anthelmintic, blocks acetylcholine, thus affecting neurotransmission and paralysing the adult worm; it has no larvicidal activity. It is effective against *Toxocara cati*, *T. canis*, *Toxascaris leonina* and *Uncinaria stenocephala*. It is ineffective against tapeworms and lung worms. High doses are required to treat hookworm infection.

Forms: *Oral:* 416 mg, 450 mg or 500 mg tablets. The above list of products may not be comprehensive. The inclusion or omission of any specific product does not indicate that the product is more or less effective.

Dose: *Cats, Dogs:* Ascarids: 100 mg/kg p.o. Repeat dose in 2–3 weeks. Hookworm: 200 mg/kg p.o.

Adverse effects and contraindications: Adverse effects are uncommon but occasionally vomiting or muscle tremors and ataxia have been reported. Puppies and kittens may be wormed from 6–8 weeks of age and should be weighed accurately to prevent overdosing. Fasting is not necessary. Piperazine may be used in pregnant animals.

Polymyxin B (Polyfax*; **Surolan**) *POM*

Indications: Polymyxin B is a cationic antibacterial effective against Gram-negative organisms; Gram-positive organisms are usually resistant. It is rapidly bactericidal (concentration-dependent mechanism) by disrupting the outer membrane of Gram-negative bacteria. It is particularly effective in the treatment of external pseudomonal infections, e.g. keratoconjunctivitis, otitis externa. Polymyxins are too toxic for systemic use and because of their strongly basic nature are not absorbed from the GI tract.

Forms: *Topical:* Surolan 5,500 IU polymyxin/ml suspension combined with miconazole and prednisolone for dermatological and otic use. Polyfax: 10,000 IU polymyxin/g ointment combined with bacitracin for dermatological and ophthalmic use.

Dose: *Cats, Dogs:*
- Skin: Apply a few drops and rub in well q12h.
- Otic: Clean ear and apply a few drops into affected ear q12h.
- Ophthalmic: Apply ointment q6–8h.

Drug interactions: Polymyxins act synergistically with a number of **other antibacterial agents** because they disrupt the outer and cytoplasmic membranes, thus improving penetration of other agents into bacterial cells. **Cationic detergents** (e.g. **chlorhexidine**) and **chelating agents** (e.g. **EDTA**) potentiate the antibacterial effects of polymyxin B against *Pseudomonas aeruginosa*.

Polysulphated glycosaminoglycan (Adequan*) POM

Indications: Polysulphated glycosaminoglycan is based on hexosamine and hexuronic acid. It binds to damaged cartilage matrix consisting of aggregated proteoglycans and stimulates the synthesis of new glycosaminoglycan molecules and may inhibit proteolytic enzymes. It is used in the management of non-infectious and non-immune-mediated arthritides.

Forms: *Injectable:* 100 mg/ml solution.

Dose: *Dogs:* 0.5 ml/joint i.m. or intra-articularly.

Adverse effects and contraindications: Do not use if the dog has renal or hepatic impairment.

Polyvinyl alcohol (Hypotears*; Liquifilm*; Sno–tears*) POM

Indications: Polyvinyl alcohol is a synthetic resin tear substitute (lacromimetic) used for lubrication of dry eyes. In cases of keratoconjunctivitis sicca (dry eye) it will improve ocular surface lubrication, tear retention and patient comfort while lacrostimulation therapy (e.g. ciclosporin) is initiated. It is more adherent and less viscous than hypromellose.

Forms: *Topical:* 1%, 1.4% drops.

Dose: *Cats, Dogs:* 1 drop/eye q1h.
Note: Patient compliance may be poor if dosing is more frequent than q4h, consider using longer acting tear replacement.

Potassium bromide (Epilease; Potassium bromide*) POM

Indication: Bromide salts have been used for their anticonvulsant effect for many years. Bromide ions suppress neuronal excitability, probably by replacing intracellular chloride and hyperpolarizing nerve cell membranes. Potassium bromide (KBr) may be used as an add-on therapy with other anticonvulsants (e.g. phenobarbital) if seizure control is inadequate, or as monotherapy especially if toxicity is encountered with other anticonvulsants (e.g. hepatic toxicity). In a behavioural context potassium bromide is used in combination with phenobarbital during the treatment of the behavioural signs of limbic epilepsy, such as sudden-onset aggressive responses and fear reactions. A long elimination half time makes KBr useful when clients are unable to provide medication at prescribed times. Potassium bromide is favoured over the sodium or ammonium salt because of its greater water solubility and bromide content. The slow rise of plasma bromide levels after enteral administration limits its usefulness in status epilepticus. Bromide is well absorbed from the GI tract and eliminated slowly by the kidney in competition with chloride.

Forms: *Oral:* 325 mg tablet; 985 mg capsules/tablets; 250 mg/ml solution.

Dose: *Dogs:* The initial daily maintenance dose if used alone is 50–80 mg/kg/day p.o., which may be divided into 2 doses given 12h apart. If administered with phenobarbital the initial daily dose is 20–40 mg/kg p.o.

Ideally, plasma drug levels should be monitored and therapy aimed at achieving values of approximately 1.0–1.5 mg/ml (values vary with laboratories). Bromide has a long half-life (>20 days) and steady state plasma concentrations may not be achieved for 3–4 months if daily therapy is used alone. To rapidly achieve therapeutic plasma concentrations, a loading dose of 450–600 mg/kg p.o. is commonly given. A dose of 450 mg/kg should achieve a plasma concentration of 1.0 mg/ml, and 600 mg/kg should achieve 1.5 mg/ml. To avoid vomiting caused by gastric irritation, the loading dose is commonly divided over 5 days and given with the maintenance dose, after which the daily maintenance dose is continued. Serum samples should be taken 2 days after the end of loading and again 3–4 weeks later. If the second sample shows a lower serum level, then the immediate post-loading dose of 250 mg/ml can be given to rapidly raise serum levels by 0.5 mg/ml. High levels of dietary salt increase renal elimination of bromide. Consequently, it is important that the diet be kept constant once bromide therapy has started. Sudden withdrawal of the drug may precipitate seizures.

Adverse effects and contraindications: Adverse neurological reactions usually reflect overdose and include ataxia, sedation and somnolence. Skin reactions have been reported in animals with pre-existing skin diseases, e.g. flea bite dermatitis. Severe coughing due to eosinophilic bronchitis, which may be fatal, has been reported in cats. Vomiting may occur after oral administration if high concentrations (>250 mg/ml) are used. Polyphagia, polydipsia and pancreatitis (rare) have also been reported. In the case of acute bromide toxicity 0.9% NaCl i.v. is the treatment of choice.

Drug interactions: The following may increase the likelihood of seizures: **tricyclic** antidepressants, **metoclopramide**, **fluoroquinolones** and possibly **glucocorticoids**.

Potassium chloride (Kay-Cee-L*; Potassium Chloride*; Slow-K*) *POM*

Indications: Used to treat hypokalaemia.

Forms:
Injectable: 15% KCl solution (150 mg KCl/ml; 2 mmol/ml K^+ and Cl^-). Dilute with at least 25 times its own volume before i.v. administration.
Oral: 600 mg KCl (8 mmol K^+ and Cl^-) tablets (Slow-K); 7.5% KCl (75 mg/ml; 1 mmol/ml K^+ and Cl^-) syrup (Kay-Cee-L).
Note: 1 mmol/l ≡ 1 mEq/l.

Dose: Intravenous doses must be titrated for each patient; dilute concentrated solutions prior to use.

Serum potassium	Amount to add to 250 ml 0.9% NaCl
<2 mmol/l	20 mmol
2–2.5 mmol/l	15 mmol
2.5–3 mmol/l	10 mmol
3–3.5 mmol/l	7 mmol

Rate of i.v. infusion should not exceed 0.5 mEq/kg body weight/h.

Cats: 2–6 mmol/cat/day p.o.
Dogs: 0.2–0.5 mmol/kg p.o. q8h or 1–3g/dog p.o. q24h.

Adverse effects and contraindications: Adverse effects include GI irritation with the oral preparations. As potassium is primarily an intracellular electrolyte, serum levels do not adequately reflect its total body store. Acid–base imbalances may also mask the actual extent of any alterations in potassium levels. Patients with systemic acidosis may appear to be hyperkalaemic when in fact they may have a significantly low total body potassium content. Alkalosis may falsely indicate a low serum potassium.

Drug interactions: ACE inhibitors and **potassium-sparing diuretics** (e.g. **spironolactone**) increase the risk of hyperkalaemia.

Potassium citrate (Potassium citrate BP*; Cystopurin*) *GSL*

Indications: Potassium citrate enhances renal tubular reabsorption of calcium and alkalinizes urine. It is used in the management of calcium oxalate and urate urolithiasis, and fungal urinary tract infections. It may be used to treat hypokalaemia, although potassium chloride/gluconate are preferred.

Forms: *Oral:* 30% oral solution. Various preparations are available.

Dose: *Cats, Dogs:* 75 mg/kg or 2 mmol/kg p.o. q12h.

Adverse effects and contraindications: Avoid its use in animals with renal impairment or cardiac disease.

Potentiated sulphonamides – see Trimethoprim/sulphonamide

Povidone–iodine (Betadine*; **Pevidine**) *GSL*

Indications: Povidone–iodine is a topical bactericidal and viricidal agent, which liberates approx 10% free iodine. It is used to treat localized bacterial infections, to reduce colonic bacterial numbers in acute cases of hepatic encephalopathy (HE) and as an ophthalmic surface irrigant prior to extraocular and intraocular surgical procedures. Its action is not impaired by blood, serum, purulent or necrotic tissue.

Forms: *Topical:* 1% (Pevidine), 10% (Betadine) solutions.

Dose: *Dogs:*
- Wound cleanser and antibacterial wash: Apply 0.5% solution to affected area.
- Hepatic encephalopathy: 10% solution per rectum as a retention enema prn.
- Otitis: Apply 1% solution to external and middle ear; rinse well with sterile saline.
- Ophthalmic: 0.2–0.5% aqeous solution. Note: do not use the alcoholic solution or surgical scrub. Aqueous solution is only stable for a few days.

Adverse effects and contraindications: It can be irritating to skin and the external ear. A 1% solution has been used in the management of otitis externa and otitis media associated with resistant bacteria (e.g. *Pseudomonas*, *Proteus*). It is ototoxic and other agents such as saline are safer. Its use is not recommended in cats.

Pralidoxime (Pralidoxime*) *POM*

Indications: Pralidoxime is a cholinesterase reactivator, allowing resumption of the destruction of accumulated acetylcholine. It is used with atropine in the management of organophosphate (OP) toxicity. It is only effective if given within 24 hours of poisoning. Additionally, pralidoxime detoxifies certain organophosphates by direct chemical inactivation and retards the 'ageing' of phosphorylated cholinesterase to a non-reactive form. Pralidoxime does not appreciably enter the CNS, thus CNS toxicity is not reversed.

Forms: *Injectable:* 200 mg/ml solution.

Dose:
Cats, Dogs: Effective if given within 24 hours of exposure. Dilute to a 20 mg/ml solution and administer 20–50 mg/kg slowly i.v. (over 2 minutes at least – 500 mg/min max.) i.m., s.c. Use with concomitant atropine therapy. Repeat doses prn.
Birds: 10–100 mg/kg i.m. q8–12h as needed.

Adverse effects and contraindications: Pralidoxime is ineffective and contraindicated for poisoning due to carbamate or OP compounds without anticholinesterase activity. If given within 24 hours of exposure, treatment is usually only required for 24–36 hours. Respiratory support may be necessary.

Drug interactions: Avoid the use of **aminophylline**, **morphine**, **phenothiazines** or **theophylline** in organophosphate-intoxicated patients. The effects of **barbiturate** may be potentiated by organophosphates, therefore use with caution when treating seizures.

Praziquantel (Droncit injectable *POM*; Droncit Spot-on *POM*; Droncit tablets *GSL*; Drontal plus *PML*; Drontal cat tablets *PML*; Milbemax *POM*)

Indications: Praziquantel is a cestocide that increases cell membrane permeability of susceptible worms, resulting in loss of intracellular calcium and paralysis. This allows the parasites to be phagocytosed or digested. Praziquantel is indicated for the treatment of *Dipylidium caninum, Taenia* spp., *Echinococcus granulosus* and *Mesocestoides* spp. in dogs and cats. Because it kills all intestinal forms of *Echinococcus,* it is the preferred drug in most *Echinococcus* control programmes. The PETS travel scheme requires animals to be treated with praziquantel prior to entry into the UK. The inclusion of pyrantel (effective against *Toxocara cati* and *Toxascaris leonina*) and febantel, which is metabolized to fenbendazole (effective against *Toxocara cati* and *Toxascaris leonina, Uncinaria stenocephala, Ancylostoma caninum* and *Trichuris vulpis*) in some preparations increases the spectrum of efficacy.

Forms:
Injectable: Droncit injectable: 56.8 mg praziquantel/ml solution.
Oral: Droncit tablets: 50 mg praziquantel; Drontal plus: 50 mg praziquantel, 144 mg pyrantel and 150 mg febantel; Drontal cat: 20 mg praziquantel and 230 mg pyrantel. Droncit Spot-on: 20 mg praziquantel.

Dose:
Dogs, Cats: 3.5–7.5 mg/kg i.m., s.c.; 5 mg/kg p.o. (Drontal plus: 1 tablet/10 kg. Drontal cat tablets: 1 tablet/4 kg); 8 mg/kg Spot-on.
Birds: 7.5 mg/kg i.m., s.c. or 5–10 mg/kg p.o. q2–4 weeks.
Reptiles: 8–20 mg/kg i.m.

Adverse effects and contraindications: Do not use in unweaned puppies or kittens, as they are unlikely to be affected by tapeworms. Drontal plus can be used from 2 weeks of age. Drontal cat tablets can be used from 6 weeks of age. Do not use the Spot-on preparation in animals <1 kg. Re-treatment is usually unnecessary unless reinfection takes place. The injection may cause localized tissue sensitivity, particularly in cats.

Prazosin (Prazosin*) *POM*

Indications: Prazosin is a post-synaptic alpha$_1$ blocking agent causing vasodilation. It is used in the management of congestive heart failure although it may lose its effectiveness with prolonged use. It may be useful in promoting urine flow in patients with benign prostatic hyperplasia (relaxes smooth muscle) and in the management of hypertension associated with cardiac or renal disease.

Forms: *Oral:* 0.5 mg, 1 mg, 2 mg, 5 mg tablets.

Dose:
Cats: 0.25–1 mg p.o. q8–12h.
Dogs: <15 kg: 1 mg p.o. q8–12h; >15 kg: 2 mg p.o. q8–12h.

Adverse effects and contraindications: These include hypotension, drowsiness and weakness.

Drug interactions: Concomitant use of **beta-blockers** (e.g. **propranolol**) or **diuretics** (e.g. **furosemide**) may increase the risk of a first dose hypotensive effect. Calcium channel-blockers may cause additive hypotension. Prazosin is highly protein-bound and so may be displaced by or displace other highly protein-bound drugs (e.g. warfarin, sulphonamide) from plasma proteins.

Prednisolone (**PLT**; Pred forte*; **Prednicare**; **Prednidale**; **Prednisolone**) *POM*

Indications: Prednisolone is a synthetic corticosteroid used as an anti-inflammatory, immunosuppressive and anti-fibrotic drug and in the management of hypoadrenocorticism and lymphoproliferative and other neoplasms. Prednisolone has approx 4 times the anti-inflammatory potency and half the relative mineralocorticoid potency of hydrocortisone. It, like methylprednisolone, is considered to have an intermediate duration of activity and is suitable for alternate-day use. In combination with cinchophen (PLT) it is used in the management of osteoarthritis.

Forms:
Ophthalmic: Prednisolone acetate 0.5%, 1% solution (Pred forte).
Topical: Prednisolone is a component of many topical dermatological, otic and ophthalmic preparations.
Injectable: Prednisolone sodium succinate 10 mg/ml solution; 7.5 mg/ml suspension plus 2.5 mg/ml dexamethasone.
Oral: 1 mg, 5 mg, 25 mg tablets.
PLT is a compound preparation containing cinchophen.

Dose:
Cats, Dogs:
- Ophthalmic: Dosage frequency and duration of therapy is dependent upon type of lesion and response to therapy. Usually 1 drop in affected eye(s) q4–8h tapering in response to therapy.
- Allergy: 0.5–1 mg/kg p.o. q12h initially, tapering to lowest q48h dose.
- Anti-inflammatory: *Cats*: 1.1 mg/kg p.o. q12h, taper to 1.1–2.2 mg/kg q48h; *Dogs*: 0.5–1 mg/kg p.o. q12h, taper to 0.5–1 mg/kg q48h.
- Immunosuppression: *Cats*: 2.2–6.6 mg/kg p.o. q12h, tapering to 2.2–4.4 mg/kg q48h; *Dogs*: 1.1–3.3 mg/kg p.o. q12h, tapering to 0.5–2.2 mg/kg q48h.
- Hypoadrenocorticism: 0.2–0.3 mg/kg with fludrocortisone. The use of prednisolone may be discontinued in most cases once the animal is stable.
- Lymphoma: *see pages 295–296.*

Small mammals: Anti-inflammatory: 1.25–2.5 mg/kg p.o. q24h.

Adverse effects and contraindications: Prolonged use of glucocorticoids suppresses the hypothalamic–pituitary axis (HPA) causing adrenal atrophy, and may cause significant proteinuria and glomerular changes in the dog. Catabolic effects of glucocorticoids leads to weight loss and cutaneous atrophy. Iatrogenic hyperadrenocorticism may develop with chronic use. Vomiting, diarrhoea and GI ulceration may develop; the latter may be more severe when corticosteroids are used in animals with neurological injury. Hyperglycaemia and decreased serum T4 values may be seen in patients receiving prednisolone. Do not use in pregnant animals. Systemic corticosteroids are generally contraindicated in patients with renal disease and diabetes mellitus. Impaired wound healing and delayed recovery from infections may be seen. Topical corticosteroids are contraindicated in ulcerative keratitis. Animals on chronic therapy should be tapered off their steroids when discontinuing the drug.

Drug interactions: There is an increased risk of GI ulceration if used concurrently with **NSAIDs**. Hypokalaemia may develop if **acetazolamide**, **amphotericin B** or **potassium-depleting diuretics** (e.g. **furosemide**, **thiazides**) are administered concomitantly with corticosteroids. Glucocorticoids may antagonize the effect of **insulin**. The metabolism of corticosteroids may be enhanced by **phenytoin** or **phenobarbital**.

Primidone (Mysoline Veterinary Tablets) *POM*

Indications: Primidone is an antiepileptic drug that raises electrically induced seizure thresholds and alters seizure patterns. The exact mechanism of seizure prevention is unknown but is thought to involve facilitating inhibitory GABA receptors. Primidone is rapidly metabolized to the active metabolites phenobarbital and phenylethylmalonamide (PEMA). In dogs approximately 85% of anti-seizure activity is thought to be due to phenobarbital, with some potentiation by PEMA. Efficacy of primidone in patients refractory to phenobarbital may be the result of improved conversion following induction of hepatic microsomal enzymes.

Forms: *Oral:* 250 mg tablet.

Dose: *Dogs:* 5–28 mg/kg p.o. q12h. Start at the lower dose if adding primidone to a treatment regimen using phenobarbital. Monitor for signs of phenobarbital toxicity and/or serum phenobarbital levels.

Adverse effects and contraindications: Adverse effects of primidone include PU/PD, polyphagia, personality changes, sedation and ataxia. The latter two signs are often seen early in therapy and may subside with time. They may indicate the development of toxic serum levels. Chronic therapy induces progressive hepatic injury; liver enzymes should be monitored every 6 months. As neutropenia, thrombocytopenia, anaemia and splenomegaly have been reported to develop in dogs receiving phenobarbital, there is the potential for such adverse effects to develop in dogs receiving primidone. Dose reduction or monitoring of serum levels is indicated if any adverse effects are present. Therapeutic barbiturate serum levels vary with different laboratories. but are in the region of 65–172 μmol/l. When withdrawing primidone reduce the dose gradually. If switching from primidone to phenobarbital, 3.8 mg primidone is equivalent to 1 mg of phenobarbital.

Drug interactions: Oral **acetazolamide** may decrease the GI absorption of primidone. As the primary active metabolite for primidone is phenobarbital the following drug interactions may be of clinical significance. The effect of primidone may be increased by other **CNS depressants** (e.g. **antihistamines**, **opoids**, **phenothiazines**). Primidone may enhance the metabolism of and therefore decrease the effect of **beta-blockers**, **corticosteroids**, **metronidazole** and **theophylline**. Primidone may decrease the absorption of **griseofulvin**; avoid giving them together. Barbiturates may enhance the toxic effect of **anti-epileptics**.

Procainamide (Pronestyl*) *POM*

Indications: Procainamide is a class 1A anti-arrhythmic agent. It acts by stabilizing the cell membrane of cardiac myocytes, thereby decreasing their excitability. Electrical conduction is slowed through the bundle of His, atrium and ventricle. The refractory period is prolonged in the atrium when compared to the ventricle. At therapeutic doses cardiac output is usually unaffected unless there is pre-existing myocardial damage, whilst slight vagolytic effects, associated with mild increases in heart rate, may be seen. Higher doses lead to the development of AV block and ventricular extrasystoles. This drug is used in the management of ventricular tachycardia and ventricular premature complexes in the dog.

Forms: *Injectable:* 100 mg/ml.

Dose:
Cats: 3–8 mg/kg i.m. q6–8h.
Dogs: Initially 6–8 mg/kg i.v. over 5 minutes or 6–20 mg/kg i.v. as 2 mg/kg/min boluses, then a constant rate infusion of 0.025–0.05 mg/kg/min. Do not exceed 0.03 mg/kg/min rate for longer than 3 hours. Dilute in normal saline when giving i.v. Thereafter, 6–20 mg/kg i.m. q4–6h.

Adverse effects and contraindications: Adverse effects include weakness, vomiting, diarrhoea, hepatotoxicity (rare), pyrexia, hypotension (particularly with too rapid i.v. administration) and myocardial depression (widening of QRS and QT intervals, AV block and decreased contractility). Solutions darker than a light amber colour should be discarded.

Drug interactions: Increased myocardial depression may develop if procainamide is used concurrently with other **anti-arrhythmic agents**. The effects of **pyridostigmine** (or other anticholinesterases) may be antagonized by procainamide. The effects of other **hypotensive drugs** may be potentiated by procainamide. Its use in patients with **digoxin** intoxication should be reserved for those where treatment with potassium, lidocaine or phenytoin has been ineffective. **Cimetidine** inhibits the metabolism of procainamide and decreases the renal clearance of procainamide and NALA (active metabolite), thereby increasing serum levels. The neuromuscular blocking activity of muscle relaxants such as **suxamethonium** may be potentiated or prolonged by procainamide.

Prochlorperazine (Buccastem*; Prochlorperazine*; Stemetil*) *POM*

Indications: Prochlorperazine is a piperazine phenothiazine compound that is used for its anti-emetic and neuroleptic qualities. Prochlorperazine blocks dopamine in the CNS. It is used predominantly to control motion sickness.

Forms:
Injectable: 12.5 mg/ml solution.
Oral: 3 mg, 5 mg, 25 mg tablets.

Dose: *Cats, Dogs:* 0.1–0.5 mg/kg i.v., i.m., s.c. q6–8h; 0.5–1 mg/kg p.o. q8–12h.

Adverse effects and contraindications: Adverse effects include sedation, depression, hypotension and extrapyramidal reactions (rigidity, tremors, weakness, restlessness, etc.).

Drug interactions: CNS depressant agents (e.g. **anaesthetics, narcotic analgesics**) may cause additive CNS depression if used with prochlorperazine. **Antacids** or **antidiarrhoeal** preparations (e.g. **bismuth subsalicylate** or **kaolin/pectin** mixtures) may reduce GI absorption of oral phenothiazines. Increased blood levels of both drugs may result if **propranolol** is administered with phenothiazines. Phenothiazines block alpha-adrenergic receptors, which may lead to unopposed beta activity causing vasodilation and increased cardiac rate if **adrenaline** is given.

Progesterone (Progesterone) *POM*

Indications: Progesterone is indicated for the treatment of threatened or habitual abortion, induction of parturition and postponement of oestrus.

Forms: *Injectable:* 25 mg/ml oily solution.

Dose:
Cats: 0.2–2 mg/kg i.m., s.c.
Dogs: 1–3 mg/kg i.m., s.c.

Doses of 2 mg/kg i.m. q48h will maintain plasma progesterone values above 2 ng/ml, the level required to maintain pregnancy. Parturition can be expected 72 hours after the last injection. Parturition should be planned for day 57 after the onset of cytological dioestrus in the bitch or 64 days after mating in the queen.

Adverse effects and contraindications: Do not use in animals with diabetes mellitus. Prolonged therapy may result in pathological uterine changes in bitches. Reversible masculization of the external genitalia may occur in female puppies born to bitches treated during pregnancy.

Proligestone (Delvosteron) *POM*

Indications: Proligestone is a progestogen used in the postponement of oestrus in the bitch, queen and jill ferret, in the treatment and prevention of false pregnancy in the bitch, and in the control of miliary dermatitis in the cat.

Forms: *Injectable:* 100 mg/ml suspension.

Dose:
Cats:
- Oestrus postponement: 100 mg/cat s.c.
- Miliary dermatitis: 33–50 mg/kg s.c. repeated once after 14 days if the response is inadequate.

Dogs:
- Suppression of oestrus and prevention/treatment of false pregnancy: 10–33 mg/kg s.c. once.
- Permanent postponement of oestrus: 10–33 mg/kg during pro-oestrus, 2nd dose 3 months later, 3rd dose 4 months after the second, and subsequent doses given q5months thereafter. Once dosing ceases bitches will come into oestrus, on average, 6–7 months later.
  The recommended dosages for bitches are:

Body weight (kg)	Dose (ml)
<5	1–1.5
5–10	1.5–2.5
10–20	2.5–3.5
20–30	3.5–4.5
30–45	4.5–5.5
45–60	5.5–6.0
thereafter 10 mg/kg	

Small mammals: Ferrets: 50 mg/ferret s.c. once
For all species see data sheet for further dosage advice.

Adverse effects and contraindications: Proligestone does not appear to be associated with as many or as serious adverse effects as other progestins (e.g. megestrol acetate, medroxyprogesterone acetate). However, adverse effects associated with long-term progestin use, e.g. temperament changes (listlessness and depression), increased thirst or appetite, cystic endometrial hyperplasia/pyometra, diabetes mellitus, acromegaly, adrenocortical suppression, mammary enlargement/neoplasia and lactation, may be expected. If proligestone is used in diabetic animals, monitor closely to ensure that insulin requirements do not change. It is recommended that proligestone is not given to bitches before or at first oestrus. Irritation at site of injection may occur and calcinosis circumscripta at the injection site has been reported. As coat colour changes may occasionally occur; injection into the medial side of the flank fold in thin-skinned or show animals is recommended.

Promethazine (Phenergan*) *P/POM*

Indications: Phenergan is an antihistamine used in the management of allergies and anaphylactic reactions. It has a duration of activity of approximately 12 hours.

Forms:
Oral: 10 mg, 25 mg tablets; 1 mg/ml elixir.
Injectable: 25 mg/ml solution.

Dose: *Cats, Dogs:* 0.2–0.4 mg/kg i.v., i.m., p.o. q6–8h (maximum dose 1 mg/kg).

Adverse effect and contraindications: CNS depression (sedation) often occurs.

Drug interactions: There may be enhancement of the sedative effects with concurrent administration of other **sedative drugs**.

Propantheline bromide (Pro-Banthine*) *POM*

Indications: Propantheline is a quarternary antimuscarinic agent used for the treatment of incontinence caused by detrusor hyperreflexia, as a peripherally acting anti-emetic and as an adjunctive therapy to treat GI disorders associated with smooth muscle spasm. In man other drugs, e.g. oxybutyrin, propiverine and trospium are more likely to be used to treat incontinence because of fewer adverse effects. Data is lacking as to their efficacy/safety in dogs/cats.

Forms: *Oral:* 15 mg tablet.

Dose:
Cats, Dogs: GI indications: 0.25 mg/kg p.o. q8–12h (round dose to nearest 3.75 mg).
Cats: Incontinence: 7.5 mg/cat p.o. q3d
Dogs: Incontinence: 0.4 mg/kg p.o. q6–8h.

Adverse effects and contraindications: Antimuscarinics may cause constipation and paralytic ileus with resultant bacterial overgrowth. Other adverse effects include sinus tachycardia, ectopic complexes, mydriasis, photophobia, cycloplegia, increased intraocular pressure, vomiting, abdominal distension, urinary retention and drying of bronchial secretions.

Drug interactions: The following may enhance the activity of propantheline and its derivatives: **antihistamines** and **phenothiazines**. The following drugs may potentiate the adverse effects of propantheline and its derivatives: chronic **corticosteroid** use (may increase intraocular pressure) and **primidone**. Propantheline and its derivatives may enhance the actions of **sympathomimetics** and **thiazide diuretics**. Propantheline and its derivatives may antagonize the actions of **metoclopramide**.

Propentofylline (Vivitonin) *POM*

Indications: Propentofylline is a xanthine derivative that increases blood flow to the heart, muscle, and CNS. This improvement in oxygenation reportedly improves demeanour in animals who are dull and lethargic. It also has an anti-arrhythmic action, positive inotropic and chronotropic effects on the heart, inhibitory effects on platelet aggregation and reduces peripheral vascular resistance. In a behavioural context propentofylline is used in the treatment of age-related behaviour problems and can be administered in combination with selegeline as well as dietary considerations for the condition of canine cognitive dysfunction.

Forms: *Oral:* 50 mg, 100 mg tablets.

Dose: *Dogs:* 2.5–5 mg/kg p.o. q12h. Administer 30 minutes prior to food.

Propofol (Rapinovet) *POM*

Indications: Propofol is an ultra-short-acting phenolic compound used for the i.v. induction of anaesthesia in dogs and cats. Duration of action in cats is longer than in dogs. Unlike thiopental, the drug is relatively non-cumulative and so anaesthesia may be maintained in dogs by repeated injection or infusion. Excitatory neurological phenomena, e.g. twitching, tremors, may be seen during anaesthesia and recovery. Despite this, propofol may be used to control benzodiazopine-resistant seizures. Recovery is normally rapid. Propofol is not irritant to tissues but a pain response may be evident during i.v. administration. Propofol is preferred to thiopental in 'sight hounds'.

Forms: *Injectable:* 10 mg/ml emulsion. Shake well before use and do not mix with other therapeutic agents or infusion fluids prior to administration. The current preparation contains no bacteriostat: opened vials must be used as rapidly as possible, or discarded.

Dose:
Cats: Unpremedicated 8 mg/kg i.v., premedicated 6 mg/kg i.v.
Dogs: Unpremedicated 6.5 mg/kg i.v., premedicated 4 mg/kg i.v.
Small mammals: 10 mg/kg i.v.; Mice: 20 mg/kg i.v.
Reptiles: Chelonians: 14 mg/kg i.v.; Lizards, Snakes: 10 mg/kg i.v.

Anaesthesia may be maintained by incremental doses of approximately 10 mg/4–8 kg as required, or by inhalational agents.

Adverse effects and contraindications: The rapid injection of large doses causes apnoea, cyanosis and severe hypotension. Problems are less likely when injection is made over 30–60 seconds. Other adverse effects include occasional vomiting and excitation during recovery. The notion that propofol is safer than thiopental in certain categories of 'high risk' cases is without foundation, and considerable care must be taken with its administration in hypovolaemic animals, and those with diminished cardiopulmonary, hepatic and renal reserves.

Propranolol (Inderal*; Propranolol*) *POM*

Indications: Propranolol is a beta adrenoceptor antagonist. It antagonizes beta$_1$ adrenoceptors, blocking their chronotropic and inotropic effects on the heart, and beta$_2$ adrenoceptors, blocking their vasodilatory actions. Propranolol is highly lipid-soluble and crosses into the CNS. It is rapidly metabolized by the liver (high first-pass effect). Propranolol is indicated for the management of cardiac arrhythmias (sinus tachycardia, atrial fibrillation or flutter, supraventricular tachycardia, premature ventricular depolarization), hypertrophic cardiomyopathy or obstructive heart disease. It is also an effective antihypertensive drug, acting through reducing cardiac output, altering the baroreceptor reflex sensitivity and blocking peripheral adrenoceptors. Propranolol is used to reverse some of the clinical features of thyrotoxicosis prior to surgery in patients with hyperthyroidism. Propranolol may be used to control the pulse rate in patients with phaeochromocytoma; always use with phenoxybenzamine for this indication, as beta blockade without concurrent alpha blockade may lead to a hypertensive crisis. Propranol may be used in behavioural therapy to reduce somatic signs of anxiety and is therefore useful in the management of situational anxieties and behavioural problems where contextual anxiety is a component. Some authors suggest using propranolol in combination with phenobarbital for the management of fear- and phobia-related behaviour problems.

Forms:
Injectable: 1 mg/ml solution.
Oral: 10 mg, 40 mg, 80 mg, 160 mg tablets.

Dose:
Cats:
- Cardiac indications: 0.04–0.06 mg/kg i.v. slowly (i.e. dilute 0.25 mg in 1 ml of saline and administer 0.2 ml boluses i.v. to effect); 2.5–5 mg/cat p.o. q8h.
- Behavioural modification: 0.2–1.0 mg/kg p.o. as required up to 3 times a day.

Dogs:
- Cardiac indications: 0.02–0.08 mg/kg i.v. slowly over 5 minutes q8h; 0.2–1 mg/kg p.o. q8h. Usual maintenance doses 5–40 mg/dog p.o. q8h (may need 80 mg q8h in large dogs).
- Phaeochromocytoma: Dogs: 0.15–0.5 mg/kg p.o. q8h in conjunction with an alpha blocker.
- Behavioural modification: 0.5–3.0 mg/kg p.o. as required up to 2 times a day.

Note: There is a significant difference between i.v. and p.o. doses. This is a consequence of propranolol's lower bioavailability when administered orally as a result of decreased absorption and a high first-pass effect.

Adverse effects and contraindications: Adverse effects are most frequent in geriatric patients with chronic heart disease or in patients with rapidly decompensating cardiac failure. They include bradycardia, impaired AV conduction, myocardial depression, heart failure, syncope, glucose intolerance, bronchospasm, diarrhoea and peripheral vasoconstriction. The use of propranolol is contraindicated in patients with supraventricular bradycardia and AV block and relatively contraindicated in animals with congestive heart failure. Although the use of propranolol is not contraindicated in patients with diabetes mellitus, insulin requirements should be monitored as propranolol may enhance the hypoglycaemic effect of insulin. Depression and lethargy are occasionally seen and are a result of propranolol's high lipid solubility and its penetration into the CNS. Propranolol may reduce the glomerular filtration rate and therefore exacerbate any pre-existing renal impairment. Sudden withdrawal of propranol may result in a noradrenaline rush that can trigger a reaction of intense fear.

Drug interactions: As the beta effects of **sympathomimetics** (e.g. **adrenaline, phenylpropanolamine, terbutaline**) may be blocked by propranolol, the unopposed alpha effects may result in severe hypertension and a decreased heart rate. The hypotensive effect of propranolol is enhanced by **anaesthetic agents** (those that depress myocardial activity), **phenothiazines, antihypertensive** drugs (e.g. **hydralazine, prazosin**), **diazepam, diuretics** and other **anti-arrhythmics**. There is an increased risk of bradycardia, severe hypotension, heart failure and AV block if propranolol is used concurrently with **calcium-channel blockers** (e.g. **diltiazem, verapamil**). Concurrent **digoxin** administration potentiates bradycardia. The metabolism of propranolol is accelerated by **thyroid hormones** thus reducing its effect. The dose of propranolol may need to be decreased when initiating **carbimazole** therapy. Oral **aluminium hydroxide** preparations reduce propranolol absorption. **Cimetidine** may decrease the metabolism of propranolol, thereby increasing its blood levels. Propranolol enhances the effects of **muscle relaxants** (e.g. **suxamethonium, tubocurarine**). Hepatic enzyme induction by **phenobarbital** or **phenytoin** may increase the rate of metabolism of propranolol. There is an increased risk of **lidocaine** toxicity if administered with propranolol due to a reduction in lidocaine clearance. The bronchodilatory effects of **theophylline** may be blocked by propranolol.

Prostaglandin $F_{2\alpha}$ – see Dinoprost tromethamine

Protamine sulphate (Protamine sulphate*) POM

Indications: Protamine is indicated for the treatment of heparin overdosage. It is an anticoagulant, that when administered in the presence of heparin forms a stable salt, causing the loss of anticoagulant activity of both compounds. The effects of heparin are neutralized within 5 minutes of protamine administration with the effect persisting for approximately 2 hours.

Forms: *Injectable:* 10 mg/ml solution.

Dose: *Cats, Dogs:* 1 mg of protamine inactivates 80–100 IU of heparin. Heparin disappears rapidly from the circulation. Decrease the dose of protamine by half for each 30-minute period since the heparin was administered. Give protamine i.v. very slowly over 1–3 minutes. Do not exceed 50 mg in any 10-minute period. Dilute protamine in 5% dextrose or normal saline.

Adverse reactions and contraindications: Adverse effects in man include anaphylaxis, hypotension, bradycardia, nausea, vomiting and lassitude. Do not store diluted solutions.

Proxymetacaine (Minims Proxymetacaine*) POM

Indications: Proxymetacaine is an amide-linked local anaesthetic used on the conjunctival sac, the external auditory meatus and the nares. It acts rapidly (within 10 seconds) and its effects last for 10–20 minutes in the conjunctival sac.

Forms: 0.5% solution.

Dose: *Cats, Dogs:* Ophthalmic: 1–2 drops/eye; apply 4–5 drops/eye over 2–3 minutes for maximum analgesia.
Aural/nasal: 5–10 drops/ear or nose q5–10 minutes (maximum 3 doses if used intranasally).

Adverse effects and contraindications: Occasionally local irritation may occur for several hours after administration. Topical anaesthetics block reflex tear production and should not be applied before a Schirmer tear test. All topical anaesthetics are toxic to the corneal epithelium, delay healing of ulcers and should not be used for therapeutic purposes.

Pyrantel (Drontal cat; Drontal plus; Drontal puppy; Strongid paste for dogs) PML

Indications: Pyrantel is a tetrahydropyrimidine that acts as a cholinergic agonist thereby interfering with neuronal transmission in parasites. It is used to control infestations of *Toxocara canis*, *Toxascaris leonina*, *Uncinaria stenocephala*, *Ancylostoma caninum* and *A. braziliensis*. The addition of febantel has a synergistic effect.

Forms: *Oral:* Strongid: 7.5 mg/g paste; 5 mg/ml suspension; Drontal plus: praziquantel 20 mg, pyrantel 144 mg, febantel 150 mg/tablet; Drontal puppy suspension: pyrantel 14.4 mg/ml, febantel 15 mg/ml; Drontal cat: 230 mg pyrantel, 20 mg praziquantel.

Dose:
Cats: 20 mg/kg p.o. repeated in 7–10 days. Note it is not licensed for use in the cat.
Dogs: Strongid: 5 mg/kg p.o. repeated in 7–10 days. Drontal plus: 1 tablet/10 kg; Drontal puppy suspension: 1 ml/10 kg repeated q2wks from 2–12 weeks of age.

Caution: Avoid contact with human skin.

Drug interactions: Administration of pyrantel with other drugs with cholinomimetic properties (e.g. **levamisole**) may potentiate toxicity. There is no evidence that simultaneous use of organophosphates enhances toxicity. Do not use Drontal products simultaneously with products containing **piperazine** as it reduces efficacy.

Pyridostigmine (Mestinon*) POM

Indications: Pyridostigmine is a long-acting anticholinesterase drug. By inhibiting acetylcholinesterase it prolongs the action of acetylcholine. It is used in the treatment of myasthenia gravis.

Forms: *Oral:* 60 mg tablets.

Dose: *Dogs:* 0.2–5 mg/kg p.o. q8–12h.

Adverse effects and contraindications: Adverse effects include vomiting, diarrhoea, increased salivation, involuntary defecation, miosis, nystagmus, bradycardia, hypotension and micturition (cholinergic SLUD syndrome). The dosage should be reduced by 25% if cholinergic signs appear. Treat cholinergic crises with atropine (0.05 mg/kg). Glucocorticoids or other immunosuppressants (e.g. azathioprine) may provide effective adjunctive therapy. However, the use of glucocorticoids is controversial as they may decrease the effectiveness of pyridostigmine. Animals with megaoesophagus should receive injectable therapy until able to swallow liquid or tablets.

Drug interactions: Aminoglycosides, clindamycin, lincomycin and **propranolol** may antagonize the effect of pyridostigmine. Pyridostigmine may enhance the effect of **suxamethonium** but antagonize the effect of **non-depolarizing muscle relaxants**.

Pyrimethamine (Daraprim*; Fansidar*) P

Indications: Pyrimethamine is a folate antagonist used in combination with sulphonamides to treat infections caused by *Toxoplasma gondii* and *Neospora caninum*. Used in birds to treat atoxoplasmosis, sarcocystis, leucocytozoonosis and avian malaria (*Plasmodium* spp.)

Forms: *Oral:* 25 mg tablet.
Fansidar contains pyrimethamine and sulphadoxine.

Dose: *Cats, Dogs:* 1 mg/kg p.o. q24h for 3 days, then 0.5 mg/kg p.o. q24h.
Birds: 0.5–1 mg/kg p.o. q12h for 30 days.

Adverse effects and contraindications: Adverse effects include depression, anorexia and reversible bone marrow suppression (within 6 days of the start of therapy). Folate supplementation (5 mg/day) may prevent bone marrow suppression. These drugs should not be used in pregnant or lactating animals without adequate folate supplementation. However, folate supplementation will reduce the efficacy of the drug if given concomitantly. Administer folate a few hours before pyrimethamine.

Drug interactions: Increased anti-folate effect if given with **phenytoin** or **sulphonamides**.

Pyriproxyfen (Cyclio) *POM*

Indications: Pyriproxyfen is a contact growth inhibitor, blocking the development of flea eggs and larvae. The drug has little if any effect on adult fleas. It can be used as part of a treatment strategy for flea allergy dermatitis.

Forms: *Topical:* Spot-on in tubes: 12 mg, 30 mg, 60 mg.

Dose:
Cats: 10.0 mg/kg.
Dogs: 2.0 mg/kg.

Adverse effects and contraindications: Do not use on kittens <1kg, puppies <1 month old, in pregnant bitches or queens, or in sick or convalescent animals.

Quinalbarbitone – see Secobarbital

Quinidine (Kinidin Durules*; Quinidine sulphate*) *POM*

Indications: Quinidine is a class 1A anti-arrhythmic agent. It depresses conduction velocity, myocardial contractility and excitability, and prolongs the refractory period. Thus, conduction time is increased and the re-entry phenomenon is prevented. Quinidine has indirect antimuscarinic effects, decreases vagal tone and may improve conduction at the AV junction. It is used in the management of ventricular arrhythmias (VPCs), refractory supraventricular tachycardias (with caution) and acute atrial fibrillation.

Forms: *Oral:* Quinidine sulphate 200 mg tablets; quinidine bisulphate (Kinidin) 250 mg sustained release tablets.

Dose: *Dogs:* 6–11 mg/kg i.m., 6–20 mg/kg p.o. q6–8h.

Adverse effects and contraindications: Adverse effects include weakness, vomiting, diarrhoea, hypotension (especially with too rapid i.v. administration), widening of QRS and QT interval, AV block and decreased contractility. Patients exhibiting signs of toxicity or a lack of response should have their serum levels measured. Serum therapeutic levels are 0.0025 to 0.005 mg/ml in dogs. Toxic effects are not usually evident when serum levels are <0.01 mg/ml.

Drug interactions: Digoxin levels may be increased by quinidine. It is recommended that the dose of digoxin be decreased by half when adding quinidine and that serum drug levels of both quinidine and digoxin be assessed. The effect of neuromuscular blockers (e.g. **atracurium**, **suxamethonium**, **tubocurarine**) may be enhanced by quinidine. Drugs that alkalinize urine (e.g. **antacids**, **carbonic anhydrase inhibitors**, **sodium bicarbonate**, **thiazide diuretics**) reduce the excretion of quinidine, thus prolonging its half-life. The half-life of quinidine may be reduced by as much as 50% as a consequence of hepatic enzyme induction by **phenobarbital** or **phenytoin**. **Cimetidine** inhibits the metabolism of quinidine by inhibiting hepatic microsomal enzymes, thereby increasing its effect. Additive cardiac depressant effects and an increased risk of ventricular arrhythmias may result if quinidine is used with **anti-arrhythmic drugs** (e.g. **procainamide**). There is an increased risk of hypotension if quinidine is used with **verapamil**.

Ramipril (Vasotop) *POM*

Indications: Ramipril is an ACE inhibitor. The indications for its use are as for enalapril. Ramipril is converted in the liver to ramiprilat. Ramiprilat is more potent and has a longer duration of action that enalaprilat and, because it is highly lipophilic, has a potentially better inhibition of tissue ACE.

Forms: *Oral:* 1.25 mg, 2.5 mg, 5 mg tablets.

Dose: *Dogs:* 0.125 mg/kg p.o. q24h.

Adverse effects and contraindications: These are the same as for enalapril.

Drug interactions: These are the same as for enalapril.

Ranitidine (Zantac*) *POM*

Indications: Ranitidine is a histamine (H_2) receptor antagonist that reduces gastric acid production. It is used to treat gastric and duodenal ulcers (including NSAID-induced ulceration), prophylactically to prevent stress ulcers and as an adjunct therapy for reversing metabolic alkalosis. It has minimal effects on hepatic enzymes (in contrast to cimetidine). Ranitidine may have a gastric prokinetic effect.

Forms:
Injectable: 25 mg/ml solution.
Oral: 150 mg, 300 mg tablets; 15 mg/ml syrup.

Dose:
Cats: 2 mg/kg/day constant i.v. infusion, 2.5 mg/kg i.v. slowly q12h, 3.5 mg/kg p.o. q12h.
Dogs: 2 mg/kg slow i.v., s.c., p.o. q8–12h.

Adverse effects and contraindications: Adverse effects are rarely reported but include cardiac arrhythmias and hypotension, particularly if ranitidine is administered by the i.v. route.

Drug interactions: Ranitidine retards oxidative hepatic drug metabolism by binding to the microsomal cytochrome P450. Administer ranitidine at least 30 minutes before **sucralfate**, as the latter may reduce the absorption of ranitidine. Stagger oral doses of ranitidine when used with **antacids**, **digoxin**, **ketoconazole** or **metoclopramide** by 2 hours as it may reduce their absorption or effect.

Retinol – see Vitamin A

Rifampin (Rifampicin) (Rifadin*; Rifampicin*; Rimactane*) *POM*

Indications: Rifampin is a rifamycin antibiotic, a product of *Amycolaptopis mediterranei*. It is a bactericidal drug binding to the beta subunit of RNA polymerase and causing abortive initiation of RNA synthesis. It has a wide spectrum of antimicrobial activity being active against bacteria (particularly Gram-positive organisms), *Chlamydophila, Rickettsia,* some protozoans and poxviruses. Rifampin is one of the most active drugs known against *Staphylococcus aureus* and is very active against *Mycobacterium tuberculosis*, the treatment of which is its main indication in human medicine. Gram-negative aerobic bacteria are usually innately resistant to rifampin as it is not able to cross the outer cell membrane of these organims. Obligate anaerobic bacteria (Gram-positive or -negative) are usually susceptible. Chromosomal mutations readily lead to resistance in many bacteria and are stable; do not use alone to treat infections. Rifampin is highly lipophilic, attaining high concentrations within cells in many tissues. Penetration into phagocytic cells is excellent, achieving concentrations several times those in serum. Exact indications for small animal veterinary practice remain to be fully established. It has been suggested as part of the combination of treatments for atypical mycobacterial infections. It may also have a place in the management of chlamydophilosis, erhlichiosis and bartonellosis. Rifampin should be used in combination with other antimicrobial drugs to prevent the emergence of resistant organisms during treatment. Clarithromycin, enrofloxacin and doxycycline have been used with rifampin in the management of mycobacteriosis. Until controlled studies are conducted to investigate the value of rifampin in these infections, recommendations remain empirical.

Forms: *Oral:* 150, 300 mg capsules; 20 mg/ml syrup.

Dose: *Cats, Dogs:* 10–15 mg/kg p.o. q24h.

Caution: Women of child-bearing potential should not handle crushed or broken tablets or the syrup without the use of gloves.

Adverse effects and contraindications: Rifampin may be teratogenic at high doses and should not be administered to pregnant animals. Clearance of the drug is heavily dependent on hepatic metabolism. It should not be administered to animals with liver disease. In dogs, increases in serum levels of hepatic enzymes are commonly seen and this can progress to clinical hepatitis. More information is needed on the adverse effects in dogs and cats. Rifampin metabolites may colour urine, saliva and faeces orange red.

Drug interactions: Rifampin is a potent hepatic enzyme inducer and increases the rate of metabolism of other drugs in man, including **barbiturates, theophylline** and **ketaconazole**. Increased dosages of these drugs may be required if used in combination with rifampin.

Ringer's solution (Aqupharm No. 9) *POM*

Indications: Ringer's solution is an isotonic solution used as a water/ electrolyte replacement fluid where there has been some intracellular potassium loss.

Forms: *Injectable:* Calcium chloride 0.322 mg/ml, potassium chloride 0.3 mg/ml and sodium chloride 8.6 mg/ml solution.
See Parenteral fluids table on page 294.

Dose: *Cats, Dogs:* Fluid requirements depend upon the degree of dehydration and ongoing losses. In uncomplicated cases administer at a dose of 50–60 ml/kg/day i.v. Higher doses are required if the animal is dehydrated.

Rocuronium (Esmeron*) *POM*

Indications: Rocuronium is an amino-steroid non-depolarizing neuromuscular blocking agent. It has intermediate (30–40 minutes) duration of action in dogs and does not appear to accumulate with repeat doses. In most aspects it is similar to vecuronium except it occasionally produces mild transient hypertension. Its availability in aqueous solution and a longer shelf-life increases convenience.

Forms: *Injectable:* 10 mg/ml solution.

Dose: *Dogs*: 0.4 mg/kg i.v. followed, when required, by maintenance doses of 0.16 mg/kg i.v.

Adverse effects and contraindications: Neuromuscular blocking agents must not be used if the provision of adequate analgesia and anaesthesia cannot be guaranteed and the means of adequate lung ventilation are unavailable. Neuromuscular blockade with rocuronium should be antagonized with an antimuscarinic/anticholinesterase drug combination.

Drug interactions: The following agents antagonize the effects of cis-atracurium, **anticholinesterases** (**edrophonium, neostigmine**), **azathioprine, potassium** and **theophylline**. The action of cis-atracurium may be prolonged and intensified by **aminoglycosides**, **clindamycin, lincomycin, inhalation anaesthetics, magnesium salts**, and **quinidine**.

Secobarbital (Quinalbarbitone/Cincochaine) (Somulose)
POM Schedule 2 Controlled Drug

Indications: Somulose is a compound preparation for euthanasia only. Secobarbital is a derivative of barbituric acid that causes loss of consciousness and cessation of respiration. Cincochaine depresses cardiac conduction resulting in rapid cardiac arrest. Since cardiac arrest is not dependent upon hypoxia, euthanasia is not accompanied by gasping.

Forms: *Injectable:* 400 mg/ml secobarbital and 25 mg/ml cincochaine solution.

Dose: *Cats, Dogs:* 0.25 ml/kg i.v. Inject over 10–15 seconds to minimize premature cardiac arrest.

Caution: This combination is not an anaesthetic agent and being extremely potent should only be used in the presence of an assistant in case of self-injection. In that event, the assistant should provide cardiac and respiratory support until an ambulance arrives; no specific antidote is available.

Selamectin (Stronghold) *POM*

Indications: Selamectin is a semi-synthetic avermectin. It is a systemic parasiticide active against *Ctenocephalides* spp., *Otodectes cynotis*, *Trichodectes canis*, *Felicola subrostratus*, *Dirofilaria immitis*, *Sarcoptes scabiei* and adult *Toxocara canis*, *T. cati* and *Ancyclostoma tubaeforme*. Regular treatment will reduce the incidence of flea allergy dermatitis. Used to prevent dirofilariasis. In rabbits it is effective against *Psoroptes cuniculi*, *Cheyletiella parasitovorax* and *Spillopsyllis cuniculi*.

Forms: *Topical:* Spot-on: 15 mg, 30 mg, 45 mg, 60 mg, 120 mg, 240 mg tubes.

Dose: *Cats, Dogs, Ferrets, Rabbits:* 6 mg/kg monthly.
For ear mite treatment, do not apply directly to the ear canal.
If used to prevent heartworm, administer within one month of first exposure to mosquitos. The last dose must be given within one month of last exposure to mosquitos.

Adverse reactions and contraindications: Use in cats has been associated with mild transient hair loss at the application site.

Selegiline hydrochloride (Selgian) *POM*

Indications: Selegiline (L-deprenyl) is a selective and irreversible inhibitor of monoamine oxidase B (MAO B). It is indicated in the treatment of canine cognitive dysfunction and may be used for behavioural disorders of emotional origin such as depression and anxiety, as well as in combination with behavioural therapy for problems such as overactivity, separation problems, phobias and unsocial behaviour. Selegeline is specifically indicated for the support of long-term behavioural therapy for canine sound phobias in cases where the dog is withdrawn, pacing and attention seeking as a result of the phobic reaction. It is also advocated in the management of fear-related behaviour problems in cats. Inhibition of MAO B downregulates dopamine production, which may reduce ACTH production. It has been suggested as a treatment for canine hyperadrenocorticism with reports of 20% of dogs showing a response. However, a recent publication casts doubt on its effectiveness.

Forms: *Oral:* 4 mg, 10 mg tablets.

Dose:
Cats: 1 mg/kg p.o. q24h.
Dogs: Behaviour modifier: 0.5 mg/kg p.o. q24h for a minimum of 2 months. Treatment can be stopped suddenly without gradual dose reduction.
Pituitary-dependent hyperadrenocorticism: 2 mg/kg p.o. q24h.

Adverse effects and contraindications: Selegiline should not be administered to lactating or pregnant bitches as it may act on prolactin secretion. Medication with selegeline can increase the risk of expression of defensively motivated aggression. Adverse effects reported in humans include postural hypotension, stereotypic behaviour, pruritus, trembling, vomiting, lethargy, disorientation and, rarely, arrhythmias.

Drug interactions: Selegiline should not be administered with **alpha$_2$ antagonists** (or within 24 hours before or after their use), **pethidine**, **fluoxetine**, **tricyclic antidepressants** (e.g. **amitryptiline**, **doxepin**, **clomipramine**), **ephedrine**, potential **monoamine oxidase inhibitors** (e.g. **amitraz**) or **phenothiazines**. The effect of **morphine** is potentiated when used simultaneously.

Sertraline (Lustral*) *POM*

Indications: Sertraline is a selective serotonin (5-hydroxytryptamine) reuptake inhibitor used in the treatment of canine anxiety, phobia and panic attacks and compulsive disorders. It is advocated for the support of long-term behavioural therapy for canine sound phobias in cases where the dog displays signs of panic.

Forms: *Oral:* 50 mg, 100 mg tablets.

Dose: *Dogs:* 1–3 mg/kg p.o. q24h.
It is advisable to give a dose of 1 mg/kg p.o. q24h for the first week of treatment, before increasing to 2 mg/kg p.o. q24h in the second week and increasing further to 3 mg/kg p.o. q24h if necessary.

Adverse effects and contraindications: Adverse effects include tachycardia, bradycardia, ataxia, pancreatitis, hepatitis and liver failure. Gastrointestinal adverse effects may be seen during the first few days of treatment. Gradually increasing the dose significantly reduces this effect. Do not use in pregnant and lactating animals or in patients with epilepsy, cardiovascular disease or renal or hepatic compromise. Use in cases involving aggression should be undertaken with care due to the risk of disinhibition.

Drug interactions: Not to be used in combination with **MAOIs**, **anti-epileptics**, **anti-arrhythmic** drugs or **propranolol**.

Serum gonadotrophin (Equine chorionic gonadotrophin) (Folligon; PMSG-Intervet*) *POM*

Indications: Serum gonadotrophin is a complex glycoprotein obtained from the serum of pregnant mares. It mimics the action of follicle stimulating hormone (FSH). It is indicated for the induction of oestrus (stimulates development of the ovarian follicle) and to increase spermatogenesis (degree of efficacy is low).

Forms: *Injectable:* 1000 IU freeze-dried plug.

Dose: *Dogs:*
• Oestrus induction: 20 IU/kg s.c. q24h for 10 days, followed by 500 IU hCG i.m. on day 10.
• To stimulate spermatogenesis: 400–800 IU i.m. twice weekly for 4–8 weeks.

Adverse effects and contraindications: Anaphylactoid reactions may occur rarely.

Sevoflurane (Sevoflo) *POM*

Indications: Sevoflurane, a volatile branch-chained fluorinated ether, is suitable for the induction and maintenance of anaesthesia for all types of surgery and in all species, irrespective of age. It is currently licensed for use in dogs >12 weeks of age. Sevoflurane is relatively impotent compared with halothane, but is highly volatile and must be delivered from a suitable, calibrated vaporizer.

Forms: 250 ml bottles.

Dose: *Cats, Dogs:* The expired concentration of sevoflurane required to maintain surgical anaesthesia in 50% of recipients is about 2.5% in animals, but depends to a large part on other drugs used (see *Drug interactions*). Sevoflurane is less soluble in blood than isoflurane and so changes in vaporizer setting cause more rapid changes in the level of anaesthesia, provided other physiological variables remain constant. The cessation of administration results in rapid recovery, which may occasionally be associated with signs of agitation.

Adverse effects and contraindications: Sevoflurane has a less pungent smell than isoflurane and induction of anaesthesia using chambers or masks is usually well tolerated in small dogs and cats. It causes a dose-dependent hypotension that does not wane with time. The effects of sevoflurane on respiration are dose-dependent and comparable to isoflurane, i.e. more depressant than halothane. Sevoflurane does not 'sensitize' the myocardium to catecholamines to the extent that halothane does. Sevoflurane is degraded by soda-lime into compounds that are nephrotoxic in rats. Conditions accelerating degradation, i.e. low gas flows, high absorbent temperatures and high sevoflurane concentrations should be avoided in long operations. Sevoflurane crosses the placental barrier and will affect neonates delivered by caesarean operation.

Drug interactions: The effects of sevoflurane on the duration of action of **non-depolarizing neuromuscular blocking agents** are similar to those of isoflurane, i.e. greater potentiation compared with halothane. **Opioid** agonists, **benzodiazepines** and **nitrous oxide** reduce the concentration of sevoflurane required to achieve surgical anaesthesia.

Sildenafil (Viagra*) POM

Indications: Phosphodiesterase type V inhibitor, causing arterial vasodilation. Indicated for the treatment of pulmonary arterial hypertension. Very limited use in dogs so far, but results appear promising.

Forms: *Oral:* 25 mg, 50 mg, 100 mg tablets.

Dose: *Dogs:* 0.3–3 mg/kg/dose p.o. q6–8h. The very limited clinical experience with this drug in dogs suggests that the upper end of dose range is safe and efficacious.

Adverse effects and contraindications: Contraindicated in patients with systemic hypotension, significant hepatic or renal impairment or bleeding disorders. Adverse effects include vomiting, dizziness and raised intraocular pressure.

Drug interactions: Cimetidine, erythromycin, itraconazole and **ketoconazole** increase plasma sildenafil concentration. Avoid concomitant use of **nitrates,** which significantly enhance its hypotensive effect.

Silver sulfadiazine (Flamazine*) POM

Indications: Silver sulfadiazine is a topical antibacterial and antifungal drug particularly active against Gram-negative organisms such as *Pseudomonas aeruginosa*. It is used in the management of 2nd and

3rd degree burns. It slowly releases silver in concentrations that are toxic to bacteria and yeasts. The sulfadiazine component has anti-infective qualities. Up to 10% may be absorbed, depending on the size of area treated.

Forms: *Topical:* 1% cream (water-soluble).

Dose: *Cats, Dogs:*
- Burns/skin infection: Apply antiseptically to the affected area to a thickness of approximately 1.5 mm. Initially, apply as often as necessary to keep wound covered then reduce as healing occurs to once a day applications. Dressings may be applied if necessary. Keep the affected area clean.
- Otitis (resistant *Pseudomonas*/refractory *Malassezia*): Dilute 1:1 with water and apply topically.

Caution: Wear gloves.

Adverse effects and contraindications: Patients hypersensitive to sulphonamides may react to silver sulfadiazine. It may accumulate in patients with impaired hepatic or renal function. Its use is contraindicated in pregnancy and should be avoided, if possible, in neonates.

Sodium acetate/acetic acid (Walpole's solution) *POM*

Indications: Walpole's solution is used to flush out and dissolve struvite urethral calculi in cats.

Forms: *Topical:* 1.17% sodium acetate and glacial acetic acid.

Dose: *Cats, Dogs:* Flush the urethra with 1 ml of solution, repeating prn until the obstruction is breached.

Sodium alkylsulphoacetate – see Sodium citrate

Sodium bicarbonate (Sodium bicarbonate*) *POM*

Indications: Sodium bicarbonate is used in the treatment of metabolic acidosis, to alkalinize urine and as an adjunctive therapy in the treatment of hypercalcaemic or hyperkalaemic crises. If sodium depletion is present, correct this first with isotonic saline provided the kidneys are not primarily affected.

Forms:
Injectable: 1.26%, 4.2%, 8.4% solutions for i.v. infusion. 8.4% solution $\equiv$ 1 mmol/ml.
Oral: 300 mg, 500 mg, 600 mg tablets.

Dose: *Cats, Dogs:*
- Severe metabolic acidosis:
  mmol $NaHCO_3$ required = base deficit x 0.5 x BW (kg)
  (Note: 0.3 is recommended instead of 0.5 in some references).
  Give half the dose slowly over 3–4 hours i.v. Recheck blood
  gases and assess the clinical status of the patient. Avoid
  over-alkalinization. If blood gases are unavailable administer
  0.5–1 mmol/kg slowly over 30 minutes.
- Acutely critical situations (e.g. cardiac arrest): 1 mmol/kg i.v. over
  1–2 minutes, followed by 0.5 mmol/kg at 10 minute intervals during
  the arrest. Data are conflicting regarding compatability in lactated
  Ringer's solution; do not use if precipitate forms.
- Adjunctive therapy of hypercalcaemia: 0.5–1 mmol/kg i.v. over
  30 minutes.
- Adjunctive therapy of hyperkalaemia: 2–3 mmol/kg i.v. over
  30 minutes.
- Metabolic acidosis secondary to renal failure or to alkalinize the
  urine: Initial dose 8–12 mg/kg p.o. q8h then adjust dose to maintain
  total blood CO_2 concentrations at 18–24 mEq/l. The dose may be
  increased to 50 mg/kg p.o. to adjust urine pH in patients with
  normal renal, hepatic and cardiac function.

Adverse effects and contraindications: 1 g of sodium bicarbonate
provides 11.9 mEq of Na^+ and 11.9 mEq of bicarbonate. Excessive use
of i.v. sodium bicarbonate can lead to metabolic alkalosis, hypernatraemia,
congestive heart failure, a shift in the oxygen dissociation curve
causing decreased tissue oxygenation, and paradoxical CNS acidosis
leading to respiratory arrest. In hypocalcaemic patients, use sodium
bicarbonate cautiously and administer very slowly. As oral sodium
bicarbonate (especially at higher doses) may contribute significant
amounts of sodium, use it with caution in patients on salt restricted
intakes, e.g. those with congestive heart failure.

Drug interactions: Sodium bicarbonate is incompatible with **many
drugs** and **calcium salts**; do not mix unless checked beforehand.
Alkalinization of urine by sodium bicarbonate decreases the excretion
of **quinidine** and **sympathomimetic drugs**, and increases the excretion
of **aspirin**, **phenobarbital** and **tetracyclines** (especially doxycycline).

Sodium chloride (Aqupharm No 1, No. 3, No. 18; Sodium
chloride*; Slow sodium*) *POM*

Indications: Sodium chloride solutions are used as water/electrolyte
replacement fluids, in the management of hypotension/shock
(hypertonic saline), a drug diluent and a hypertonic ophthalmic solution
for corneal oedema. When used for fluid replacement dilute saline
solutions primarily replace interstitial volume whereas hypertonic saline
replenish intravascular volume.

Forms:
Ophthalmic: 5% ointment (compounded by an ocular pharmacy).
Injectable: 0.45–7% NaCl solutions; 0.18% NaCl with 4% glucose and 0.9% NaCl with 5% glucose solutions.
Oral: 300 mg, 600 mg tablets.

Dose: *Cats, Dogs:*
- Corneal oedema: Apply ointment q8–24h.
- Fluid therapy: Fluid requirements depend upon the degree of dehydration and ongoing losses. In uncomplicated cases 0.45–3% NaCl solutions should be administered at a dose of 50–60 ml/kg/day i.v., p.o. Higher doses are required if the animal is dehydrated. Solutions containing 0.9–3% NaCl are suitable for replacing deficits. Solutions containing 0.45% NaCl (with added potassium) are indicated for longer term maintenance.
- Hypotension/shock: 5–7.5% NaCl solutions (hypertonic saline) at doses of 3–8 ml/kg i.v. Solutions of this concentration are hypertonic; they should therefore be used with caution and in conjunction with other appropriate fluid replacement strategies. NaCl may be combined with 6% Dextran 70.
- Salt-wasting syndromes (hypoadrenocorticism): 1–5 g p.o. q24h.

Adverse effects and contraindications: Oral enteric coated products may not be adequately absorbed by dogs. Hypertonic saline may cause cellular dehydration if used alone; always administer isotonic electrolyte solutions concurrently. Bradyarrhythmias may develop following administration of hypertonic saline. Ophthalmic ointment may cause stinging.

Sodium citrate (Micolette*; Micralax*; Relaxit*) *P*

Indications: Sodium citrate is a component of Micralax, a faecal softener/lubricant used to treat constipation and to prepare the lower GI tract for proctoscopy and radiography.

Forms: Rectal micro-enemas containing 450 ml sodium citrate, 45 mg sodium alkylsulphoacetate (Micralax) or 75 mg sodium laurylsulphate (Micolette, Relaxit) and 5 mg/5 ml sorbic acid.

Dose: *Cats, Dogs:* 1 enema inserted per rectum to full length of nozzle.

Adverse effects and contraindications: Not recommended for use in cases with inflammatory bowel disease.

Sodium cromoglicate (Sodium cromoglycate)
(Nalcrom*; Rynacrom*; Sodium cromoglicate*) *P/POM*

Indications: Sodium cromoglycate prevents mast cell degranulation, even after exposure to an allergen. It is indicated for the control of ocular, nasal and food allergies.

Forms:
Topical: 2%, 4% nasal/ocular drops.
Oral: 100 mg capsules (Nalcrom); 20 mg/ml solution.

Dose: *Cats, Dogs:* 1–2 drops/eye or nose q6h; 5–10 mg/kg p.o. q6h.

Adverse effects and contraindications: In man, occasional nausea, rashes and joint pain are reported following oral administration. Intranasal application may cause local irritation and, rarely, bronchospasm.

Sodium stibogluconate (Pentostam*) *POM*

Indications: Sodium stibogluconate is a pentavalent antimony compound indicated for the treatment of leishmaniasis in dogs. Pentavalent antimony compounds are active against the amastigote stages of the parasite but their exact mode of action is unknown. Animals may be clinically normal after treatment but remain carriers, and follow-on treatment with allopurinol may be beneficial.

Forms: *Injectable:* 100 mg/ml solution.

Dose: *Dogs:* 30–50 mg/kg i.v., s.c. q24h for 3–4 weeks.
If giving i.v., administer slowly (over at least 5 minutes) to avoid cardiac toxicity.
Seek expert advice before treating leishmaniasis.

Adverse effects and contraindications: Adverse effects include pain and inflammation at the injection site, anorexia and vomiting and myalgia. Meglumine antimonate is said to be less toxic than sodium stibogluconate. Sodium stibogluconate is contraindicated in the face of significant renal impairment and in lactating animals. It should be used with caution in the face of hepatic impairment.

Somatropin (Growth hormone) (Genotropin*; Humatrope*; Norditropin*) *POM*

Indications: Somatropin is a recombinant growth hormone of human sequence. It is used in the treatment of growth hormone deficiency.

Forms: *Injectable:* 2–16 IU vials for reconstitution.

Dose: *Cats, Dogs:* 0.3–0.7 IU/kg weekly divided into 3–5 doses s.c., i.m. (painful). Continue for at least 6 weeks to evaluate response. Serum IGF-1 measurements may be helpful to monitor therapy.

Adverse effects and contraindications: Growth hormone is diabetogenic; monitor blood glucose. Antibody formation may limit its effectiveness in the long term. Local reactions may be seen; rotate injection sites.

Sotalol (Sotacor*; Sotalol*) *POM*

Indications: Sotalol is a combined class III antidysrhythmic and beta-blocker. It is used to treat both supraventricular and ventricular dysrhythmias and produces a marked prolongation of action potential duration and refractoriness.

Forms:
Oral: 40 mg, 80 mg, 160 mg tablets.
Injectable: 10 mg/ml solution.

Dose: *Dogs:* 0.5–2 mg/kg p.o. q12h.

Adverse effects and contraindications: The non-selective beta-blocking effects can decrease heart rate, stroke volume and cardiac output in dogs and may precipitate congestive cardiac failure. The drug is eliminated in urine and faeces and elimination half-life may increase greatly with renal insufficiency, leading to accumulation at standard doses. Adverse effects include hypotension, bradydysrhythmias, depression, nausea, vomiting and diarrhoea. The drug is potentially pro-arrhythmic and can cause torsades de pointes, especially in hypokalaemia.

Drug interactions: Concomitant administration of **sympathomimetics** (e.g. **adrenaline, phenylpropanolamine, terbutaline**) may lead to uncontrolled alpha effects (hypertension and bradycardia). Hypotensive effects are enhanced by anaesthetic agents, **phenothiazines, antihypertensive drugs, diazepam, diuretics** and other **anti-arrhythmics**. Negative inotropic and chronotropic effects may be enhanced with concurrent administration of **calcium-channel blockers** (e.g. **diltiazem, verapamil**). **Digoxin** may enhance bradycardia. There is an increased risk of ventricular dysrhythmias when co-administered with **amiodarone**. Diuretics that cause hypokalaemia (e.g. **thiazides, furosemide** and other **loop diuretics**) may be pro-arrhythmic.

Spironolactone (Spironolactone*) *POM*

Indications: Spironolactone is a potassium-sparing diuretic that competitively inhibits aldosterone, preventing sodium reabsorption in the distal tubule. It also potentiates thiazide and loop diuretics. Spironolactone is useful in hyperaldosteronism or when hypokalaemia develops with other diuretics. It is particularly useful in the treatment of oedema associated with congestive heart failure (when hypokalaemia may potentiate digoxin toxicity) and hepatic failure (when hypokalaemia can precipitate hepatic encephalopathy).

Forms: *Oral:* 25 mg, 50 mg, 100 mg tablets; 1 mg/ml, 2 mg/ml, 5 mg/ml syrup.

Dose: *Cats, Dogs:* 2–4 mg/kg p.o. q24h.

Adverse effects and contraindications: Hyponatraemia and hyperkalaemia may develop. Discontinue if hyperkalaemia develops. Hepatotoxicity is reported in man.

Drug interactions: Hyperkalaemia may result if **ACE inhibitors** (e.g. **captopril, enalapril**), **NSAIDs, ciclosporin** or **potassium supplements** are administered in conjunction with spironolactone. However, in practice spironolactone and **ACE inhibitors** appear safe to use concurrently. There is an increased risk of nephrotoxicity if spironolactone is administered with **NSAIDs**. The plasma concentration of **digoxin** may be increased by spironolactone.

Sterculia (Normacol*; **Peridale**) *GSL*

Indications: Sterculia is a bulk-forming agent that increases faecal mass and stimulates peristalsis. It is used in the management of impacted anal sacs, diarrhoea and constipation.

Forms: *Oral:* granules containing 98% sterculia; 118 mg capsule; 120 mg/unit dose paste in a syringe.

Dose: *Cats, Dogs:* <5 kg: 1.5 g p.o. q24h; 5–15 kg: 3 g p.o. q12–24h; >15 kg: 4 g p.o. q12–24h. Sprinkle over feed or place on tongue.

Adverse effects and contraindications: Do not use in cases of intestinal obstruction or where enterotomy or enterectomy is to be performed. During treatment, fluid should be provided or a moist diet given. Preparations that swell in contact with water should be administered with plenty of water.

Streptokinase (Streptokinase*) *POM*

Indications: Streptokinase is a fibrinolytic drug. It activates plasminogen to form plasmin, which degrades fibrin and leads to thrombin dissolution. It is indicated for the management of life-threatening thrombosis and pulmonary thrombosis. Alteplase (Actilyse*) and anistreplase (Eminase*) are similar, but very expensive, drugs that have more specific actions and result in less bleeding.

Forms: 250,000 IU, 750,000 IU, 1,500,000 IU powders for reconstitution.

Dose: *Cats, Dogs:* 90,000–250,000 IU by i.v. infusion over 30–60 minutes followed by 45,000–100,000 IU/h by i.v. infusion. There is little information on the use of this drug. These doses are empirical, based on those used in man.

Adverse effects and contraindications: Nausea, vomiting and bleeding are the main adverse effects. If bleeding is severe, stop administration and use antifibrolytic drugs (e.g. aprotonin). Anaphylaxis may be seen. Contraindications to use include recent haemorrhage, trauma, surgery or coagulopathies.

Streptomycin (Depomycin Forte; Devomycin) *POM*

Indications: Streptomycin is an aminoglycoside antibiotic active against a wide range of Gram-~~negative~~ and ~~some~~ Gram-positive pathogens. It is particularly indicated in the treatment of infections caused by *Leptospira* spp. and *Mycobacterium tuberculosis* (in combination with other drugs). Aminoglycosides require an oxygen-rich environment to be effective, thus they are ineffective in sites of low oxygen tension (abscesses, exudates) and all obligate anaerobes are resistant. Aminoglycosides are bactericidal and their mechanism of killing is concentration-dependent, leading to a marked post-antibiotic effect allowing pulse-dosing regimens to be used to limit toxicity.

Forms: *Injectable:* 250 mg/ml solution (Devomycin). Depomycin contains dihydrostreptomycin (200 mg/ml) and procaine penicillin (200 mg/ml).

Dose:
Dogs: 25 mg/kg i.m. q24h. Dosing 2–3 times a week is used to treat mycobacteriosis in man.
Small mammals: Rabbits, Hamsters: 25–50 mg/kg i.m., s.c. q24h.
Birds: 15–30 mg/kg i.m. q24h.
Reptiles: 10 mg/kg i.m., s.c. q48h @ 24°C.

Adverse effects and contraindications: Streptomycin is ototoxic, interfering with balance and hearing, which can be permanent. Nephrotoxicosis may be a problem but is less likely than with other aminoglycosides. This drug should not be used in cats. Use with caution in birds as it is toxic, especially in raptors.

Drug interactions: There is an increased risk of nephrotoxicity with **cephalosporins** (notably **cephalothin**) and **cytotoxic drugs**. Ototoxicity is increased with **cisplatin** and **loop diuretics**. The effects of **neostigmine** and **pyridostigmine** may be antagonized by aminoglycosides. The effect of non-depolarizing muscle relaxants, e.g. **pancuronium**, may be enhanced. **Penicillin** and streptomycin act synergistically. Aminoglycosides may be chemically inactivated by **beta-lactam antibiotics** (e.g. **penicillins**, **cephalosporins**) or **heparin** when mixed *in vitro*.

Sucralfate (Antepsin*) POM

Indications: Sucralfate is a complex of aluminium hydroxide and sulphated sucrose. In an acidic medium an aluminium ion detaches from the compound, leaving a very polar, relatively non-absorbable ion. This ion then binds to proteinaceous exudates in the upper GI tract forming a 'bandage' over ulcer sites, preventing further erosion from acid, pepsin and bile salts. However, its major action appears to relate to stimulation of mucosal defences and repair mechanisms. These effects are produced by prostaglandin-dependent and prostaglandin-independent pathways and are seen at neutral pH. Sucralfate is indicated for the treatment of oesophageal, gastric and duodenal ulceration, usually with an H_2 antagonist (e.g. ranitidine) but given separately.

Forms: *Oral:* 1g tablet; 0.2 g/ml suspension.

Dose:
Cats: 250 mg/cat p.o. q8–12h.
Dogs: <20 kg: 500 mg/dog p.o. q6–8h; >20 kg: 1–2 g/dog p.o. q6–8h.

Preferably administer on an empty stomach at least 1 hour before feeding.

Adverse effects and contraindications: Adverse effects with sucralfate appear to be minimal, with constipation being the main problem in man.

Drug interactions: Sucralfate may decrease the bioavailability **of H_2 antagonists** (e.g. **cimetidine**), **phenytoin** and **tetracycline**. Although, there is little evidence to suggest that this is of clinical importance it may be a wise precaution to administer sucralfate at least 2 hours before these drugs. It interferes significantly with the absorption of **fluoroquinolones** and **digoxin**.

Sulfadiazine – see Trimethoprim/sulphonamide and Silver sulfadiazine

Sulfasalazine (Salazopyrin*; Sulphasalazine*) POM

Indications: Sulfasalazine is a chemical combination of 5-aminosalicylic acid (5-ASA) and sulphapyridine connected by an azo bond. 5-ASA is probably the primary active ingredient, having a local anti-inflammatory effect in the colon. Most adverse effects are probably related to the sulphapyridine moiety. Sulfasalazine is indicated for the treatment of chronic colitis. In man, approximately one third of the oral dose is absorbed as the parent compound from the small intestine, whilst the other two thirds is cleaved by bacteria in the colon into 5-ASA and sulphapyridine. In the cat it has been suggested that <1% of the 5-ASA is absorbed. Balsalazide and olsalazine are related compounds. *See Olsalazine*. No safety data published for the use of balsalazide in dogs or cats.

Forms: *Oral:* 500 mg tablet; 250 mg/ml oral suspension.

Dose:
Cats: 10–20 mg/kg p.o. q8–12h.
Dogs: 15–30 mg/kg p.o. q8–12h, maximum 6 g/day.

Adverse effects and contraindications: Adverse effects are uncommon but include keratoconjunctivitis sicca (KCS), vomiting, allergic dermatitis and cholestatic jaundice. Owners should be made aware of the seriousness of KCS and what signs to monitor. The cause of the KCS is not clear. Historically sulphapyridine has been blamed. Olsalazine, a dimer of 5-ASA has been recommended as the incidence of KCS is less with its use, but it is not completely abolished. It is possible that 5-ASA or the combination may sometimes be responsible.

Drug interactions: The absorption of **digoxin** may be inhibited by sulfasalazine.

Sulphonamides – see Trimethoprim/sulphonamide

Suxamethonium (Suxamethonium*) *POM*

Indications: Suxamethonium is a depolarizing neuromuscular blocking agent. It prevents neuromuscular transmission by depolarizing the motor endplate in a similar manner to acetylcholine. However, depolarization persists for longer because its disengagement from receptors and subsequent metabolism is slower. It has no effect on consciousness or pain perception and should only be used in conjunction with anaesthetics. Suxamethonium is rapidly hydrolysed by plasma cholinesterase (pseudocholinesterase) and so is ultra short-acting in species with effective plasma cholinesterase activity, i.e. cats, pigs and primates. It has a variable duration of action and effect in dogs. Its very rapid onset of action (5–15 seconds) and short duration (3–5 minutes) make it suitable for facilitating endotracheal intubation in cats and primates. There are few, if any, indications for suxamethonium in dogs. Atracurium or vecuronium produce a similar duration of action without the adverse effects.

Forms: *Injectable:* 50 mg/ml solution.

Dose: *Cats:* 1.0 mg/kg i.v. A total dose of 3.5 mg is satisfactory in cats weighing >3.5 kg.

Adverse effects and contraindications: Suxamethonium must be used with caution in patients with pre-existing hepatic disease as plasma cholinesterase is produced in the liver. Neuromuscular blocking agents **must not be used** if the provision of adequate anaesthesia and analgesia cannot be guaranteed and the means for adequate lung ventilation are unavailable. Suxamethonium should not be used in animals that have been exposed to organophosphate compounds, as these inhibit plasma cholinesterase activity. Unexpectedly long activity must not be antagonized with anticholinesterase drugs as these are likely to aggravate blockade. Prolonged neuromuscular block should be treated by the infusion of fresh cross-matched blood containing active plasma cholinesterase. The risk of over-transfusion is lowered if recipient blood is removed, i.e. replaced, on a ml for ml basis. Suxamethonium may elevate plasma potassium levels and may cause arrythmias in hyperkalaemic animals. The drug also raises intraocular, intragastric and intracranial pressure in man and so should not be used where these changes are undesirable.

Drug interactions: The actions of suxamethonium may be enhanced by **beta-adrenergic blockers** (e.g. **propranolol**), **furosemide**, **isoflurane**, **lidocaine**, **magnesium salts**, **phenothiazines** and **procainamide**. **Diazepam** may reduce the duration of action of suxamethonium. Suxamethonium may cause a sudden outflux of potassium from muscle cells, which may initiate arrhythmias in **digitalized** patients. **Neostigmine** and **pyridostigmine** should not be administered with suxamethonium as they inhibit pseudocholinesterases, thereby enhancing suxamethonium's effect.

Tepoxalin (Zubrin) *POM*

Indications: Tepoxalin is a NSAID that inhibits both cyclooxygenase and lipoxygenase activity, making it a dual inhibitor of arachidonic acid metabolism. Tepoxalin is indicated for the control of musculoskeletal pain and inflammation in dogs, particularly associated with osteoarthritis. Tepoxalin has reduced gastrointestinal ulcerogenic activity compared to some other NSAIDs, possibly due to a protective effect caused by 5-lipoxygenase inhibition.

Forms: *Oral:* 30 mg, 50 mg, 100 mg, 200 mg tablets.

Dose: *Dogs:* 10 mg/kg p.o. q24h. Give with food as this leads to more effective absorption.

Note: A single initial dose of 20 mg/kg may be given if rapid pain relief is desired. After administration, keep the patient's mouth closed for approximately 4 seconds to ensure the tablet is fully dispersed. Do not administer with wet hands as tablets dissolve readily in water.

Adverse effects and contraindications: Rare adverse effects include diarrhoea, vomiting, incoordination, anorexia and incontinence. Overdosage (>100 mg/kg) may result in gastric irritation and haemorrhage. Use is contraindicated in animals with cardiovascular disease, hepatic dysfunction, renal insufficiency, GI ulceration or previous hypersensitivity to tepoxalin. Do not use in animals with hypovolaemia, hypotension or dehydration as there is an increased risk of renal toxicity. Do not use in pregnant or lactating bitches or in dogs less than 6 months of age as safety has not been evaluated.

Drug interactions: Do not administer with other **NSAIDs** or **corticosteroids** as this may greatly increase the occurrence of adverse effects.

Terbinafine (Lamisil*) *POM*

Indications: Terbinafine is an allylamine antifungal drug, used in human medicine in dermatophytosis where oral therapy is considered necessary and where the nail beds are infected. It has been used orally and by nebulization in birds for the treatment of aspergillosis. Like griseofulvin, terbinafine is keratophilic but, unlike griseofulvin, it is fungicidal. Terbinafine inhibits ergosterol synthesis but its target is the enzyme squalene epoxidase rather than the cytochrome P450 system.

Forms:
Oral: 250 mg tablet.
Topical: 1% terbinafine hydrochloride cream.

Dose: *Cats, Dogs:* At the present time there is insufficient experience to recommend a dose rate in dogs. The human dose is 4–8 mg/kg. A dose of 8.25 mg/kg p.o. q24h for 3 weeks has been used in cats to eradicate *Microsporum canis* from asymptomatic carriers. In other trials in cats dose rates of 30–40 mg/kg for up to 4 months in some cases were required to achieve a mycological cure of cats infected with *M. canis.*
Birds: 10–15 mg/kg p.o. q12–24h, or nebulization of 1 mg/ml for 20 minutes q8h.

Adverse effects and contraindications: Care should be taken with this drug in the face of hepatic or renal impairment and in pregnant or lactating animals. Adverse effects in man include loss of appetite, nausea, diarrhoea and skin reactions.

Drug interactions: The plasma concentrations of terbinafine will be increased by concomitant administration of **cimetidine** and decreased by **rifampin**. Because terbinafine does not inhibit cytochrome P450 systems, the potential drug interactions seen are likely to be fewer than with the antifungal azoles, such as **ketoconazole**.

Terbutaline (Bricanyl*; Monovent*) *POM*

Indications: Terbutaline is a selective beta$_2$ adrenoceptor stimulant (beta$_2$ agonist) used as a bronchodilator and to maintain the heart rate in animals with sick sinus syndrome.

Forms:
Injectable: 0.5 mg/ml solution.
Oral: 5 mg tablets; 1.5 mg/5 ml syrup.

Dose:
Cats: 0.312–1.25 mg/cat p.o. q8–12h, 0.015 mg/kg i.m., s.c. q4h.
Dogs: 1.25–5 mg/dog p.o. q8–12h, 0.01 mg/kg i.m., s.c. q4h.

Adverse effects and contraindications: Adverse effects include fine tremor, tachycardia, hypokalaemia, hypotension and hypersensitivity reactions. I.m. administration may be painful. Use with caution in patients with diabetes mellitus, hyperthyroidism, hypertension or seizure disorders.

Drug interactions: There is an increased risk of hypokalaemia if **theophylline** or high doses of **corticosteroids** are given with high doses of terbutaline. Use with digitalis glycosides or inhalational anaesthetics may increase the risk of cardiac arrhythmias. Beta blockers may antagonize its effects. Other sympathomimetic amines may increase the risk of adverse cardiovascular effects.

Testa triticum tricum (Trifyba*) *GSL*

Indications: Testa triticum tricum is a high fibre supplement that bulks up faeces and is used to assist in the maintenance of normal bowel function.

Forms: *Oral:* 3.5 g sachets.

Dose: *Cats, Dogs:* 1.75–7 g sprinkled on food.

Testosterone (Durateston) *POM*

Indications: Testosterone is the main male androgenic steroid. It is used in the management of feminization associated with oestrogen-producing testicular tumours, suppression of oestrus in the bitch, false pregnancy and testosterone-responsive incontinence and alopecia in male dogs.

Forms: *Injectable:* 50 mg/ml comprising 6 mg/ml testosterone propionate, 12 mg/ml testosterone phenylpropionate, 12 mg/ml testosterone isocaproate and 20 mg/ml testosterone decanoate.

Dose:
Cats: 2.5–5 mg/kg (0.05–0.1 ml) i.m., s.c. monthly.
Dogs: 2.5–10 mg/kg (0.05–0.2 ml) i.m., s.c. monthly.

Adverse effects and contraindications: Contraindications to the use of testosterone include prostatic enlargement, perineal hernia, recurrence or exacerbation of perianal adenomas, cardiac insufficiency, liver or renal disease. Do not use in pregnant animals. Use of testosterone in male cats may cause spraying. Administration of androgens to prepubertal animals may result in early closure of epiphyseal growth plates.

Drug interactions: Insulin requirements may be decreased in diabetic patients receiving androgenic therapy.

Tetanus antitoxin (Tetanus antitoxin behring) POM

Indications: Tetanus antitoxin is indicated as a preventive measure in animals at risk of developing tetanus from wounds. It may be used in established tetanus cases but is less effective as it does not displace bound toxin.

Forms: Injectable: 500–1500 IU/ml solution.

Dose: Cats, Dogs: Prophylactic administration: 500–1000 IU i.m., s.c. once. Therapy of established tetanus: 100–500 IU/kg s.c. once, max. 20,000 IU.

Adverse effects and contraindications: All antisera have the potential to produce anaphylactoid reactions, particularly if the patient has previously received products containing horse protein. Repeated doses may lead to hypersensitivity reactions. Adrenaline or antihistamines may be used to manage these adverse effects.

Tetracaine (Amethocaine) (Minims amethocaine hydrochloride*) POM

Indications: Tetracaine is an ester-linked topical ophthalmic anaesthetic of the procaine group. Although effective it is now rarely used in veterinary ophthalmology.

Forms: Topical: 0.5%, 1% solutions.
Store in refrigerator.

Dose: Dogs, Cats: 1–2 drops per eye, once.

Adverse effects and contraindications: Tetracaine often causes marked conjunctival irritation, chemosis and pain on application. An alternative ophthalmic anaesthetic, such as proxymetacaine, is advised. Topical anaesthetics block tear production and should not be applied before a Schirmer tear test. All topical anaesthetics are toxic to the corneal epithelium, delay healing of ulcers and should not be used for therapeutic purposes.

Tetracosactide (Tetracosactrin, ACTH) (Synacthen*) POM

Indications: Tetracosactide is an analogue of adrenocorticotrophic hormone (ACTH). It is used to stimulate cortisol production for the diagnosis of hyperadrenocorticism (Cushing's syndrome) and hypoadrenocorticism (Addison's disease).

Forms: *Injectable:* 0.25 mg/ml solution.

ACTH stimulation test:
Cats: Assess cortisol levels at 0, 60 and 120–180 minutes. Administer tetracosactide (Synacthen), 0.125 mg i.v. at 0 hours. The low-dose dexamethasone suppression test may be more sensitive and specific. Interpretation:
• Normal animals: Post-ACTH cortisol concentrations are 2–3 times higher than basal levels in normal animals and values are within the normal ranges.
• Pituitary-dependent HAC (PDH): An exaggerated response is seen, with pre-ACTH cortisol values often in the normal range but post-ACTH values above the normal range.
• Adrenal-dependent HAC: Exaggerated response or high basal level that fails to increase post-ACTH administration may be seen.
• Stress: Cortisol levels may rise by more than 3 times the basal level in animals stressed due to concomitant diseases. On some occasions this may take the post-ACTH value above the normal range.
• Hypoadrenocorticism: No or very little rise in cortisol levels.
Dogs: Assay cortisol levels at 0 and 2 hours. Administer tetracosactide (Synacthen), 0.125 mg i.v. (<5 kg BW) or 0.25 mg i.v. (>5 kg) at 0 hours. Doses as low as 0.005 mg/kg have been shown to be effective in stimulating cortisol production.

Theophylline (Corvental-D) POM

Indications: Theophylline is a methylxanthine. It causes bronchodilation (smooth muscle relaxation), enhanced mucociliary clearance, stimulation of the respiratory centre and increased sensitivity to $PaCO_2$, increased diaphragmatic contractility, stabilization of mast cells, a mild inotropic effect and a mild diuretic action. Its mechanisms of action are thought to include: inhibition of phosphodiesterase enzyme, alteration of intracellular calcium, catecholamine release and adenosine and prostaglandin antagonism. It is useful as a bronchodilator and in the management of pulmonary oedema.

Forms: *Oral:* 100 mg, 200 mg, 500 mg sustained-release capsules.

Dose:
Cats: 10 mg/kg p.o. q24h (sustained release preparation).
Dogs: 15–20 mg/kg p.o. q12–24h. Note: Manufacturer only recommends q24h dosing. Some texts indicate q12h dosing of the sustained release preparation is required to maintain therapeutic serum levels. Consider q12h dosing where the response to q24h dosing is inadequate.

Therapeutic plasma theophylline values are 5–20 µg/ml.

Adverse effects and contraindications: Adverse effects include vomiting, diarrhoea, polydipsia, polyuria, reduced appetite, tachycardia, arrhythmias, nausea, twitching, restlessness, agitation, excitement and convulsions. The severity of these effects may be decreased by the use of modified release preparations. They are more likely to be seen with twice daily dosing.

Drug interactions: Phenobarbital and **phenytoin** may decrease theophylline's effect. Plasma theophylline levels may be increased by **cimetidine, diltiazem, erythromycin, fluroquinolones** and **verapamil**. Theophylline and **beta-adrenergic blockers** (e.g. **propranolol**) may antagonize each other. The concurrent use of theophylline with **beta sympathomimetics** is contraindicated, as additive or synergistic interactions may result in exaggerated adverse effects. There is an increased risk of dysrrhythmias if theophylline is administered with **halothane** and an increased incidence of seizures if administered with **ketamine**. Hyperaesthesia is seen in cats.

Thiabendazole – see Tiabendazole

Thiamine – see Vitamin B1

Thiopental (Thiopentone) (Intraval; Thiovet) *POM*

Indications: Thiopental is an ultra-short-acting thiobarbiturate used by the i.v. route for the induction of anaesthesia.

Forms: *Injectable:* 943 mg/g powder for reconstitution. Aqueous solutions are unstable, particularly when exposed to air.

Dose:
Cats, Dogs: 5–20 mg/kg i.v. without hesitation. Dose depends mainly on the degree of depression caused by pre-anaesthetic medication. Reduce dose after premedication.
Small mammals: Ferrets: 10 mg/kg i.v.; Others: 30 mg/kg rapidly i.v.
Reptiles: 20–30 mg/kg i.p.

Use 1.25% (12.5 mg/ml) or 2.5% (25 mg/ml) solutions.

Adverse effects and contraindications: Thiopental solutions >1.25% should not be used if venous access cannot be guaranteed. Extravascular injections (of 2.5% and higher concentrations) are very likely to cause extensive tissue damage. Extravascular injections must be enthusiastically diluted using large volumes of sterile water or saline solutions followed by massage and dispersal. The dose of thiopental is reduced in animals that are hypovolaemic, hypoalbuminaemic and acidaemic. Normal doses are safe for use in 'sight hounds' but cause prolonged recoveries.

Thiostrepton (Panolog) POM

Indications: Thiostrepton is a thioazole-containing antibiotic. It inhibits ribosome function and is active against Gram-positive bacteria.

Forms: Ointment 2,500 IU/ml.

Dose: Topical: Apply to affected area q6–12h.

Thyroid hormones – see Levothyroxine and Liothyronine

Thyroid stimulating hormone (Thyrotropin, TSH)/ Thyrotropin releasing hormone (TRH) (Protirelin*; TSH*) POM

Indications: TSH and TRH stimulate thyroid hormone production; TRH acts through the pituitary by stimulating TSH production. They are used to assess thyroid function. The TSH stimulation test is considered to be the 'gold standard' in the diagnosis of hypothyroidism. The TRH stimulation test is considered to be of limited value in the diagnosis of hypothyroidism.

Forms:
TSH: No licensed preparation of TSH is currently available in the UK. Recombinant human TSH may be imported on a STA.
TRH: 100 µg/vial (Protirelin) (keep refrigerated).

Thyroid stimulation test:
Cats:
Assess serum T4 at 0 and 4 hours. Administer 4 µg/kg TRH (Protirelin) i.v. at time 0.
Interpretation: Normal cats and those with non-thyroid disease show at least a 60% rise in T4. Hyperthyroid cats have a <50% rise in T4.

Dogs:
Assess serum T4 at 0 and 6 hours. Administer 200 μg/dog TRH (Protirelin) i.v. at time 0.
Interpretation: In normal animals following TRH administration the T4 concentration should increase by 6.5 nmol/l in all cases and doubles in most normal patients. Cases of primary hypothyroidism will fail to respond. Cases with sick euthyroid syndrome will respond but concentrations remain low.

Drug interactions: Anabolic or **androgenic steroids, carbimazole, barbiturates, corticosteroids, diazepam, heparin, mitotane (op'-DDD), nitroprusside, phenylbutazone, phenytoin** and **salicylates** may all decrease serum T4 levels. **Fluorouracil, insulin, oestrogens, propranolol** and **prostaglandin F$_{2\alpha}$ (Dinoprost)** may cause T4 levels to be increased.

Adverse effects and contraindications: Chemical grade TSH may be associated with anaphylactic responses; do not use.

L—Thyroxine – see Levothyroxine

Tiabendazole (Thiabendazole) (Auroto) POM

Indications: Tiabendazole is an acaricide used in the treatment of ear mites (*Otodectes cynotis*) infestation.

Forms: *Topical:* 4% w/v solution.

Dose: *Cats, Dogs:* 3–5 drops/ear q12h for 7 days.

Ticarcillin (Timentin*) POM

Indications: Ticarcillin is a carboxypenicillin. It is a member of the beta-lactam group, and is susceptible to beta-lactamase enzymes but is co-formulated with clavulanic acid, the beta-lactamase inhibitor. Beta-lactam antibiotics bind penicillin-binding proteins involved in cell wall synthesis, decreasing bacterial cell wall strength and rigidity, and affecting cell division, growth and septum formation. As animal cells lack a cell wall the beta-lactam antibiotics are extremely safe. Ticarcillin is indicated for the treatment of serious (usually but not exclusively life-threatening) infections caused by *Pseudomonas aeruginosa*, although it also has activity against certain other Gram-negative bacilli including *Proteus* spp. and *Bacteroides fragilis*. For *Pseudomonas* septicaemias anti-pseudomonal penicillins are often given with an aminoglycoside (e.g. gentamicin) as there is a synergistic effect.

Forms: *Injectable:* 1.5 g ticarcillin and 100 mg clavulanic acid (Timentin); 3 g ticarcillin and 200 mg clavulanic acid powder for reconstitution.

Dose:
Cats, Dogs: 40–100 mg/kg i.v., i.m. q4–6h.
Birds: 200 mg/kg i.v., i.m. q8h.

As ticarcillin kills bacteria by a time-dependent mechanism, dosing regimens should be designed to maintain tissue concentration above the MIC for the bacteria throughout the interdosing interval.

Adverse effects and contraindications: Nausea, diarrhoea and skin rashes may be seen. After reconstitution it is stable for 48–72 hours. **Do not administer penicillins to hamsters, gerbils, guinea pigs, chinchillas or rabbits.**

Drug interactions: Do not mix with **aminoglycosides** in the same syringe because there is mutual inactivation.

Timolol maleate (Timolol*; Timoptol*) *POM*

Indications: Timolol is a non-selective beta-blocker used to reduce intraocular pressure.

Forms: *Ophthalmic:* 0.25%, 0.5% solutions – 0.5% solution usually used in veterinary medicine.

Dose:
Cats: One drop/eye(s) q12h.
Dogs: One drop/eye(s) q8–12h.

Adverse effects and contraindications: Ocular adverse effects include miosis, conjunctival hyperaemia and local irritation. Systemic absorption may occur following topical application and the most common adverse effect seen is bradycardia.

Drug interactions: Additive adverse effects may develop if given concurrently with oral **beta-blockers**. Concomitant administration of timolol with **verapamil** may cause a bradycardia and asystole. Prolonged AV conduction times may result if used with **calcium antagonists** or **digoxin**.

Tobramycin (Nebcin*; Tobramycin*) *POM*

Indications: Tobramycin is an aminoglycoside antibiotic used to treat Gram-negative infections. It is less active against most Gram-negative organisms than gentamicin, but appears to be more active against

Pseudomonas aeroginosa. Aminoglycosides are ineffective at sites of low oxygen tension (e.g. abscesses) and all obligate anaerobic bacteria are resistant. They are bactericidal and operate concentration-dependent cell killing, leading to a marked post-antibiotic effect and allowing pulse-dosing to be used.

Forms: *Injectable:* 10 mg/ml, 40 mg/ml solution (Nebcin).

Dose: More pharmacokinetic work is necessary to be sure of the dose rate, particularly in cats. The doses below are for general guidance only, and should be assessed according to the clinical response.
Cats, Dogs: Systemic: 2–4 mg/kg i.v., i.m., s.c. q8–24h. Pulse dosing (q24h) may be more effective (as for gentamicin).
Birds: 5 mg/kg s.c., i.m. q12h.
Reptiles: 2 mg/kg i.m. q24h.

Adverse effects and contraindications: Geriatric animals or those with decreased renal function should only be given this drug systemically when absolutely necessary and then every 12 hours or less frequently. Cellular casts found in the urine sediment are an early sign of nephrotoxicity. Tobramycin is considered to be less nephrotoxic than gentamicin. Do not use ophthalmic product where corneal ulceration is present.

Drug interactions: Avoid the concurrent use of other nephrotoxic, ototoxic or neurotoxic agents (e.g. **amphotericin B**, **cisplatin**, **furosemide**). Increase monitoring and adjust dosages when these drugs must be used together. Aminoglycosides may be chemically inactivated by **beta-lactam antibiotics** (e.g. **penicillins**, **cephalosporins**) or **heparin** when mixed *in vitro*. The effect of **non-depolarizing muscle relaxants** (e.g. **pancuronium**) may be enhanced by aminoglycosides. Synergism may occur when aminoglycosides are used with **penicillins** or **cephalosporins**.

Toldimphos – see Phosphate

Tolfenamic acid (Tolfedine) *POM*

Indications: Tolfenamic acid is an NSAID that inhibits COX, thereby limiting prostaglandin production. Tolfenamic acid has antipyretic and analgesic effects and is used to control mild to moderate pain and inflammation.

Forms:
Injectable: 40 mg/ml solution. Do not mix with other substances in the same syringe.
Oral: 6 mg, 20 mg, 60 mg tablets.

Dose: *Cats, Dogs:* 4 mg/kg s.c., i.m. (i.m. only in dogs) repeated once after 24h if necessary, or p.o. q24h for a maximum of 3 days.

Adverse effects and contraindications: Adverse effects are dose-related and reflect reduced prostaglandin synthesis. As with other NSAIDs possible adverse effects include GI irritation and ulceration and renal papillary necrosis, particularly if hypotension, dehydration or other nephrotoxic drugs are present. Although tolfenamic acid does not appear to be associated with such adverse effects to the same extent as other NSAIDs, its use where gastric or duodenal ulceration is suspected, in haemorrhagic syndromes or in cases of cardiac, hepatic or renal failure should be considered carefully. Severe toxicity following an acute overdose may result in vomiting, pyrexia, metabolic acidosis, depression, coma, seizures and GI bleeding. Treatment of acute toxic ingestion includes emptying the gut, treating the acidosis, alkalinizing the urine with sodium bicarbonate and supportive therapy.

Drug interactions: Do not use with **corticosteroids** or with **other NSAIDs** (increased risk of GI ulceration). In man there is an increased risk of convulsions if NSAIDs are administered with **fluoroquinolones**. NSAIDs may antagonize the hypotensive effects of **anti-hypertensives** (e.g. **beta-blockers**). The concomitant use of **diuretics** may increase the risk of nephrotoxicity. NSAIDs may cause false low **T3** and **T4** values and displace a variety of protein-bound drugs including **anaesthetics**, thereby potentiating their effects.

Tretinoin – see Vitamin A

Triamcinolone acetonide (Kenalog*; **Panolog**) *POM*

Indications: Triamcinolone is an intermediate-acting glucocorticoid, with approx 1.25 times the anti-inflammatory potency of prednisolone. On a dose basis, 0.8 mg triamcinolone is equivalent to 1 mg prednisolone. It has negligible mineralocorticoid activity. It is used in the management of inflammatory arthritides and dermatoses. It is unsuitable for alternate-day use because of its duration of activity.

Forms:
Injectable: 40 mg/ml (Kenalog) suspension for deep i.m., intra-articular or intralesional use.
Topical: 1 mg/g or ml cream or ointment (Panolog also contains neomycin).

Dose: *Cats, Dogs:*
- Systemic: 0.1–0.2 mg/kg i.m. initially then 0.02–0.04 mg/kg maintenance. A single i.m. dose of the long-acting preparations is effective for 3–4 weeks.

- Intralesional: 1.2–1.8 mg (total dose) injected intralesionally. Maximum 0.6 mg at any one site; separate injections by 0.5–2.5 cm.
- Topical: Apply small amount to affected area q6–8h.
- Intra-articular: Cats: 1–3 mg; Dogs: 6–18 mg.

Adverse effects and contraindications: Prolonged use of glucocorticoids suppress the hypothalamic–pituitary axis (HPA) and cause adrenal atrophy. Animals on chronic therapy should be tapered off their steroids when discontinuing the drug. Catabolic effects of glucocorticoids leads to weight loss and cutaneous atrophy. Iatrogenic hyperadrenocorticism may develop with chronic use. Vomiting and diarrhoea may be seen in some patients. GI ulceration may develop. Glucocorticoids may increase urine glucose levels and decrease serum T3 and T4 values. Do not use in pregnant animals. Systemic corticosteroids are generally contraindicated in patients with renal disease and diabetes mellitus. Impaired wound healing and delayed recovery from infections may be seen.

Drug interactions: There is an increased risk of GI ulceration if systemic glucocorticoids are concurrently with **NSAIDs**. Hypokalaemia may develop if **potassium-depleting diuretics** (e.g. **furosemide**, **thiazides**) are administered with corticosteroids. **Insulin** requirements may increase in patients taking glucocorticoids. Metabolism of corticosteroids may be enhanced by **phenobarbital** or **phenytoin**.

Trientine (Trientine dihydrochloride*) POM

Indications: Trientine is a copper chelator used to aid the elimination of copper in dogs with copper hepatotoxicosis.

Forms: *Oral:* 300 mg capsule.

Dose: *Dogs:* 10–15 mg/kg p.o. q12h.

Adverse effects and contraindications: Adverse effects include nausea, gastritis, abdominal pain, melaena and weakness.

Trifluorothymidine (F3T*) POM

Indications: Trifluorothymidine (trifluridine) is a nucleoside analogue topical anti-viral drug. It does not depend on viral thymidine kinase for phosphorylation. It is clinically the most effective anti-viral available for feline herpesvirus infection. Its use is usually reserved for corneal ulceration due to herpetic disease. It is safe to combine with topical interferon solution and is available in the UK if compounded by an ophthalmic pharmacy (e.g. Moorfields Eye Hospital, London). It has a short shelf-life of 12 weeks from the manufacturer, even unopened and is expensive.

Forms: 1% ophthalmic solution in 10 ml bottle.

Dose: *Cats:* 1 drop/eye q4–6h for a maximum of 3 weeks. More frequent application q1–2h for acute infection is safe if tolerated.

Adverse effects and contraindications: Ocular irritation may occur and the frequency of application should be reduced if this develops. Treatment should not be continued for more than 3 weeks.

Trilostane (Vetoryl) *POM*

Indications: Trilostane is a synthetic steroid with no innate hormonal activity. It acts as a competitive and, therefore, reversible inhibitor of the 3-β-hydroxysteroid-dehydrogenase enzyme system that converts pregnenolone to progesterone. Trilostane blocks adrenal synthesis of glucocorticoids, mineralocorticoids and sex hormones, such as testosterone and oestradiol. It is authorized for the treatment of canine pituitary- and adrenal-dependent hyperadrenocorticism. It has been reported in the treatment of feline hyperadrenocorticism and sex hormone excess.

Forms: *Oral:* 60 mg, 120 mg capsules.

Dose:
Cats: 30 mg/cat p.o. q 24h, adjusting dose according to clinical signs and 4–6 hour post-treatment ACTH stimulation tests.
Dogs: 2–12 mg/kg p.o. once daily.
Initial dose with a body weight of 5–20 kg, 60 mg; 21–40 kg, 120 mg; and >40 kg, 120–240 mg. Perform ACTH stimulation tests (4–6 hours post-dosing) and haematology/biochemistry screens at 10 days, 4 weeks, 12 weeks and then every three months. Aim for a post-ACTH cortisol of <150 nmol/l. In cases where clinical signs persist or polydipsia appears within the 24-hour period, ACTH stimulation tests performed later in the day and/or sequential cortisol determinations may be needed for dose adjustment (either mg/kg or frequency). Dosage adjustments may be necessary even after prolonged periods of stability.

N.B. Optimal treatment and monitoring regimes are not established.

Adverse reactions and contraindications: In man, idiosyncratic reactions include diarrhoea, colic, muscle pain, nausea, hypersalivation and rare cases of skin changes (rash or pigmentation). Reported adverse effects in dogs include mild increases in serum potassium, bilirubin and calcium. Clinical hypoadrenocorticism can be seen. Adrenal necrosis has been reported. Adrenal hyperplasia has been noted. Prolonged adrenal suppression after drug withdrawal has been noted in some cases.

Renal and hepatic insufficiency should be excluded before commencing therapy.

Drug interactions: In general, trilostane should not be administered concurrently with other drugs that suppress adrenal function, e.g. **mitotane**, **ketoconazole**. A month gap between ceasing **mitotane** and commencing trilostane is suggested.

Trimeprazine – see Alimemazine

Trimethoprim/Sulphonamide (Chanoprim; Delvoprim; Duphatrim; Monotrim*; Norodine; Tribrissen; Trimacare; Trimedoxine; Trimethoprim*) POM

Indications: Trimethoprim and sulphonamides block sequential steps in the synthesis of tetrahydrofolate, a cofactor required for the synthesis of many molecules, including nucleic acids, the building blocks for DNA synthesis. Sulphonamides block the synthesis of dihydropteroic acid and subsequently dihydrofolic acid by competing with para-aminobenzoic acid, and trimethoprim inhibits the enzyme dihydrofolate reductase, preventing the reduction of dihydrofolic acid to tetrahydrofolic acid. This two-step mechanism ensures that bacterial resistance develops more slowly than to either agent alone. Many organisms are susceptible, including *Nocardia, Brucella,* Gram-negative bacilli, some Gram-positive organisms (*Streptococcus* spp.), plus *Pneumocystis carinii, Toxoplasma gondii* and other coccidians. *Pseudomonas* spp. and *Leptospira* spp. are usually resistant. Trimethoprim/sulphonamide is useful in the management of urinary, respiratory tract and prostatic infections, but ineffective in the presence of necrotic tissue. Trimethoprim alone may be used for urinary, prostatic, systemic salmonellosis and respiratory tract infections. Fewer adverse effects are seen with trimethoprim alone. Trimethoprim is a weak base which becomes ion-trapped in fluids that are more acidic than plasma (e.g. prostatic fluid and milk). Sulphonamides are weak acids.

Forms:
Injectable: trimethoprim 40 mg/ml and sulfadiazine 200 mg/ml (240 mg/ml total) suspension for s.c. use; trimethoprim 40 mg and sulfadoxine 200 mg/ml (240 mg/ml total) solution for s.c. use in dogs, s.c. or i.m. use in other species.
Oral: trimethoprim 5 mg and sulfadiazine 25 mg (30 mg total) tablet; trimethoprim 20 mg and sulfadiazine 100 mg (120 mg total) tablet; trimethoprim 40 mg/5ml and sulfamethoxazole 200 mg/5ml (240 mg/ 5 ml total) oral suspension (co-trimoxazole); trimethoprim 80 mg and sulfadiazine 400 mg (480 mg total) tablet; trimethoprim alone 100 mg, 200 mg tablets, 10 mg/ml suspension (Trimethoprim, Monotrim).

Dose: Doses (mg) of <u>total</u> product (trimethoprim + sulphonamide):
Cats, Dogs:
* Mastitis: 30 mg/kg p.o. q12h for 7 days.
* CNS and *Pneumocystis carinii* infections: 15 mg/kg s.c., p.o. q8h for 14 days.
* Other susceptible bacteria and coccidiosis: 15 mg/kg p.o. q12h for 10–14 days.

Small mammals: Ferrets, Rabbits, Chinchillas, Guinea pigs, Hamsters: 30 mg/kg i.m., s.c. q24h, 100 mg/kg p.o. q24h; Rats, Gerbils, Mice: 120 mg/kg i.m., s.c. q24h, 100 mg/kg p.o. q24h.
Birds: 10 mg/kg i.m., s.c. q12h; 20–50 mg/kg p.o. q12h.
Reptiles: 15–30 mg/kg i.m. q24h @ 24°C.

Trimethoprim alone:
Cats, Dogs: 4–5 mg/kg p.o. q12h.

Adverse effects and contraindications: Adverse effects in cats include anorexia, leucopenia, anaemia and hypersalivation. Adverse effects in dogs include acute hepatitis, vomiting, cholestasis, immune-mediated thrombocytopenia and an immune-mediated polyarthritis. Acute hypersensitivity reactions are possible with sulphonamide products; they may manifest as a type III hypersensitivity reaction. Haematological effects (anaemias, agranulocytosis) are possible but rare in dogs. Sulphonamides may reversibly suppress thyroid function. Dermatological reactions (e.g. toxic epidermal necrolysis) have been associated with the use of sulphonamides in some animals. Keratoconjunctivitis sicca (KCS) has been reported in dogs treated with sulphapyridine and other sulphonamides. Sulphonamide crystal formation can occur in the urinary tract, particularly in animals producing very concentrated acidic urine. Ensure patients receiving sulphonamides are well hydrated and are not receiving urinary acidifying agents. Trimethoprim/sulphonamide combinations should be used with caution in patients with pre-existing hepatic or renal disease.

Drug interactions: The anticoagulant effect of **warfarin** may be enhanced by trimethoprim/sulphonamide. **Antacids** may decrease the bioavailability of sulphonamides if administered concomitantly. Urinary acidifying agents will increase the tendency for sulphonamide crystals to form within the urinary tract. Concomitant use of drugs containing **procaine** may inhibit the action of sulphonamides since procaine is a precursor for para-amino benzoic acid. When using the Jaffe alkaline picrate reaction assay for **creatinine** determination, trimethoprim/sulphonamide may cause an over-estimation of approximately 10%.

Tri-iodothyronine – see Liothyronine

Tropicamide (Mydriacyl*) *POM*

Indications: Tropicamide is a short-acting antimuscarinic used for mydriasis (dilate pupil) and cycloplegia (paralyse the ciliary muscle). It has a duration of action of 4–12 hours and is used mainly as a mydriatic to facilitate intraocular examination.

Forms: *Ophthalmic:* 0.5%, 1% solutions.

Dose: *Cats, Dogs:* 1 drop/eye, repeat after 20–30 mins if necessary.

Tylosin (Bilosin*; Tylan*; Tyluvet*) *POM*

Indications: Tylosin is a bacteriostatic macrolide antibiotic that binds to the 50S ribosomal subunit, suppressing bacterial protein synthesis. Tylosin has good activity against mycoplasms and has the same antibacterial spectrum of activity as erythromycin but is generally less active against bacteria. Although, rarely indicated in small animal medicine, it has been used for the treatment of chronic colitis (mechanism of action is unknown although it is active against *Clostridium perfringens* and spirochaetes that may play a role in colitis), antibiotic-responsive diarrhoea and cryptosporidiosis.

Forms:
Injectable: 200 mg/ml solutions (Bilosin, Tylan, Tyluvet).
Oral: 100 g/bottle soluble powder (Tylan).

Dose:
Cats, Dogs: 2–10 mg/kg i.m. q24h, 7–11 mg/kg p.o. q6–8h. May need higher dosages for dogs with chronic colitis and in the treatment of cryptosporidiosis.
Small mammals: 10 mg/kg i.m., s.c. q12h (not recommended in Guinea pigs or Rabbits).
Birds: 20–40 mg/kg i.m. q8–12h or by nebulization of 100 mg diluted in 5 ml DMSO and 10 ml saline solution.
Reptiles: 25 mg/kg i.m. q24h @ 30°C.

Adverse effects and contraindications: Adverse effects include GI disturbances. The activity of tylosin is enhanced in an alkaline pH. Tylosin can cause pain at the site of injection.

Drug interactions: These are not well documented for tylosin in small animals. It does not appear to inhibit the same hepatic enzymes as erythromycin.

Ursodeoxycholic acid (Ursodiol) (Destolit*; Urdox*; Ursodeoxycholic acid*; Ursofalk*) *POM*

Indications: Ursodeoxycholic acid is a relatively hydrophilic bile acid with cytoprotective effects in the biliary system. It inhibits ileal absorption of hydrophobic bile acids, thereby reducing their concentration in the body pool; hydrophobic bile acids are toxic to hepatobiliary cell membranes and may potentiate cholestasis. Ursodeoxycholic acid is used in patients with cholestatic liver disease.

Forms: *Oral:* 150 mg, 300 mg tablet, 250 mg capsule, 50 mg/ml suspension.

Dose: *Cats, Dogs:* 10–15 mg/kg p.o. q24h.

Adverse effects and contraindications: Vomiting is a rare effect. Serious hepatotoxicity has been recognized in rabbits and non-human primates, but not in dogs or cats.

Vasopressin (ADH) (Pitressin*) *POM*

Indications: Vasopressin is a posterior pituitary hormone with vasopressive and antidiuretic properties. It is used in the diagnosis and treatment of central diabetes insipidus.

Forms: *Injectable:* 20 IU/ml of argipressin (synthetic vasopressin) in aqueous solution.

Dose: *Cats, Dogs:* 0.5 IU/kg i.m., s.c. prn; maximum dose 5 IU.

Adverse effects and contraindications: Adverse effects in man include nausea, muscle cramp, hypersensitivity reactions and constriction of myocardial arteries. Do not use if cardiac disease is present.

Vecuronium (Norcuron*) *POM*

Indications: Vecuronium is a non-depolarizing neuromuscular blocking agent with an intermediate and dose-dependent duration of action of (20–30 minutes). Vecuronium has no cardiovascular effects. Repeated doses are non-cumulative and solutions may be infused for the long-term maintenance of neuromuscular block.

Forms: *Injectable:* 10 mg powder for reconstitution.

Dose: *Cats, Dogs:* 0.1 mg/kg i.v. initially produces neuromuscular block for 25–30 minutes. Block is then maintained using increments of 0.03 mg/kg.
Lower loading doses of 0.05 mg/kg i.v. produce neuromuscular block lasting 16–19 minutes. Duration of action is longer with isoflurane than halothane.

Adverse effects and contraindications: Vecuronium **must not be used** if the provision of adequate anaesthesia and analgesia cannot be guaranteed and the means for adequate lung ventilation are unavailable. Although vecuronium has an intermediate duration of action, its antagonism with antimuscarinic/anticholinesterase mixtures is recommended.

Drug interactions: Aminoglycosides, **clindamycin** and **lincomycin** may enhance the effect of vecuronium.

Vedaprofen (Quadrisol) *POM*

Indications: Vedaprofen is an aryl-propionic acid NSAID that inhibits prostaglandin synthesis. It has antipyretic, analgesic and anti-inflammatory effects and is used to control mild to moderate pain.

Forms: *Oral:* 5 mg/ml gel.

Dose: *Dogs:* 0.5 mg/kg p.o. q24h with food for a maximum of 28 days.

Adverse effects and contraindications: Adverse effects reflect reduced prostaglandin synthesis. The commonest adverse effects associated with NSAIDs are GI irritation and ulceration, and renal papillary necrosis (renal failure). These effects are more likely to develop in anaesthetized patients or if hypotension, dehydration or other nephrotoxic drugs are present. Do not use if GI, renal or cardiac disease is suspected, in haemorrhagic syndromes, where previous reactions to NSAIDs have occurred, or in anorectic dogs. Blood dyscrasias, hepatotoxicity and exacerbation of heart failure may be seen rarely following NSAID usage. Severe toxicity (usually with an acute overdose) may present with vomiting, pyrexia, metabolic acidosis, depression, coma, seizures and GI bleeding. Treatment of acute toxic ingestion includes emptying the gut, treating the acidosis, alkalinizing urine with sodium bicarbonate and supportive therapy. Do not use in animals less than 6 weeks of age or in aged animals.

Drug interactions: Do not use with **corticosteroids** or **other NSAIDs** (increased toxicity). In man there is an increased risk of convulsions if NSAIDs are administered with **fluoroquinolones**. NSAIDs may antagonize the hypotensive effects of **anti-hypertensives** (e.g. **beta-blockers**). The concomitant use of **diuretics** may increase the risk of nephrotoxicity. Do not mix with other substances in the same syringe.

Verapamil (Securon*; Verapamil*) *POM*

Indications: Verapamil is a calcium-channel blocker. It acts by interfering with the inward movement of calcium ions through the slow channels in myocardial cells and cells within the specialized conduction system in the heart and vascular smooth muscle; vascular smooth muscle is as equally sensitive to verapamil as myocardial tissues (relative activity of 1:1). Systemic resistance vessels and large arteries respond to calcium-channel blockers more readily than venous capacitance vessels and pulmonary vasculature. Verapamil causes a reduction in myocardial contractility (negative inotrope), depressed electrical activity (retards AV conduction) and vasodilation (cardiac vessels and peripheral arteries and arterioles). It is primarily used to control supraventricular tachyarrhythmias, sustained and paroxysmal ventricular tachycardias particularly in cases of hypertrophic cardiomyopathy and the heart rate in dogs with atrial fibrillation as an adjunct to digoxin. Verapamil is often used as a second-choice calcium-channel blocker behind diltiazem as it has a more pronounced negative inotropic effect. Calcium-channel blockers are preferred to propranolol for the management of feline hypertrophic cardiomyopathy by some authors because they improve myocardial relaxation, increase ventricular filling and dilate coronary vasculature. Verapamil is also effective in the management of hypertension, but to a lesser degree than amlodipine. In rabbits verapamil can be used perioperatively to minimize formation of surgical adhesions.

Forms:
Injectable: 2.5 mg/ml solution.
Oral: 40 mg, 80 mg, 120 mg, 160 mg tablets; 8 mg/ml syrup.

Dose:
Cats: 0.5–1 mg/kg p.o. q8h or 0.025 mg/kg slowly i.v. over 3 minutes (with ECG monitoring). Up to 8 repeat i.v. administrations at 3–5 minute intervals may be made if necessary.
Dogs: 0.5–1 mg/kg p.o. q8h or 0.05 mg/kg slowly i.v. over 10 minutes (with ECG monitoring). Up to 4 repeat i.v. administrations at a reduced dose of 0.025 mg/kg at 5 minute intervals may be made if necessary.
Small mammals: Rabbits: Prevention of adhesions: 0.2 mg/kg slow i.v. or p.o. after surgery and repeated q8h for 9 doses.

Adverse effects and contraindications: Verapamil can cause hypotension, bradycardia, tachycardia, dizziness, exacerbation of CHF, nausea, constipation and fatigue. Its use is contraindicated in patients with 2nd or 3rd degree heart block, hypotension, sick-sinus syndrome or with severe left ventricular dysfunction. Patients with severe hepatic disease may have a reduced ability to metabolize the drug; reduce the dose by 70%.

Drug interactions: If verapamil is administered with **beta-adrenergic blockers** (e.g. **propranolol**), there may be additive negative inotropic and chronotropic effects. The activity of verapamil may be adversely affected by **calcium** or **vitamin D**. Plasma concentrations of **digitoxin** and **digoxin** are increased by verapamil; monitor serum levels if used with verapamil. Verapamil enhances the effects of **non-depolarizing muscle relaxants**. **Cimetidine** inhibits the metabolism of verapamil, increasing plasma concentrations. Verapamil enhances the effect of **theophylline,** possibly leading to toxicity. Verapamil may displace protein-bound agents (e.g. **warfarin**) from plasma proteins. Verapamil may increase intracellular **vincristine** levels by inhibiting the drugs outflow from the cell.

Vetrabutine (Monzaldon) POM

Indications: Vetrabutine is a specific uterine relaxant and musculotropic stimulator used in bitches to dilate the cervix and coordinate uterine contractions to ease and shorten parturition.

Forms: *Injectable:* 100 mg/ml solution.

Dose: *Dogs:* 2 mg/kg i.m. repeated at 30–60 minute intervals up to 3 times.

Caution: Pregnant women should exercise great care when administering the drug to avoid self-injection.

Adverse effects and contraindications: Do not use in cats.

Vinblastine (Velbe*)

Indications: Vinblastine is a vinca alkaloid with cell-cycle specific activity. It interferes with microtubule assembly during mitosis, resulting in an arrest of cell division leading to cell death. In veterinary medicine vinblastine is used less frequently than vincristine for treatment of lymphoproliferative disorders, but it has been used with prednisolone for treatment of high-grade canine mast cell tumours.

Forms: *Injectable:* 1 mg/ml solution.

Dose: *Cats, Dogs:* 2.0–2.5 mg/m^2 q7–14d.
See page 293 for conversion of bodyweight to surface area (m^2).

Adverse effects and contraindications: Unlike vincristine the main dose-limiting toxicity is myelosuppression with neutropenia. Mucositis, stomatitis and GI tract toxicity may also occur. Use with care in patients with abnormal liver function, dose reduction recommended.

Drug interactions: Any drugs that inhibits metabolism via hepatic cytochrome P450 system may reduce metabolism and thus increase toxicity of vinblastine, e.g. **calcium-channel blockers**, **cimetidine**, **ciclosporin**, **erythromycin**, **metoclopramide**, **ketoconazole**.

Vincristine sulphate (Vincristine*) *POM*

Indications: Vincristine, an alkaloid, interferes with microtubule assembly, causing metaphase arrest. It is used with other neoplastic agents in the treatment of canine and feline neoplastic diseases, particularly lymphoproliferative disorders. It may be used in the management of thrombocytopenia to stimulate release of platelets.

Forms: *Injectable:* 1 mg, 2 mg, 5 mg vials.

Dose: *Cats, Dogs:*
- Transmissible venereal tumours: 0.025 mg/kg i.v. q7d for 4 weeks.
- Other neoplastic diseases: usual doses are 0.5–0.75 mg/m^2.
  See lymphoma chemotherapy protocols on pages 295–296.
  See page 293 for conversion of body weight to surface area (m^2).
- To increase circulating platelet numbers: 0.01–0.025 mg/kg i.v. q7d prn.

Adverse effects and contraindications: These include peripheral neuropathy, constipation and severe local irritation if administered perivascularly. Wear gloves when using vincristine solutions. Wash off from exposed skin with large volumes of water.

Drug interactions: Concurrent administration of vincristine with **drugs that inhibit cytochromes of the CYP3A family** may result in decreased metabolism of vincristine and increased toxicity. If vincristine is used in combination with **crisantaspase** (asparaginase) it should be given 12–24 hours before the enzyme. Administration of crisantaspase with or before vincristine may reduce clearance of vincristine and increase toxicity.

Vitamin A (Isotretinoin, Retinol, Tretinoin) (Isotrex*; Isotreninoin*; Retin-A*; Roaccutane*) *POM*

Indications: Tretinoin is the acid form of vitamin A and isotretinoin is an isomer of tretinoin. Vitamin A is used to treat hypovitaminosis A. Topical application of tretinoin or isotretinoin modifies keratinization to reduce pilosebaceous duct occlusion, whilst oral administration reduces sebum secretion. It is used in the management of dermatological disorders, e.g. sebaceous adenitis, seborrhoea, keratinization disorders and follicular dysplasia. It has been used in the treatment of the diffuse form of epitheliotropic lymphoma.

Forms:
Injectable: Vitamin A (retinol) 50,000 IU/ml.
Oral: 5 mg, 20 mg isotretinoin capsules (Roaccutane).
Topical: 0.05% isotretinoin gel (Isotrex); 0.025% tretinoin cream; 0.01% tretinoin gel (Retin-A).

Dose:
Cats, Dogs:
- Hypovitaminosis A: 10,000–100,000 IU i.m. q3d.
- Dermatological: Apply isotretinoin/tretinoin gel/cream to clean skin q12h; 1 mg isotretinoin/kg p.o. q12h for 1 month, reducing the dosage to 1 mg/kg p.o. q24h if improvement is seen.
Birds: 20,000 IU/kg i.m. maximum.
Reptiles: 1,000–5,000 IU i.m. weekly for 4 consecutive weeks.

Adverse effects and contraindications: Avoid contact with eyes, mouth or mucous membranes. Do not use topical preparations simultaneously with other topical drugs. Minimize exposure to sunlight. Redness and skin pigmentation may be seen after several days. Animals receiving oral dosing should be monitored for vitamin A toxicity. Many adverse effects are reported in man following the use of oral isotretinoin, predominantly involving the skin, haematological parameters, nervous system and bone changes.

Vitamin B Complex (Anivit 4BC *POM*; Bimavite *POM*; Combivit *POM*; Duphafral* *POM*; Vitamin B tablets *GSL*)

Indications: There are several B vitamins. Multiple deficiencies of B vitamins may occur in patients with renal or hepatic disease.

Forms: Various preparations containing varying quantities of vitamins are available. Most are for parenteral use.

Dose: Dosages and routes vary with individual products. Check manufacturer's recommendations prior to use. In general:
Cats: 1 ml s.c., i.m., i.v.
Dogs: BW up to 15 kg: 1–5 ml; >15 kg: 5–10 ml s.c., i.m., i.v.
Birds: Up to 1 ml i.m. q7d.

Vitamin B1 (Thiamine) (Thiamine* *GSL*; **Vitamin B1** *POM*)

Indications: Thiamine supplementation is required in deficient animals. Although uncommon this may occur in animals fed fish diets. Thiamine may be beneficial in alleviating signs of lead poisoning.

Forms:
Injectable (Vitamin B1)*:* 100 mg/ml solution.
Oral: Thiamine: 25 mg, 100 mg, 300 mg tablets.

Dose:
Cats, Dogs:
- Vitamin B1 deficiency: 50 mg p.o., i.m. q12–24h.
- Lead poisoning: 2 mg/kg i.m., s.c. q12h.
Reptiles: Snakes: Cerebrocortical necrosis: 25 mg/kg q24h.

Vitamin B12 (Cyanocobalamin/Hydroxocobalamin)
(Anivit B12*; Cobalin-H*; Hydroxocobalamin*; Neo-Cytamen*; Vitbee*) *POM*

Indications: Cyanocobalamin is used to treat vitamin B12 deficiency. Such a deficiency may develop in patients with small intestinal bacterial overgrowth (SIBO), ileal disease or exocrine pancreatic insufficiency. In man hydroxocobalamin has almost completely replaced cyanocobalamin as the form of vitamin B12 choice for therapy. Hydroxocobalamin is retained longer in the body and thus for maintenance therapy need only be administered at 3-monthly intervals. Information as to its use in dogs is lacking.

Forms: *Injectable:* cyanocobalamin: 0.25 mg/ml, 0.5 mg/ml, 1 mg/ml; hydroxocobalamin: 1 mg/ml solutions.

Dose: *Cats, Dogs:* Deficiency states: 0.02 mg/kg i.m., s.c. monthly (cyanocobalamin) or q3months (hydroxocobalamin), until serum concentration is normalized.

Vitamin C (Ascorbic acid) (Vitamin C*) *GSL*

Indications: Vitamin C is used to reduce methaemoglobinaemia associated with acetaminophen toxicity. Supplemental vitamin C may be required by working dogs or those with pain or hepatic disease.

Forms:
Injectable: 100 mg/ml.
Oral: Various tablet strengths.

Dose:
Cats, Dogs:
- Methaemoglobinaemia: 30–40 mg/kg s.c. q6h for 7 treatments.
- Other indications: 50–80 mg/kg p.o. q24h.

Small mammals: Guinea pigs: Maintenance: 10 mg/kg/day or 200–400 mg/l drinking water. Treatment of hypovitaminosis C 100 mg/kg p.o. q24h.

Vitamin D (Alfacalcidol*; AT 10*; Calciferol*; Calcijex*; One-alpha*; Pet-Cal; Rocaltrol*) *POM*

Indications: Vitamin D is a general term used to describe a range of compounds that influence calcium and phosphorus metabolism. They include vitamin D2 (ergocalciferol or calciferol), vitamin D3 (colecalciferol), dihydrotachysterol, alfacalcidol and calcitriol (1,25-dihydroxy-colecalciferol). These different drugs have differing rates of onset and durations. Vitamin D2 (ergocalciferol) requires 5–14 days before serum calcium concentrations rise, whilst therapy may have to be discontinued for 1–4 weeks (up to 18 weeks reported in man) before serum calcium concentrations return to normal following overdosage. Dihydrotachysterol raises serum calcium within 1–7 days with a discontinuation time of 1–3 weeks for serum calcium levels to normalize. Calcitriol and alfacalcidol (1-alpha-hydroxycolecalciferol) have a rapid onset of action (1–4 days) and a short half-life of <1 day; they are the preferred forms for use. Vitamin D requires hydroxylation by the kidney to its active form and therefore the hydroxylated derivatives alfacalcidol and calcitriol should be used in patients with renal failure. Vitamin D is used to control hypocalcaemia associated with chronic renal failure, hypoparathyroidism or following thyroidectomy. It is also useful in the management of vitamin D deficiency associated with intestinal malabsorption or chronic liver disease. Calcitriol has been used in the management of renal secondary hyperparathyroidism; it reduces serum parathyroid hormone concentrations.

Forms:
Oral: Alfacalcidol 2 μg/ml solution (One-alpha), 0.25–1 μg capsules (Alfacalcidol; One-alpha).
Calcitriol 0.25–0.5 μg capsules (Calcitriol; Rocaltrol).
Dihydrotachysterol 0.25 mg/ml solution (AT 10).
Ergocalciferol 0.25 mg tablet (Calciferol).
Vitamin D, calcium, phosphate tablets (Pet-Cal).
Injectable: Alfacalcidol 2 μg/ml solution (One-alpha).
Calcitriol 1–2 μg/ml solution (Calcijex).

Dose: *Cats, Dogs:*
- Hypocalcaemia/vitamin D deficiency:
  ergocalciferol: 4000–6000 IU/kg p.o. q24h initially, then 1000–2000 IU/kg p.o. q1–7d for maintenance; dihydrotachysterol: 0.02–0.03 mg/kg p.o. q24h initially, then 0.01–0.02 mg/kg p.o. q24–48h for maintenance; calcitriol: 0.01–0.06 μg/kg p.o. q24h for 2–3 days, then decrease to 0.02–0.03 μg/kg p.o. q24h for 2–3 days then give 0.01 mg/kg p.o. q24h; alfacalcidol: 0.05 μg/kg p.o. q24h.

- Renal secondary hyperparathyroidism: calcitriol: 1.5–6.6 ng/kg p.o. q24h; some authors recommend higher doses if ionized serum calcium concentrations can be assessed.
  Note: These doses are lower than those recommended for the management of hypocalcaemia. Assess serum calcium and phosphate levels serially and maintain total calcium x phosphate product below 4.2 (calcium and phosphate in mmol/l). Do not use if this is not possible.
- Oral supplement: Pet-Cal: up to 9 kg 1/2 tablet/day, >9 kg BW 1 tablet/day.

Adverse effects and contraindications: Serum phosphorus and calcium levels should be monitored weekly. Use vitamin D analogues in normophosphataemic patients only.

Drug interactions: The concurrent use of **magnesium-containing antacids** may lead to the development of hypermagnesaemia. Hypercalcaemia is more likely to develop if **thiazide diuretics** are given concomitantly with vitamin D. Hypercalcaemia may potentiate the toxic effects of **verapamil** or **digoxin**; monitor carefully.

Vitamin E **(Alpha tocopheryl acetate)** (Vitamin E*); *GSL*

Indications: Vitamin E supplementation is required in deficient animals. However, vitamin E deficiency is rarely recognized in small animal medicine, although many animals with exocrine pancreatic insufficiency may have a subclinical deficiency.

Forms: *Oral:* 100 mg/ml suspension.

Dose: *Cats, Dogs:* 1.6–8.3 mg/kg p.o. q24h.

Vitamin K1 **(Phytomenadione)** (Konakion*) *POM*

Indications: Vitamin K1 is used in the management of vitamin K1 deficiency in patients with fat malabsorption, hypoprothrombinaemia secondary to the ingestion of anticoagulant rodenticides, or other vitamin K1-dependent clotting factor abnormalities.

Forms:
Injectable: 2 mg/ml, 10 mg/ml solutions.
Oral: 10 mg tablets.

Dose:
Cats, Dogs, Ferrets:
- Known warfarin or other 1st generation coumarin toxicity or vitamin K1 deficiency: Initially 2.5 mg/kg s.c. in several sites, then 0.25–2.5 mg/kg in divided doses p.o. q8–12h for 5–7 days.

- Known inandione (diphacinone) or 2nd generation coumarin (brodifacoum) toxicity: Initially 5 mg/kg s.c. in several sites, then 5 mg/kg p.o. divided q8–12h for 2 weeks, then re-evaluate coagulation status. The patients activity should be restricted for 1 week following treatment. Evaluate the coagulation status 3 weeks after cessation of treatment.
- Unknown anticoagulant toxicity: Initially 2.5 mg/kg s.c. over several sites. Then 2.5 mg/kg p.o. divided q8–12h for 7 days. Re-evaluate coagulation status 2 days after stopping therapy. If the OSPT time is elevated, continue therapy for 2 additional weeks. If not elevated repeat OSPT in 2 days. If normal, the animal should be rested for 1 week, if abnormal then continue therapy for an additional week and re-check OSPT times as above. Use a small gauge needle when injecting s.c. or i.m.
- Liver disease: cholestatic hepatopathy: 0.5 mg/kg s.c. q12h, i.m. for 3 days; chronic liver disease: 0.5 mg/kg p.o. q7–20 days.

Small mammals: 1–10 mg/kg i.m. as needed depending upon clinical signs/clotting times
Birds: 0.2–2.2 mg/kg i.m. q4–8h until stable, then q24h.

Adverse effects and contraindications: Adverse effects include anaphylactoid reactions following i.v. administration of vitamin K1, therefore use with extreme caution when using by this route. One stage prothrombin times are the best method of monitoring therapy.

Drug interactions: The absorption of oral vitamin K is reduced by **mineral oil**.

Warfarin (Warfarin*) *POM*

Indications: Warfarin is a vitamin K antagonist used in the management of thromboembolic disorders.

Forms: *Oral:* 1 mg, 3 mg, 5 mg tablets.

Dose:
Cats: 0.2–0.5 mg/cat p.o. q24h.
Dogs: 0.2 mg/kg p.o. q24h.
Monitor the one stage prothrombin time regularly. The dose should be titrated to maintain the OSPT at 1.5 times normal.

Adverse effects and contraindications: Haemorrhage is the major adverse effect. Other adverse effects reported in man include hypersensitivity, diarrhoea, skin necrosis, hepatic dysfunction, vomiting and pancreatitis. Its use is contraindicated in patients with hepatic or renal disease or in those undergoing surgery.

Drug interactions: Warfarin is highly protein-bound and therefore its activity may increase if serum protein levels drop or drugs which are themselves protein-bound are administered concomitantly. In particular **NSAIDs, cimetidine, clarithromycin, erythromycin, fluoroquinolones, ketoconazole, metronidazole, potentiated sulphonamides, tetracyclines** and **thyroxine** may enhance the anticoagulant effect of warfarin. **Barbiturates** and **griseofulvin** accelerate warfarin metabolism. Anti-coagulant effect of warfarin may be enhanced or reduced by **corticosteroids**.

Xylazine (Chanazine; Rompun; Virbaxyl; Xylacare; Xylazine) *POM*

Indications: Xylazine is an alpha$_2$-adrenergic receptor agonist. It is a potent sedative and muscle relaxant; although it provides good visceral analgesia, somatic analgesia is poor. Sedation tends to last longer than its analgesic effects; duration of analgesia is approx 20 minutes to 1 hour. Xylazine is used alone for chemical restraint, sedation and pre-anaesthetic medication. In combination with other drugs surgical anaesthesia may be produced. Pre-anaesthetic medication with xylazine has a marked sparing effect on the dose of induction and maintenance agents used subsequently. It counteracts the muscle rigidity associated with 'dissociative anaesthesia'. It can be used in conjunction with acepromazine and opioids to improve the 'stopping power' of chemical restraint mixtures for dangerous animals. It can be used to promote emesis in emergency situations where more suitable emetics are unavailable. Xylazine also stimulates growth hormone production and may be used to assess the pituitary's ability to produce this hormone.

Forms: *Injectable:* 20 mg/ml solution.

Dose:
Cats: 3 mg/kg i.m.
Dogs: 1-3 mg/kg i.v., i.m.
Small mammals: Rabbits, Ferrets, Chinchillas: 1–3 mg/kg i.v., 3–5 mg/kg i.m., s.c.; Gerbils, Guinea pigs, Hamsters, Rats: 5 mg/kg i.m., 10 mg/kg i.p.; Mice: 10 mg/kg i.m., i.p. Used in combination with ketamine to provide general anaesthesia. In ferrets, use in combination with butorphanol to provide sedation.
Birds: 1–2.2 mg/kg i.v., i.m.
See Sedation protocols, pages 297–301.

Xylazine stimulation test (to assess growth hormone production): Take EDTA blood sample for growth hormone estimation at 0 and 20 minutes. Administer 100 µg/kg xylazine i.v. after taking the basal sample. Separate plasma as soon as possible and store at −20°C.

Send samples on dry ice to Faculty of Veterinary Medicine, University of Utrecht, Dept of Clinical Science of Companion Animals, Biochemical Lab, PO 80154, 3508 TD Utrecht, The Netherlands. Interpretation: Normal baseline values 1–4 ng/ml. Following stimulation, ratios of peak to basal values range from 3.4 to 111.7. Note: Assessment of plasma insulin growth factor in a single sample is an alternative useful screening test for a growth hormone disorder. Low IGF is seen with growth hormone deficiency, whilst elevated IGF levels are seen with acromegaly, diabetes mellitus, hyperadrenocorticism.

Adverse effects and contraindications: Adverse effects include bradycardia, hypotension, bradydysrhythmias, hypoventilation, hyperglycaemia, salivation and vomiting. Xylazine may initiate (occasionally fatal) ventricular arrhythmias in the presence of exogenous and endogenous catecholamines. It should not be used in animals with diminished cardiopulmonary reserve. Small dogs and cats are particularly sensitive to the adverse effects of xylazine on thermoregulation, and must be protected from extreme environmental temperatures. Atipamezole may be used to reverse the effects of xylazine if an overdose is given (unlicensed use of atipamezole).

Zidovudine (Azidothymidine; AZT) (Retrovir*) POM

Indications: Zidovudine is a deoxythymidine analogue. It is an antiviral drug that requires activation to the 5'-triphosphate form by cellular kinases to produce competitive inhibition of reverse transcriptase. In the FIV-positive cat that is not showing clinical signs use of zidovudine should delay the onset of the clinical phase of the infection. In human medicine it is used in combination with other nucleoside reverse transcriptase inhibitors, e.g. abacavir, didanosine, lamivudine, stavudine, tenofovir and zalcitabine. Two of these drugs are usually used with either a non-nucleotide reverse transcriptase inhibitor or a protease inhibitor. Use of drug combinations in HIV-positive patients aims to avoid the development of drug resistance. The protease inhibitors currently used in human medicine seem to lack efficacy against FIV, thus hampering this approach to manage FIV-infected acts in the clinical phase of this disease.

Forms:
Oral: 100, 250 mg capsules, 50 mg/5 ml syrup.
Injection: 10 mg/ml solution for use as i.v. infusion.

Dose: *Cats:* 5–10 mg/kg daily p.o., s.c. in 2–4 divided doses.

Adverse effects and contraindications: Hepatotoxicity and severe anaemia can occur at high doses. Haematological monitoring is recommended. Animals that are severely anaemic or leucopenic should not be given this drug. Long-term adverse effects of lower doses have not been ascertained.

Zinc sulphate (Z Span*) *P*

Indications: Zinc sulphate is used as a supplement for treatment of zinc deficiency or zinc-responsive disease. Zinc supplementation in copper-associated liver disease is recommended as a preventative measure or after successful 'de-coppering' with D-penicillamine or trientine, but not during chelation therapy.

Forms: *Oral:* 61.8 mg zinc sulphate (= 22.5 mg elemental zinc) capsules.

Dose: *Cats, Dogs:*
- Zinc deficiency: Initially 1 mg/kg elemental zinc/kg p.o. q24h (= 5 mg zinc sulphate/kg p.o. q24h), increasing dose by 50% if ineffective after 1 month and reducing dose gradually if a response is seen.
- Copper-associated or fibrotic liver disease: 4–20 mg elemental zinc/kg p.o. q24h for 3–6 months, then reduce the dose to 1–5 mg elemental zinc/kg p.o. q24h. Use the lower end of the dose range for larger dogs and maintain plasma zinc at 200–300 µg/dl.

Adverse effects and contraindications: Adverse effects include vomiting, diarrhoea and abdominal discomfort.

Antibiotic selection according to organ system

Bone: Most antibacterials penetrate bone, as it has a good blood supply, and are then distributed in interstitial fluid. Osteomyelitis is often caused by *Staphylococcus* spp., although obligate anaerobes and Gram-negative Enterobacteriaceae may be involved. Choice of drug therapy should be made after culture of bone fragments removed at surgery; otherwise, drugs effective against beta-lactamase-producing staphylococci and obligate anaerobes should be chosen. These include:

Amoxicillin/Clavulanate	Clindamycin
Cefalexin	Lincomycin
Cefazolin	

Urinary tract: Many antibacterials attain high concentrations in urine since this is a major route of excretion for drugs. If a drug is filtered but not reabsorbed to any extent, its urine concentration exceeds its plasma concentration by 100-fold. Some drugs are actively secreted into urine (e.g. beta-lactams) and reach concentrations that are 300 times higher than plasma concentrations. The susceptibility of uropathogens is fairly predictable; if the animal has not been treated with antibacterial drugs in the last couple of months, the following first line antibacterial drugs are successful in more than 80% of uncomplicated lower urinary tract infections according to the causative organism involved:

Organism	Drug of choice
Escherichia coli	Potentiated sulphonamide
Staphylococcus spp.	Ampicillin or amoxicillin
Streptococcus spp.	Ampicillin or amoxicillin
Proteus mirabilis	Ampicillin or amoxicillin
Klebsiella pneumoniae	Cefalexin
Pseudomonas aeruginosa	Oxytetracycline
Enterobacter	Potentiated sulphonamide

Recurrent or relapsing urinary tract infections should have cultures and sensitivity tests performed to determine the most appropriate antibacterial drug. Fluoroquinolones and clavulanate-potentiated penicillins should be reserved for the more difficult infections. Aminoglycosides may be required in some cases, but their nephrotoxic effects should always be considered in cases where renal involvement may be present.

Prostate: Many antimicrobials attain therapeutic concentrations in the prostate during acute prostatitis. Only a few penetrate the prostate in chronic prostatitis. These include highly lipophilic drugs, and those that are weak bases have the added advantage that they will be ion-trapped in the acidic prostatic fluid. Examples include:

Baquiloprim	Doxycycline	Minocycline
Chloramphenicol	Erythromycin	Trimethoprim
Clindamycin	Fluoroquinolones	

Hepatic/biliary system: Antibacterials that penetrate liver and biliary tract well include:

Aminoglycosides
Ampicillin
Amoxicillin
Amoxicillin/clavulanate
Cephalosporin

Chloramphenicol
Clindamycin
Fluoroquinolones
Metronidazole

Respiratory system: Most antibacterials penetrate the pulmonary parenchyma. Lipid-soluble drugs, however, are recommended for bronchial infections. These include:

Chloramphenicol
Difloxacin
Doxycycline

Fluoroquinolones
Minocycline
Potentiated sulphonamide

CNS: The following drugs may be useful in CNS infections:

Intermediate penetration:
Amoxicillin
Ampicillin
Flucytosine

Ketoconazole
Ticarcillin

Note: Beta-lactams are organic acids which are mainly ionized at physiological pH and will only penetrate if there is inflammation.

Good penetration:
Chloramphenicol
Fluoroquinolones

Metronidazole
Trimethoprim/sulphonamide

Modification of drug dosages in renal or hepatic insufficiency

With failure of liver or kidney, the excretion of some drugs may be impaired, leading to increased serum concentrations.

Renal failure

a Double the dosing interval or halve the dosage in patients with severe renal insufficiency. Use for drugs that are relatively non-toxic

b Increase dosing interval 2-fold when creatinine clearance (Ccr) is 0.5–1 ml/min/kg, 3-fold when Ccr is 0.3–0.5 ml/min/kg and 4-fold when Ccr is <0.3 ml/min/kg

c Precise dose modification is required for some toxic drugs that are excreted solely by glomerular filtration, e.g. aminoglycosides. This is determined by using the dose fraction K_f to amend the drug dose or dosing interval according to the following equations:

Modified dose reduction = normal dose x K_f
Modified dose interval = normal dose interval / K_f
where K_f = Patient Ccr/normal Ccr

Where Ccr is unavailable, Ccr may be estimated at 88.4/serum creatinine (μmol/l) (where serum creatinine is <350 μmol/l). K_f may be estimated at $\leq$0.33 if urine is isosthenuric or $\leq$0.25 if the patient is azotaemic.

Drug	Nephrotoxic	Dose adjustment in renal failure
Amikacin	yes	c
Amoxicillin	no	a
Amphotericin B	yes	c
Ampicillin	no	a
Cefalexin	no	b
Chloramphenicol	no	N, A
Digoxin	no	c
Gentamicin	yes	c
Kanamycin	yes	c
Nitrofurantoin	no	CI
Penicillin	no	a
Streptomycin	yes	b
Tetracycline	yes	CI
Tobramycin	yes	c
Trimethoprim/ sulphonamide	yes	b, A

a, b, c: refer to section above on dose adjustment; N = normal dose; A = avoid in severe renal failure; CI = contraindicated.

Hepatic insufficiency

Drug clearance by the liver is affected by many factors and thus it is not possible to apply a simple formula to drug dosing. The table below is adapted from information in the human literature.

Drug	DI	CI
Aspirin		✓
Azathioprine		✓
Captopril	✓	
Cefotaxime	✓	
Chloramphenicol		✓
Clindamycin		✓
Cyclophosphamide	✓	
Diazepam		✓
Doxorubicin	✓	
Doxycycline	✓	
Fluorouracil		✓
Furosemide	✓	
Hydralazine	✓	
Ketoconazole	✓	
Lidocaine	✓	
Metronidazole	✓	
Morphine	✓	
NSAIDs	✓	
Naproxen	✓	
Pentazocine		✓
Phenobarbital	✓	
Pentobarbital	✓	
Procainamide	✓	
Propranolol	✓	
Tetracycline		✓
Theophylline	✓	
Thiopental	✓	
Vincristine	✓	

DI = a change in dose or dosing interval may be required
CI = contraindicated; avoid use if at all possible

Dosing small animals including 'exotic pets'

The size of some animals, particularly 'exotic pets', makes dosing difficult and care must be taken when calculating small doses. Some points to bear in mind when dosing are:

- Where powders are to be dissolved in water, sterile water for injection should be used.
- Most **solutions** may be diluted with water for injection or 0.9% saline.
- Dilution will be necessary when volumes <0.1 ml are to be administered.
- Suspensions cannot be diluted.
- Use 1 ml syringes for greatest accuracy.
- When reformulating tablets, consider using a pharmacist.

Example: To dose a 15 g canary with dexamethasone (2 mg/ml)

Dose required is 0.023 mg.
Take 0.1 ml of dexamethasone and dilute with 0.9 ml water to produce a solution containing 0.2 mg/ml.
The canary requires 0.023 mg/0.2 ml = 0.115 ml of the diluted dexamethasone.

Body weight to body surface area (BSA) conversion tables

Dogs

Weight (kg)	BSA (m^2)	Weight (kg)	BSA (m^2)	Weight (kg	BSA (m^2)
0.5	0.06	11	0.49	24	0.83
1	0.1	12	0.52	26	0.88
2	0.15	13	0.55	28	0.92
3	0.2	14	0.58	30	0.96
4	0.25	15	0.6	35	1.07
5	0.29	16	0.63	40	1.17
6	0.33	17	0.66	45	1.26
7	0.36	18	0.69	50	1.36
8	0.4	19	0.71	55	1.46
9	0.43	20	0.74	60	1.55
10	0.46	22	0.78		

Cats

Weight (kg)	BSA (m^2)	Weight (kg)	BSA (m^2)	Weight (kg	BSA (m^2)
0.5	0.06	2.5	0.184	4.5	0.273
1	0.1	3	0.208	5	0.292
1.5	0.134	3.5	0.231	5.5	0.316
2	0.163	4	0.252	6	0.33

Percentage solutions

The concentration of a solution may be expressed on the basis of weight per unit volume (w/v) or volume per unit volume (v/v).

% w/v = number of grams of a substance in 100 ml of a liquid
% v/v = number of ml of a substance in 100 ml of liquid

% solution	g or ml/100 ml	mg/ml	solution strength
100	100	1000	1:1
10	10	100	1:10
1	1	10	1:100
0.1	0.1	1	1:1000
0.01	0.01	0.1	1:10,000
0.001	0.001	0.01	1:100,000
0.0001	0.0001	0.001	1:1,000,000

Parenteral fluids comparison table

Fluid	Na^+ (mmol/l)	K^+ (mmol/l)	Ca^{2+} (mmol/l)	Cl^- (mmol/l)	HCO_3^- (mmol/l)	Dext. (g/l)	Osmol. (mosm/l)
0.45% NaCl	77			77			155
0.9% NaCl	154			154			308
5% NaCl	856			856			1722
Ringer's	147	4	2	155			310
Hartmann's	131	5	2	111	29*		280
Darrow's	121	35		103	53*		312
0.9% NaCl + 5.5% Dext	154			154		50	560
0.18% NaCl + 4% Dext.	31			31		40	264

*Bicarbonate is present as lactate. Dext. = Dextrose. Osmol. = Osmolality
See specific monographs.

Chemotherapy protocols for lymphoma

Various protocols are described in the literature. Two examples are provided below.

Protocol 1: Combination cytotoxic therapy COP (low dose)

Induction:
Cyclophosphamide: 50 mg/m^2 p.o. on alternate days or 50 mg/m^2 p.o. for the first 4 days of each week
Vincristine: 0.5 mg/m^2 i.v. q7d
Prednisolone: 40 mg/m^2 p.o. q24h for first 7 days then 20 mg/m^2 p.o. on alternate days and given with cyclophosphamide

Maintenance after a minimum of 2 months:
Cyclophosphamide: 50 mg/m^2 p.o. on alternate days or 50 mg/m^2 p.o. for the first 4 days of each second week (alternate week therapy)
Vincristine: 0.5 mg/m^2 i.v. q14d
Prednisolone: 20 mg/m^2 p.o. on alternate days of each second week and given with cyclophosphamide

Maintenance after 6 months (if disease in remission):
Cyclophosphamide: 50 mg/m^2 p.o. q48h or 50 mg/m^2 p.o. for the first 4 days of each third week (one week in 3)
Vincristine: 0.5 mg/m^2 i.v. q21d
Prednisolone: 20 mg/m^2 p.o. on alternate days of each third week and given with cyclophosphamide

Maintenance after 12 months:
Cyclophosphamide: 50 mg/m^2 p.o. q48h or 50 mg/m^2 p.o. for the first 4 days of each fourth week (one week in 4)
Vincristine: 0.5 mg/m^2 i.v. q28d
Prednisolone: 20 mg/m^2 p.o. on alternate days of each fourth week and given with cyclophosphamide

Notes: Melphalan (5 mg/m^2 p.o.) may be administered as an alternative to cyclophosphamide after 6 months in order to reduce the risk of cystitis developing.
Chlorambucil (5 mg/m^2 p.o. on alternate days) or melphalan may be given as alternatives for cyclophosphamide if haemorrhagic cystitis develops.
Doxorubicin (30 mg/m^2 i.v. q3w) or crisantaspase (10,000–20,000 IU/m^2 i.m. q7d or as necessary) may be used to manage relapsing or recurrent disease.

Protocol 2: Combination cytotoxic therapy COP (high dose)

Induction:
Cyclophosphamide: 250–300 mg/m^2 p.o. q21d
Vincristine: 0.75 mg/m^2 i.v. q7d for 4 weeks then 0.75 mg/m^2 i.v. q21d administered with cyclophosphamide
Prednisolone: 1 mg/kg p.o. q24h for 4 weeks then 1 mg/kg p.o. on alternate days

Maintenance after 12 months:
Cyclophosphamide: 250–300 mg/m^2 p.o. q28d
Vincristine: 0.75 mg/m^2 i.v. q28 days with cyclophosphamide
Prednisolone: 1 mg/kg p.o. on alternate days

Note: Some authors recommend a maximum cyclophosphamide dose in dogs of 250 mg/m^2.

Adverse effects and contraindications: Myelosuppression, a haemorrhagic cystitis (cyclophosphamide only) or GI effects may occur. Peripheral neuropathies although reported are rare. If toxicities other than myelosuppression develop, reduce vincristine and cyclophosphamide dose by one third. Perform a complete blood count (CBC) with platelet count weekly during the induction course. Discontinue cyclophosphamide therapy for 1 week if the neutrophil count decreases to <2 x 10^9/l. If neutropenia recurs following re-institution of therapy, decrease dosage by one quarter.

Sedation protocols

Sedative combinations for dogs

Acepromazine (ACP)

Acepromazine alone is not a particularly effective sedative. Increasing the dose above 0.1 mg/kg does little to improve the predictability of achieving adequate sedation but increases the risk of incurring adverse effects, increases the severity of adverse effects and prolongs the duration of action of any effects (desirable or adverse) that arise. Doses of 0.0125 to 0.1 mg/kg may be given by slow i.v., i.m. or s.c. injection. Doses >0.025 mg/kg should not be used in Boxers or giant breeds.

Neuroleptanalgesia

Acepromazine used in combination with opioid analgesics reduces the dose requirement of both components and the incidence of adverse effects. Acepromazine (0.0125–0.05 mg/kg) can be combined with:

Pethidine	2–10 mg/kg i.m.
Morphine	0.1–1.0 mg/kg i.m.
Papaveretum	0.2–2.0 mg/kg i.m.
Buprenorphine	0.005–0.01 mg/kg i.v., i.m.
Butorphanol	0.1–0.3 mg/kg i.v., i.m.
Pentazocine	1.0–3.0 mg/kg slow i.v.

Alpha$_2$ agonists and alpha$_2$ agonist/opioid mixtures

Medetomidine may be used alone at 0.01–0.08 mg/kg i.m. Low doses (0.0025 mg/kg) may be given i.v. Adverse effects may be antagonized with i.m. atipamezole at 5 times the agonist dose rate; the (unlicensed) i.v. route is preferable in critical situations.

Xylazine (1–3 mg/kg) may be used alone, given i.m. or i.v. (unlicensed). Adverse effects may be antagonized with i.m. or i.v. atipamezole, although this use is unlicensed.

Including opioids with medetomidine or xylazine lowers the dose required to achieve a given level of sedation and limits the severe effects that alpha$_2$ agonists exert on cardiopulmonary function.

Medetomidine (0.0025–0.01 mg/kg) or xylazine (1.0 mg/kg) can be combined with:

Pethidine	2 mg/kg i.m.
Buprenorphine	0.005–0.01 mg/kg slow i.v., i.m.
Butorphanol	0.1–0.2 mg/kg slow i.v., i.m.

While alpha$_2$ agonist/opioid combinations are safer than alpha$_2$ agonists alone, they should only be used in healthy animals.

Acepromazine/alpha₂ agonist/opioid mixtures

A mixture of acepromazine (0.1 mg/kg) with any of the combinations given for alpha₂ agonists and alpha₂ agonist/opioid mixtures (higher end of dose ranges) is suitable for the chemical restraint of large, dangerously aggressive dogs. Severe depression can be antagonized, using naloxone and atipamezole.

Low doses of acepromazine (0.01 mg/kg) and medetomidine (0.0025 mg/kg) combined with opioid agonist drugs provide profound sedation without signs of severe cardiopulmonary depression.

Benzodiazepines and benzodiazepine/opioid mixtures

Benzodiazepines do not reliably sedate dogs when used alone; indeed, stimulation ranging from increased motor activity to gross excitation may be seen. The risk of excitation is proportional to the health of the recipient: the chances of producing sedation are highest (but not guaranteed) in very sick cases. Diazepam (0.1–0.25 mg/kg i.v.) or midazolam (0.05–0.25 mg/kg i.v.) given during anaesthesia can smooth recovery in animals prone to excitability, providing adequate analgesia is present.

Opioid/benzodiazepine mixtures are satisfactory and relatively safe in critically ill animals. The opioid component (listed below) is given first, and usually produces little if any effect.

Pethidine	2–10 mg/kg i.m.
Morphine	0.1–1.0 mg/kg i.m.
Papaveretum	0.2–2.0 mg/kg i.m.
Buprenorphine	0.005–0.02 mg/kg i.m.
Butorphanol	0.1–0.3 mg/kg i.m.
Fentanyl	0.01 mg/kg slow i.v.

Satisfactory sedation usually results when either diazepam (0.25 mg/kg) or midazolam (0.25 mg/kg) is given by slow i.v. injection 20–30 minutes later.

General notes

- A well managed light level of general (inhalational) anaesthesia is frequently safer than heavy sedation in sick animals.
- Neuroleptanalgesic combinations are safer than alpha₂ agonist/opioid mixtures, but are less likely to produce adequate conditions for minor operations or investigations involving abnormal body positions. Furthermore, only the opioid component can be antagonized.
- In very ill animals, benzodiazepines given 20–30 minutes after neuroleptanalgesic combinations have been injected are likely to produce the best compromise between adequate conditions and patient safety.
- Most of the aforementioned combinations will have a profound sparing effect on i.v. and inhalational anaesthetics should a general anaesthetic be required after sedation. This is particularly true of

combinations containing alpha$_2$ agonists. When given slowly i.v., atipamezole will counter severe physiological derangement in dogs which have been given medetomidine and are subsequently anaesthetized with inhalation anaesthetics. Anaesthesia may 'lighten' but a full return to consciousness will not occur if inspired concentrations are adequate.

Sedative combinations for cats

Acepromazine

Acepromazine alone is not a particularly effective sedative and increasing the dose incurs the same problems as in dogs. Doses of 0.025–0.1 mg/kg may be given by i.m. or s.c. injection.

Neuroleptanalgesia

Neuroleptanalgesic combinations confer the same advantages in cats as in dogs.
Acepromazine (0.05–0.1 mg/kg) can be combined with:

Pethidine	2–10 mg/kg i.m.
Morphine	0.1–0.2 mg/kg i.m.
Papaveretum	0.2–0.4 mg/kg i.m.
Buprenorphine	0.005–0.01 mg/kg i.m.
Butorphanol	0.1–0.3 mg/kg i.m.

Alpha$_2$ agonists and alpha$_2$ agonist/opioid mixtures

Medetomidine may be used alone at 0.025–0.08 mg/kg i.m. Adverse effects may be antagonized with i.m. atipamezole at 2.5 times the agonist dose rate.

Xylazine (1– 3 mg/kg) may be used alone given by i.m. injection. Adverse effects may be antagonized with i.m. or i.v. atipamezole, although this use is unlicensed.

Including opioids with medetomidine or xylazine lowers the dose required to achieve a given level of sedation; and limits the severe effects that alpha$_2$ agonists exert on cardiopulmonary function.

Medetomidine (0.025–0.05mg/kg) or xylazine (1.0 mg/kg) can be combined with:

Pethidine	2 mg/kg i.m.
Buprenorphine	0.005–0.02 mg/kg slow i.v., i.m.
Butorphanol	0.1–0.2 mg/kg slow i.v., i.m.

While alpha$_2$ agonist/opioid combinations are safer than alpha$_2$ agonists alone, they should only be used in healthy animals.

Benzodiazepines
Diazepam (0.25 mg/kg) or midazolam (0.25 mg/kg) i.v. can provide satisfactory sedation in very sick cats. The inclusion of opioids at doses given for alpha$_2$ agonist/opioid mixtures may improve conditions.

Ketamine and ketamine-based techniques
Ketamine is relatively safe in ill animals, but high doses cause prolonged recoveries and are associated with muscle rigidity.

Acepromazine (0.05–0.1mg/kg) with midazolam (0.25mg/kg) or diazepam (0.25 mg/kg) and ketamine at either 2.5, 5.0 or 7.5 mg/kg, mixed and injected i.m., provides good conditions with only modest cardiopulmonary depression. The higher doses of ketamine should be used in excitable animals undergoing more stimulating interventions. Lower doses of acepromazine and/or ketamine may be used in very ill animals. Excluding the benzodiazepine component or the acepromazine from this combination reduces its efficacy without increasing safety.

Alternatives:

Ketamine (2.5 mg/kg) combined with diazepam (0.25 mg/kg) and given i.v. provides profound sedation which lasts for about 15–20 minutes.

Ketamine (5 mg/kg) with medetomidine 50–75 μg (micrograms) /kg i.m. produces profound sedation but should only be used in healthy cats. Atipamezole may be given if severe problems are encountered. Xylazine (0.5–1 mg/kg) may be used instead of medetomidine, but is no safer.

Although ketamine elimination depends heavily on renal function in cats, a full recovery still occurs, albeit more slowly, in animals with renal disease or urinary tract obstruction. However, low doses should be used in such cases.

General notes
- A crush cage is useful for restraining violent cats for i.m. injection. If these are unavailable, the animal, within its cage, may be placed in a large 'bin-bag' into which inhalational anaesthetics are piped. Most of the aforementioned combinations will have a profound sparing effect on i.v.and inhalational anaesthetics should a general anaesthetic be required after sedation. This is particularly true of combinations containing alpha$_2$ agonists. When given slowly i.v., atipamezole will counter severe physiological derangement in cats which have been given medetomidine and are subsequently anaesthetized with inhalation anaesthetics.
- The high body surface area:volume ratio of cats results in rapid heat loss compared with dogs. Attention to thermoregulation must be diligent.

Sedative combinations for exotic pets

Small mammals

Ketamine 40–50 mg/kg i.m. or 200 mg/kg i.p. plus xylazine 2–5mg/kg i.m. or 10 mg/kg i.p.
or ketamine 40–50 mg/kg i.m. or 200 mg/kg i.p. plus diazepam 1 mg/kg i.m. or 2.5 mg/kg i.p.
or ketamine 40–50 mg/kg i.m. or 200 mg/kg i.p. plus medetomidine 0.5 mg/kg i.m. (not Rabbits)
or fentanyl/fluanisone 0.3 ml/kg plus diazepam 1 mg/kg i.v., i.m. or 2.5–5 mg/kg i.p.
or fentanyl/fluanisone 0.3 ml/kg plus midazolam 1–2.5 mg/kg i.v., i.m., i.p.

Rabbits: As for small mammals except ketamine 15 mg/kg s.c. plus medetomidine 0.25 mg/kg s.c., to which can be added butorphanol 0.4 mg/kg s.c.

Ferrets: Ketamine 5–8 mg/kg i.m. plus medetomidine 0.1 mg/kg i.m. or xylazine 2 mg/kg i.m. plus butorphanol 0.2 mg/kg i.m.

N.B. Reduce doses if animal is debilitated.

Birds

Ketamine 15–40 mg/kg i.m. plus acepromazine 0.5–1mg/kg i.m.
or ketamine 15–40 mg/kg i.m. plus diazepam 1–1.5mg/kg i.m.
or ketamine 15–40 mg/kg i.m. plus xylazine 4 mg/kg i.m.
or ketamine 2–10 mg/kg i.m. plus medetomidine 0.2–0.8 mg/kg i.m.

Reptiles

Ketamine 10–50 mg/kg i.m., s.c.
Alfaxalone/alfadalone 15 mg/kg i.m. or 6–9 mg/kg i.v.
Propofol 10 mg/kg (for anaesthetic induction) gives 5–10 minutes sedation/light anaesthesia.

Drugs used in the treatment of 'exotic pets'

This table lists those drugs that are used in the treatment of 'exotic pets'.
A ✓ indicates that the drug may be used.
A ✗ indicates that information concerning its use is lacking. It does not necessarily mean that the use of the drug is contraindicated, specific monographs/texts should be consulted.

Drug	Birds	Reptiles	Small mammals
Anaesthetics/analgesics			
ACP	✗	✓	✓
Alfaxalone/Alfadolone	✓	✓	✓
Atipamazole	✓	✗	✓
Atropine	✓	✓	✓
Buprenorphine	✓	✗	✓
Butorphanol	✓	✓	✓
Diazepam	✓	✗	✓
Doxapram	✓	✓	✓
Fentanyl/fluanisone (Hypnorm)	✗	✗	✓
Halothane	✗	✓	✓
Isoflurane	✓	✓	✓
Ketamine	✓	✓	✓
Medetomidine	✓	✗	✓
Methohexitone	✗	✓	✓
Midazolam	✗	✗	✓
Morphine	✗	✗	✓
Nalbuphine	✗	✗	✓
Nitrous oxide	✓	✗	✓
Paracetamol	✗	✗	✓
Pentazocine	✗	✗	✓
Pethidine	✗		
Propofol	✓	✓	✓
Thiopental	✗	✗	✓
Xylazine	✗	✗	✓
Anthelmintics			
Albendazole	✗	✓	✓ (Rabbit)
Amitraz	✗	✗	✓
Fenbendazole	✓	✓	✓
Imidaclopriol	✗	✗	✓
Ivermectin	✓	✓ (not chelonians)	✓
Levamisole	✓	✓	✗
Mebendazole	✗	✗	✓
Niclosamide	✓	✗	✓
Oxfendazole	✗	✓	✗
Praziquantel	✓	✓	✗

Drug	Birds	Reptiles	Small mammals
Antibacterials			
Amikacin	✓	✓	✗
Amoxicillin	✓	✓	✓ (not rodents or lagomorphs)
Amoxicillin/clavulanate	✓	✗	✓ (Ferrets)
Ampicillin	✓	✓	✓ (not rodents or lagomorphs)
Carbenicillin	✓	✓	✗
Cefalexin	✓	✓	✓
Cefotaxime	✓	✓	✗
Ceftazidime	✓	✓	✗
Cefuroxime	✗	✓	✗
Chloramphenicol	✓	✓	✓
Ciprofloxacin	✓	✗	✗
Doxycycline	✓	✓	✗
Enrofloxacin	✓	✓	✓
Erythromycin	✓	✗	✓ (Hamsters)
Gentamicin	✓	✓	✓
Furazolidone	✗	✗	✓
Fusidic acid	✗	✗	✓
Lincomycin	✓	✗	✗
Metronidazole	✓	✓	✓
Neomycin	✗	✗	✓
Oxytetracycline	✓	✗	✓
Piperacillin	✓	✓	✗
Streptomycin	✗	✓	✓
Ticarcillin	✓	✗	✗
Tobramycin	✓	✓	✗
Trimethoprim/sulphonamide	✓	✓	✓
Tylosin	✓	✓	✓
Antifungals			
Amphotericin	✓	✓	✓
Clotrimazole	✓	✗	✗
Enilconazole	✗	✗	✓
Fluconazole	✓	✗	✗
Flucytosine	✓	✗	✗
Griseofulvin	✗	✗	✓
Itraconazole	✓	✗	✗
Ketoconazole	✓	✓	✗
Miconazole	✓	✓	✗
Nystatin	✓	✓	✗

Drug	Birds	Reptiles	Small mammals
Antiprotozoal			
Amprolium	✓	✗	✗
Carnidazole	✓	✗	✗
Clazuril	✓	✗	✗
Pyrimethamine	✓	✗	✗
Antidotes			
Calcium EDTA	✓	✗	✓
Carprofen	✓	✗	✓
Immunoglobulin	✗	✗	✓ (Ferret)
Penicillamine	✓	✗	✗
Pralidoxime	✓	✗	✗
Anti-inflammatory drugs			
Betamethasone	✗	✗	✓
Dexamethasone	✓	✗	✓
Flunixin	✗	✗	✓
Prednisolone	✗	✗	✓
Dermatological agents			
Chlorhexidine	✗	✗	✓
Diuretics			
Furosemide	✓	✗	✓
Endocrine			
Chorionic gonadotrophin	✗	✗	✓ (Ferret)
Dinoprostone	✓	✗	✗
GnRH	✗	✗	✓ (Ferret)
Levothyroxine	✓	✗	✗
Medroxyprogesterone	✓	✗	✓ (Ferret)
Mitotane	✗	✗	✓ (Ferret)
Proligestone	✗	✗	✓ (Ferret)
Oxytocin	✓	✓	✓
Gastrointestinal			
Colestyramine	✗	✗	✓ (Rabbit)
Lactulose	✓	✗	✗
Metoclopramide	✓	✓	✓
Pancreatic enzyme	✓	✗	✗
Paraffin	✓	✗	✗
Nutritional products			
Calcium borogluconate	✓	✓	✓
Calcium chloride	✓	✗	✓
Iron	✓	✗	✗
Vitamin A	✓	✓	✗
Vitamin B complex	✓	✓	✓
Vitamin B1	✗	✓	✗
Vitamin C	✗	✗	✓ (G.pig)
Vitamin K	✗	✗	✓

Drug	Birds	Reptiles	Small mammals
Respiratory system			
Acetylcysteine	✓	✗	✓
Bromhexine	✓	✗	✓
Diphenhydramine	✓	✗	✓ (Ferret)
Naloxone	✗	✗	✓
Renal			
Allopurinol	✓	✓	✗
Behaviour			
Fluoxetine	✓	✗	✗
Clomipramine	✓	✗	✗
Delmadinone	✓	✗	✗
Doxepin	✓	✗	✗
Hydroxyzine	✓	✗	✗
Ophthalmic			
Hypromellose	✓	✗	✓

Index sorted by therapeutic class

▶

CARDIOVASCULAR SYSTEM *continued*

Blood substitute
Haemoglobin glutamer-200 133

Calcium-channel blockers
Amlodipine 24
Diltiazem 90
Verapamil 278

Cardiac glycosides
Digitoxin 89
Digoxin 89

Fluid therapy
Hartmann's solution 155
Lactated Ringer's solution 155
Ringer's solution 245
Sodium chloride solutions 252

Plasma substitutes
Dextrans 85
Etherified starch 112
Gelatine 127

Positive inotropes
Adrenaline 13

Dobutamine 95
Dopamine 97
Milrinone 183
Pimobendan 222

Shock
Adrenaline 13
Dobutamine 95
Dopamine 97
Phenylephrine 217

Vasodilators
Arteriodilators
  Hydralazine 136
  Milrinone 183
  Sildenafil 250
Arterio- and venodilators
  Enalapril 103
  Nitroprusside 195
  Pentoxifylline 212
  Pimobendan 222
  Prazosin 230
Venodilators
  Glyceryl trinitrate 131
  Isosorbide dinitrate 149

DERMATOLOGICAL DRUGS

Alopecia
  Melatonin 170

Anti-allergics
  Alimemazine 16
  Chlorphenamine 62
  Clemastine 70
  Cyproheptadine 78
  Diphenhydramine 94
  Hydroxyzine 139
  Pentoxifyline 212
  Promethazine 235
  Sodium cromoglycate 253

Antiparasitic
  Fipronil 118
  Methoprene 175
  Nitenpyram 194

  Pyriproxyfen 242
  Selamectin 247

Cleansers and sebolytics
  Benzoyl peroxide 40
  Chlorhexidine 62
  Povidone–iodine 228

Immune-mediated dermates
  Nicotinamime 193

Psychogenic dermatoses
  Amitriptyline 24
  Clomipramine 72
  Doxepin 99
  Fluoxetine 123
  Selegiline hydrochloride 247

ENDOCRINE SYSTEM

GASTROINTESTINAL DRUGS

GENITO-URINARY TRACT

►

GENITO-URINARY TRACT *continued*

Prostaglandin and analogues
Dinoprost tromethamine 93
Dinoprostone 93
Misoprostol 184

Urinary acidifiers
Methionine 174

Urinary alkalinizers
Potassium citrate 227
Sodium bicarbonate 251

Urinary antiseptic
Methenamine hippurate 173

Urinary retention
Parasympathomimetic
Bethanecol 41

Urinary incontinence
Alpha-adrenoceptor blocker
Phenoxybenzamine 214
Antimuscarinic
Propantheline bromide 236
Sympathomimetic
Phenylpropanolamine 217

Urolithiasis
Cystinuria
Penicillamine 207
Oxalate
Potassium citrate 227
Struvite
Sodium acetate/acetic acid 251
Uric acid
Allopurinol 17

Xanthine oxidase inhibitor
Allopurinol 17

HEPATIC SYSTEM

Anti-fibrotic drugs
Colchicine 75

Hepatic encephalopathy
Lactulose 156
Metronidazole 180
Neomycin 190

Cholestatic liver disease
Ursodeoxycholic acid 276

Copper toxicosis
Penicillamine 207
Trientine 271

HAEMOPOIETIC SYSTEM

Anticoagulant
Heparin 135
Warfarin 285

Antithrombotic
Streptokinase 256

Blood replacement
Haemoglobin glutamer-200 133

Bone marrow stimulant
Epoetin 107
Filgrastim 117
Lenograstim 157
Lithium carbonate 161

IMMUNE SYSTEM

Immunomodulator
Interferon alfa 144
Interferon omega 145

Immunostimulant drugs
Levamisole 157

▶

IMMUNE SYSTEM *continued*

Immunosuppressive drugs
Auranofin 36
Aurothiomalate 36
Azathioprine 36
Chlorambucil 60
Ciclosporin 65
Cyclophosphamide 77

Danazol 80
Melphalan 171
Methotrexate 175
Nicotinamide 193
Prednisolone 230
Vincristine sulphate 280

NEUROMUSCULAR SYSTEM

Alpha$_2$ adrenoceptor agonists
Medetomidine 167
Xylazine 286

Alpha$_2$ adrenoceptor antagonists
Atipamezole 33
Nicergoline 193

Anaesthetic drugs
Injectable
  Alfaxalone/Alfadolone 15
  Ketamine 151
  Propofol 237
  Thiopental 265
Inhalational agents
  Halothane 134
  Isoflurane 148
  Nitrous oxide 196
  Sevoflurane 249

Anticholinesterases
Edrophonium chloride 103
Neostigmine 191
Pyridostigmine 241

Anticonvulsants
Diazepam 86
Pentobarbital 211
Phenobarbital 213
Phenytoin 218
Potassium bromide 225
Primidone 231

Antidepressants
Amitriptyline 24
Clomipramine 72
Doxepin 99
Fluoxetine 123

Antimuscarinic drugs
Atropine 34
Glycopyrronium bromide 132

Benzodiazepines
Diazepam 86
Midazolam 182
Oxazepam 201

CNS/respiratory stimulants
Doxapram 98

Euthanasia drugs
Pentobarbital 211
Secobarbital 246

Local anaesthetic drugs
Bupivicaine 45
Lidocaine 159
Mepivacaine 172
Proxymetacaine 240
Tetracaine 263

Muscle relaxants
Non-depolarizing drugs
  Atracurium 34
  Cisatracurium 67
  Pancuronium 204
  Rocuronium 246
  Vecuronium 276
Depolarizing drugs
  Suxamethonium 259
Skeletal muscle relaxants
  Dantrolene 80
  Diazepam 86
  Methocarbamol 175

Neuroleptanalgesics
Fentanyl 116

▶

NEUROMUSCULAR SYSTEM *continued*

Non-opioid analgesics
Amantadine 19

Opioid analgesics
Agonists
  Alfentanil 16
  Fentanyl 116
  Methadone 172
  Morphine 186
  Papaveretum 205
  Pethidine 212
Agonists/antagonists
  Buprenorphine 45
  Butorphanol 47
  Nalbuphine 188
  Pentazocine 210

Opioid antagonist
Naloxone 189

Sedatives
Acepromazine maleate 10
Diazepam 86
Medetomidine 167
Xylazine 286

Sedative antagonist
Atipamezole 33

Sympathomimetics
Adrenaline 13
Terbutaline 262

NON-STEROIDAL ANTI-INFLAMMATORY DRUGS

Acetyl salicylic acid 31
Aspirin 31
Auranofin 36
Aurothiomalate 36
Carprofen 54
Cinchophen 66
Dapsone 81
Diclofenac 86
DMSO 92
Flunixin meglumine 121
Flurbiprofen 124
Ketoprofen 154
Ketorolac 155

Meloxicam 170
Metamizole 48
Olsalazine 198
Paracetamol 206
Pentosan polysulphate 211
Phenylbutazone 216
Polysulphated
  glycosaminoglycan 225
Sulfasalazine 258
Tepoxalin 260
Tolfenamic acid 269
Vedaprofen 277

NUTRITIONAL PRODUCTS

Appetite stimulants
Diazepam 86
Oxazepam 201

Minerals
Calcium borogluconate 50
Calcium chloride 51
Calcium gluconate 51
Iron 148
Magnesium sulphate 164
Mineral mixtures 184
Phosphate 221
Potassium chloride/gluconate 226
Potassium citrate 227
Sodium bicarbonate 251
Sodium chloride 252
Zinc sulphate 288

Parenteral nutrition products
Amino acids 21
Fat/Triglycerides 113
Glucose 130

Vitamins
Ascorbic acid 282
Cyanocobalamin 282
Phytomenadione 284
Thiamine 282
Vitamin A 281
Vitamin B complex 281
Vitamin B1 282
Vitamin B12 282
Vitamin C 282
Vitamin D 283
Vitamin E 284
Vitamin K1 284

OPHTHALMIC DRUGS

Anti-infective/ anti-inflammatory
Diclofenac 88
Fluorometholone 122
Ketorolac 155
Ofloxacin 198

Antiviral
Aciclovir 13
Interferon omega 145
Lysine 164

Glaucoma
Acetazolamide 11
Apraclonidine 31
Betaxolol 41
Brinzolamide 43
Dorzolamide 98
Glycerol 130
Latanoprost 156
Pilocarpine 222
Timolol maleate 268

Immunosuppressant
Ciclosporin 65

Tear substitute
Hyaluronate 136
Hypromellose 140
Polyvinyl alcohol 225

Local anaesthetic
Proxymetacaine 240
Tetracaine 263

Ophthalmic beta-blocker
Timolol maleate 268

Mydriatic
Atropine 34
Cyclopentolate 76
Phenylephrine 217
Tropicamide 275

Miotic
Pilocarpine 222

Ophthalmic irrigant
Balanced salt solution 200

OTIC DRUGS

Anti-infective
Chlorhexidine 62
Povidone–iodine 228

Cleansers
Benzoyl peroxide 40
Chlorhexidine 62

RADIOGRAPHY

Barium sulphate contrast media 38

Iodine contrast media 145

RESPIRATORY DRUGS

Antihistamines
Alimemazine 16
Chlorphenamine 62
Diphenhydramine 94
Promethazine 235

Antitussives
Butorphanol 47
Codeine 74

Bronchodilators
Beta$_2$-adrenoceptor stimulants
  Terbutaline 262

Xanthines
  Aminophylline 21
  Etamiphylline 111
  Theophylline 264

Mucolytics
Acetylcysteine 12
Bromhexine 43

Nasal decongestants
Oxymetazoline 201
Phenylpropanolamine 217

Respiratory stimulant
Doxapram 98

Drugs new to the fifth edition

Amantadine
Bisacodyl
Carvedilol
Chlortetracycline
Cinchophen
Dactinomycin D
Dapsone
Fentanyl
Hyaluronate
Imidapril
Interferon omega
Ioversol
Ioxilan

Lysine
Melatonin
Methimazole
Nicotinamide
Pentoxifylline
Rocuronium
Sevoflurane
Sildenafil
Tepoxalin
Thiostrepton
Trifluorothymidine
Vinblastine

Drugs deleted from the fifth edition

Baquiloprim
Bretylium
Brimonidine
Calcium carbonate
Carteolol
Cefadroxil
Cefazolin
Cisapride
Diethylstilbestrol
Difloxacin

Fluanisone
Idoxuridine
Isoprenaline
Levocabastine
Lodoxamide
Methoxamine
Molgramostim
Stanozolol
Terfenadine
Tetracycline

INDEX

Generic names are in plain type.
Trade names are in italics.

If you have any suggestions or comments about this publication please complete the form below and return it to:

British Small Animal Veterinary Association
Woodrow House, 1 Telford Way, Waterwells Business Park, Quedgeley, Gloucestershire GL2 2AB

If you could supply your name and address this would enable us to follow up any queries we have about your comments. We are particularly interested in learning of drugs that are not included in this publication, their indications, doses and adverse effects

Comments on the BSAVA Small Animal Formulary

Name:
Address:

Drug (generic/trade name):

Comments:

Drug (generic/trade name):

Comments:

Drug (generic/trade name):

Comments:

Department for Environment, Food & Rural Affairs
Veterinary Medicines Directorate,
FREEPOST KT4503, Woodham Lane, New Haw,
Addlestone, Surrey KT15 3BR
Tel. No: 01932 338427 Fax: 01932 336618

ASSURING THE SAFETY, QUALITY AND EFFICACY OF VETERINARY MEDICINES

IN CONFIDENCE

For Official Use Only	
Adverse Reaction No.	
SAR file	
Date received	
Date Ack.	

Suspected Adverse Reaction Surveillance Scheme (SARSS)

Animal suspected adverse reaction report

- This form should be completed in **BLOCK LETTERS** and sent to the **FREEPOST** address given above, whenever a suspected adverse reaction is observed in **animals** (including birds and fish) during or after the use of a veterinary medicine.

All reporters MUST complete this section

Full name of product

Product number (on label)*   Batch number

Full name and address of person sending this form to the VMD

County:
Postcode: Date ___/___/___

Full address where reaction(s) occurred

County: Postcode:

Full name and address of veterinarian involved

County: Postcode:

This form will be copied to the Company (Marketing Authorisation holder) in order that they are aware of any reported suspected adverse reaction to their product. They may wish to contact you for further details. If you do not want the name(s) and address(es) on the form to be revealed to the Company, please tick this box

Has the Company already been informed?   YES ☐   NO ☐

Your reference No. (if any)

MLA 252A (Rev. 8/01)

Details of animal suspected adverse reaction(s)

Reason for using product [ ]

No. of animals treated on this occasion [ ]   No. of animals reacting [ ]

No. of deaths [ ]   Actual amount of product administered [ ]

Administered by [ ]   Date of first administration [, ,]
(occupation)

Duration of treatment [ ]

Site & route of [/]   Previous use of product in this animal(s)   YES [ ]   NO [ ]
administration

If YES, number of occasions [ ]

Date of reaction(s)	Species/Breed	Weight kg	Age	Sex (M/F)	Nature of reaction **including time of onset and duration of symptoms**
__/__/__					

Full details of products given concurrently (if any)

Immediate treatment given (if any)

Previous vaccination history (if immunological product involved in suspected adverse reaction) product number* and batch number

Post mortem and/or laboratory tests:
Have any post mortems or relevant diagnostic tests been performed?   YES [ ]   NO [ ]

If **YES** please attach copies or forward to VMD in due course.

* The product number is preceded by PL, VM or MA

Comments: If you have any comments or further information please continue on a separate sheet

Extra Forms: Tick this box if extra forms are required [ ]

Receipt of this form will be acknowledged.